# Recent Results in Cance



Volume 191



For further volumes:
http://www.springer.com/series/392

Andrew T. Chan · Elmar Detering
Editors

# Prospects for Chemoprevention of Colorectal Neoplasia

## Emerging Role of Anti-Inflammatory Drugs

Springer

*Editors*
Andrew T. Chan
Division of Gastroenterology
Massachusetts General Hospital
Harvard Medical School
Boston, MA
USA

Elmar Detering
Global Medical Affairs (Primary Care)
Bayer Pharma AG, Berlin
Germany

ISSN 0080-0015
ISBN 978-3-642-43447-1 ISBN 978-3-642-30331-9 (eBook)
DOI 10.1007/978-3-642-30331-9
Springer Heidelberg New York Dordrecht London



Printed on acid-free paper

Springer is part of Springer Science+Business Media (www.springer.com)

# Contents

# An Emerging Role for Anti-inflammatory Agents for Chemoprevention

Andrew T. Chan and Elmar Detering

**Abstract**

There have been a number of promising recent developments in the prevention of colorectal cancer. This book examines in detail important aspects of the current status of and future prospects for chemoprevention of colorectal tumors, particularly using anti-inflammatory drugs. Research into the mechanisms that lead from early colorectal adenoma to colorectal cancer is discussed. The role and modes of action of available anti-inflammatory drugs, such as aspirin, celecoxib, and sulindac are described and recent data from trials of aspirin are reviewed. In addition, the possible impact of nutritional agents with anti-inflammatory properties is considered, and strategies applicable in those with a high level of genetic risk are evaluated. An important feature of the book is its interdisciplinary perspective, offering highly relevant information for gastroenterologists, internists, general practitioners, oncologists, colorectal and gastroenterological surgeons, and public health practitioners.

## Contents



*Prospects for Chemoprevention of Colorectal Neoplasia—
Emerging Role of Anti-Inflammatory Drugs.?*

A. T. Chan (✉)
Division of Gastroenterology Massachusetts General Hospital, Harvard Medical School, 55 Fruit Street, Boston, MA 02114, USA
e-mail: achan@partners.org

E. Detering
Global Medical Affairs (Primary Care), Bayer Pharma AG, 13465 Berlin, Germany

A. T. Chan and E. Detering (eds.), *Prospects for Chemoprevention of Colorectal Neoplasia*,
Recent Results in Cancer Research 191, DOI: 10.1007/978-3-642-30331-9_1,

Colorectal cancer (CRC) is a compelling example of a chronic disease for which there is a critical need for novel preventive strategies. CRC is the second most common cancer in developed countries, with about 1 million new cases and 600,000 deaths worldwide each year. The incidence rates (IR) of CRC vary markedly worldwide, being highest in Europe, North America, and Oceania. The lifetime risk of CRC in Western populations such as the United States (US) is 5%. In Europe, there were 412,900 new cases and 217,400 deaths due to CRC during 2006. While the incidence of CRC has been declining in the US since the 1980s, several countries, especially those that are economically transitioning to a more urbanized/westernized lifestyle, have been seeing important increases (GLOBOCAN 2008).

Given the poor outcomes of advanced CRC, considerable emphasis has been focused on prevention through population screening for the early detection of CRCs and adenomatous polyps, the precursor for the vast majority of cancers. Although screening modalities such as fecal occult blood testing and endoscopy are efficacious, patient uptake is often suboptimal, limiting its real-world effectiveness. Thus, there is a clear imperative to consider alternative preventative strategies, including chemoprevention.

'Chemoprevention' describes the use of drugs or other (including natural) agents to inhibit or prevent the development or progression of malignant changes in cells. An important milestone in the evolution of agents for chemoprevention was the discovery of the "inhibition of prostaglandin synthesis as a mechanism of action for aspirin-like drugs" by Sir John Vane in 1971, who received the Nobel Prize in 1982 (together with Bergstrom and Samuelsson) (Vane 1971). Their work was seminal in establishing cyclooxygenase (COX), also known as prostaglandin synthase (PTGS), as the principle target enzyme for aspirin and aspirin-like drugs now commonly known as non-steroidal anti-inflammatory drugs (NSAIDs) (Vane 1982). The COX-1 and COX-2 isoenzymes are responsible for formation of prostaglandins and related biologically active substances, important mediators of inflammation.

Historically, in vitro and animal studies with aspirin and NSAIDs as potential chemopreventive agents began early in the 1980s. In humans, sulindac was among the first drugs with demonstrated chemopreventive efficacy in studies of patients with familial adenomatous polyposis (FAP), an autosomal dominant hereditary CRC syndrome that has provided tremendous insight into the pathogenesis of sporadic colorectal cancer. The key distinguishing feature of classic FAP is the development of hundreds to thousands of adenomatous polyps throughout the colon, often beginning as early as the second decade of life. Colorectal adenocarcinomas inevitably develop in FAP patients, typically by age 40. In early studies, sulindac treatment caused marked regression of polyps in patients with FAP (Giardiello et al. 1993).

The FAP model also paved the way for further analysis of the NSAIDs celecoxib and rofecoxib, selective COX-2 inhibitors, as potential chemopreventatives in colorectal adenoma and cancer (Steinbach et al. 2000; Hallak et al. 2003; Arber et al. 2006; Bertagnolli et al. 2006). Despite their demonstrated efficacy in well-designed clinical trials of both FAP and sporadic adenoma, the occurrence of cardiovascular events associated with these agents has dampened enthusiasm for their routine use for chemoprevention.

Concerns about NSAID-associated cardiovascular toxicity have refocused attention on the chemopreventive properties of aspirin, the oldest of the "modern" anti-inflammatory drugs. Aspirin not only has a favorable cardiovascular profile but is already widely used for the prevention of cardiovascular events. Several epidemiological studies (Chan 2011), randomized controlled trials (RCTs) of colon polyp recurrence (Cole et al. 2009; Chan et al. 2007; Baron et al. 2003; Sandler et al. 2003; Benamouzig et al. 2003; Logan et al. 2008), and RCTs in patients with hereditary CRC syndromes (Burn et al. 2011a, 2011b; Chan et al. 2005, 2008, 2009), have shown that aspirin reduces incidence of colorectal neoplasia. In five cardiovascular-prevention RCTs, Rothwell and colleagues previously observed that daily aspirin at any dose reduced risk of CRC by 24 % and of CRC-associated mortality by 35 % after a delay of 8–10 years (Rothwell et al. 2010). Thus, aspirin may be currently the most promising agent considering it demonstrated effectiveness and its favorable cardiovascular safety profile. Because CRC and vascular disease have overlapping risk factors (e.g., diabetes, obesity, physical inactivity), use of aspirin for the dual purpose of cancer and vascular disease prevention has considerable appeal. Moreover, emerging data show that aspirin may be associated with a lower risk of death from cancer of sites other than the colorectum (Rothwell et al. 2011, 2012). Thus, despite aspirin's known association with gastrointestinal toxicity, the overwhelming benefits of aspirin for a wide range of the most common chronic diseases could overall tip the scales in favor of aspirin as the chemopreventive agent of choice for many individuals Chan et al. (2012) and Avivi et al. (2012)

Our knowledge about the mechanism underlying the anti-neoplastic benefit of these anti-inflammatory agents is growing, but yet incomplete. At present, the known effects of these agents in inhibiting COX-1 and COX-2 appear to play a significant role. COX-1 is considered a constitutive enzyme, found in most tissues, including gastrointestinal mucosa (Schror 2009). COX-2, on the other hand, is undetectable in most normal tissues, with expression induced in areas of inflammation. More importantly, COX-2 been shown to be upregulated in various carcinomas and to have a central role in tumorigenesis (Chan et al. 2007). Nonetheless, there have been many COX-independent mechanisms proposed for aspirin's anti-cancer benefit. Moreover, there remains a need to further elucidate downstream pathways of COX-2 that influence cancer.

In recent years, there has been a substantial new body of evidence demonstrating the potential of anti-inflammatory drugs as chemopreventive agents for colorectal cancer. This volume will review the current body of evidence for aspirin in sporadic neoplasia (Chap. 7, Rothwell) and hereditary cancers (Chap. 9, Burn) and NSAIDs (Chap. 5, Arber). We will also describe the many proposed anti-cancer mechanisms of NSAIDs and aspirin (Chap. 3, Patrigani; Chap. 2, Dixon; Chap. 4, Rodriguez; and Chap. 6, Piazza) and the evidence for the use of alternative agents with similar anti-inflammatory mechanisms of action (Chap. 8, Hull). Taken together, this volume will provide several different perspectives that demonstrate the emerging role of anti-inflammatory agents for chemoprevention for CRC and other chronic diseases.

## References

Arber N, Eagle CJ, Spicak J, Rácz I, Dite P, Hajer J et al (2006) Celecoxib for the prevention of colorectal adenomatous polyps. N Engl J Med 355(9):885–895

Avivi D, Moshkowitz M, Detering E, Arber N (2012) The role of low-dose aspirin in the prevention of colorectal cancer. Expert Opin Ther Targets PMID 22313430 1:s51–s62

Baron JA, Cole BF, Sandler RS, Haile RW, Ahnen D, Bresalier R et al (2003) A randomized trial of aspirin to prevent colorectal adenomas. N Engl J Med 348(10):891–899

Benamouzig R, Deyra J, Martin A, Girard B, Jullian E, Piednoir B et al (2003) Daily soluble aspirin and prevention of colorectal adenoma recurrence: one-year results of the APACC trial. Gastroenterology 125(2):328–336

Bertagnolli MM, Eagle CJ, Zauber AG, Redston M, Solomon SD, Kim K et al (2006) Celecoxib for the prevention of sporadic colorectal adenomas. N Engl J Med 355(9):873–884

Burn J, Bishop DT, Chapman PD et al (2011a) A randomized placebo-controlled prevention trial of aspirin and/or resistant starch in young people with familial adenomatous polyposis. Cancer Prev Res (Phila) 4(5):655–665

Burn J, Gerdes AM, CAPP2 investigators (2011b) Long-term effect of aspirin on cancer risk in carriers of hereditary colorectal cancer: an analysis from the CAPP2 randomised controlled trial. Lancet 378(9809):2081–2087.

Chan AT, Giovannucci EL, Meyerhardt JA, Schernhammer ES, Curhan GC, Fuchs CS (2005) Long-term use of aspirin and nonsteroidal anti-inflammatory drugs and risk of colorectal cancer. JAMA 294(8):914–923

Chan AT, Ogino S, Fuchs CS (2007) Aspirin and the risk of colorectal cancer in relation to the expression of COX-2. N Engl J Med 356:2131–2142

Chan AT, Giovannucci EL, Meyerhardt JA, Schernhammer ES, Wu K, Fuchs CS (2008) Aspirin dose and duration of use and risk of colorectal cancer in men. Gastroenterology 134(1):21–28

Chan AT, Ogino S, Fuchs CS (2009) Aspirin use and survival after diagnosis of colorectal cancer. JAMA 302(6):649–658

Chan AT, Hsu M, Zauber AG, Hawk ET, Bertagnolli MM (2012) The influence of UGT1A6 variants and aspirin use in a randomized trial of celecoxib for the prevention of colorectal adenoma. Cancer Prev Res PMID: 22313430 5(1):61–72

Cole BF, Logan RF, Halabi S, Benamouzig R, Sandler RS, Grainge MJ et al (2009) Aspirin for the chemoprevention of colorectal adenomas: meta-analysis of the randomized trials. J Natl Cancer Inst 101:256–266

Giardiello FM, Hamilton SR, Krush AJ, Piantadosi S, Hylind LM, Celano P et al (1993) Treatment of colonic and rectal adenomas with sulindac in familial adenomatous polyposis. N Engl J Med 328:1313–1316

Ferlay J, Shin HR, Bray F, Forman D, Mathers C and Parkin DM. GLOBOCAN 2008 v1.2, Cancer Incidence and Mortality Worldwide: IARC CancerBase No. 10 [Internet].Lyon, France: International Agency for Research on Cancer; 2010. Available from: http://globocan.iarc.fr, accessed on 02/02/2011

Hallak A, Alon-Baron L, Shamir R, Moshkowitz M, Bulvik B, Brazowski E et al (2003) Rofecoxib reduces polyp recurrence in familial polyposis. Dig Dis Sci 48:1998–2002

Logan RFA, Grainge MJ, Shepherd VC, Armitage NC, Muir KR (2008) Group uT. Aspirin and folic acid for the prevention of recurrent colorectal adenomas. Gastroenterology 134(1):29–38

Rothwell PM, Wilson M, Elwin C-E, Norrving B, Algra A, Warlow CP et al (2012) Long-term effect of aspirin on colorectal cancer incidence and mortality: 20-year follow-up of five randomised trials. The Lancet PMID 22440694 376(9754):1741–1750

Rothwell PM, Fowkes FG, Belch JF, Ogawa H, Warlow CP, Meade TW (2011) Effect of daily aspirin on long-term risk of death due to cancer: analysis of individual patient data from randomised trials. Lancet 377(9759):31–41

Sandler RS, Halabi S, Baron JA, Budinger S, Paskett E, Keresztes R et al (2003) A randomized trial of aspirin to prevent colorectal adenomas in patients with previous colorectal cancer. N Engl J Med 348(10):883–890

Schror K (2009) Acetylsalicyclic acid. Blackwell, Germany

Steinbach G, Lynch PM, Phillips RK, Wallace MH, Hawk E, Gordon GB et al (2000) The effect of celecoxib, a cyclooxygenase-2 inhibitor, in familial adenomatous polyposis. N Engl J Med 342:1946–1952

Vane JR (1971) Inhibition of prostaglandin synthesis as a mechanism of action for aspirin-like drugs. Nat New Biol 231(25):232–235

Vane JR (1982) Adventures and excursions in bioassay: the stepping stones to prostaglandins. Nobel lecture, 8 December PMID 6360277

# Mechanistic Aspects of COX-2 Expression in Colorectal Neoplasia

Dan A. Dixon, Fernando F. Blanco, Annalisa Bruno and Paola Patrignani

**Abstract**

The cyclooxygenase-2 (COX-2) enzyme catalyzes the rate-limiting step of prostaglandin formation in pathogenic states and a large amount of evidence has demonstrated constitutive COX-2 expression to be a contributing factor promoting colorectal cancer (CRC). Various genetic, epigenetic, and inflammatory pathways have been identified to be involved in the etiology and development of CRC. Alteration in these pathways can influence COX-2 expression at multiple stages of colon carcinogenesis allowing for elevated prostanoid biosynthesis to occur in the tumor microenvironment. In normal cells, COX-2 expression levels are potently regulated at the post-transcriptional level through various RNA sequence elements present within the mRNA 3′ untranslated region (3′UTR). A conserved AU-rich element (ARE) functions to target COX-2 mRNA for rapid decay and translational inhibition through association with various RNA-binding proteins to influence the fate of COX-2 mRNA. Specific microRNAs (miRNAs) bind regions within the COX-2 3′UTR and control COX-2 expression. In this chapter, we discuss novel insights in the mechanisms of altered post-transcriptional regulation of COX-2 in CRC and

D. A. Dixon (✉) · F. F. Blanco
Department of Cancer Biology, University of Kansas Medical Center, Kansas, KS 66106, USA
e-mail: ddixon3@kumc.edu

A. Bruno
Center of Excellence on Aging (CeSI) and Department of Medicine and Aging, G. d'Annunzio University, School of Medicine, Via dei, Vestini 31, 66100 Chieti, Italy

P. Patrignani (✉)
Center of Excellence on Aging (CeSI) and Department of Neuroscience and Imaging, G. d'Annunzio University, School of Medicine, Via dei, Vestini 31, 66100 Chieti, Italy
e-mail: ppatrignani@unich.it

A. T. Chan and E. Detering (eds.), *Prospects for Chemoprevention of Colorectal Neoplasia*,
Recent Results in Cancer Research 191, DOI: 10.1007/978-3-642-30331-9_2,

how this knowledge may be used to develop novel strategies for cancer prevention and treatment.

**Abbreviations**

| | |
|---|---|
| CRC | Colorectal cancer |
| CV | Cardiovascular |
| CIN | Chromosomal instability |
| APC | Adenomatous polyposis coli |
| FAP | Familial adenomatous polyposis |
| EGF | Epidermal growth factor |
| TGF | Transforming growth factor |
| COX | Cyclooxygenase |
| PG | Prostaglandin |
| (TX)$A_2$ | Thromboxane |
| $PGI_2$ | Prostacyclin |
| GI | Gastrointestinal |
| NSAIDs | Nonsteroidal anti-inflammatory drugs |
| mPGES | Microsomal Prostaglandin E Synthase |
| 15-PGDH | 15-hydroxyprostaglandin dehydrogenase |
| PPAR | Peroxisome proliferator-activated receptor |
| AU | Rich elements (AREs) |
| miRNAs | MicroRNAs |
| HuR | Hu antigen R |
| TIA-1 | T cell intracellular antigen 1 |
| RBM3 | RNA-binding motif protein 3 |

## Contents

# 1 Molecular Basis of Colorectal Adenoma and Carcinoma

Colorectal cancer (CRC) is the third most diagnosed cancer in males and the second in females worldwide. The highest incidence rates are found in Australia and New Zealand, Europe, and North America, whereas the lowest rates are found in Africa and South-Central Asia (Jemal et al. 2011). In economically developed countries, death rates for CRC have largely decreased as result of the improved treatment and use of population-based colorectal screening programs. According to a recent randomized clinical trial (RCT) in the United Kingdom, a one-time flexible sigmoidoscopy screening between 55 and 64 years of age reduced CRC incidence by 33 % and mortality by 43 % (Atkin et al. 2010). However, proximal colon cancers are not effectively prevented by screening using sigmoidoscopy or colonoscopy. It is quite interesting the finding that the use of low-dose aspirin reduces the 20-year risk of developing CRC (by 24 %) and the risk of dying from the cancer (by 35 %) and that 70 % of the reduced risk is associated with fewer cancers in the right section of the colon (proximal colon) (Rothwell et al. 2010).

An important limitation in prevention-based strategies of CRC is the lack of biomarkers of early detection and of safe and effective chemopreventive agents. The reduced risk of CRC by low-dose aspirin, if supported by the results of mechanistic studies which are ongoing (see Chap. 3), will open the way to primary prevention strategy in CRC with the drug. In fact, the possible enhanced risk of bleeding associated with low-dose aspirin administration could be overcome by the joint reduced risk of vascular events and cancers. Thus, the association of lifestyle changes, population-based colorectal screening programs, and the use of chemopreventive agents affecting early phases of tumorigenesis, such as low-dose aspirin (see Chap. 3), would lead to a sharp drop in CRC risk within the next 10 years.

Over the last 25 years, important strides have been made in the understanding of the molecular mechanisms associated with the adenoma-carcinoma sequence, which represents the bedrock of our knowledge of the colonic carcinogenesis process (Ahnen 2011). In fact, the study of molecular mechanisms underlying this sequence has had a profound impact on the understanding of the initiation and progression of colon cancer, thus allowing for the development of improved strategies to identify high-risk patients and provide clinical care to patients with colonic polyps and cancer.

## 1.1 Genetic Basis of Adenoma-Carcinoma Sequence

Molecular analyses of colorectal adenomas and carcinomas have led to the development of a genetic model of colon carcinogenesis wherein colon tumorigenesis arises from an accumulation of genetic alterations that promote tumor initiation and disease progression. There are at least three distinct molecular pathways to CRC: (1) the chromosomal instability (CIN) pathway, which is largely driven by mutational events in oncogenes and tumor suppressor genes; (2) the microsatellite instability (MSI) pathway, which is driven by mutations in DNA repair genes, and (3) the epigenetic pathway, which is driven in large part by hypermethylation-induced silencing of tumor suppressor genes (Kulendran et al. 2011). Among them, the CIN pathway is the most commonly observed in CRC accounting for up to 80 % of cases (Grady and Carethers 2008).

## 1.2 Adenomatous Polyposis Coli

Inactivating mutations in the adenomatous polyposis coli (APC) tumor suppressor gene occur early in the adenoma stages of CRC (Kulendran et al. 2011). The absence of functional APC leads to an inappropriately and constitutively activation of the Wnt signaling pathway, thereby promoting CRC tumor initiation (Kulendran et al. 2011; Markowitz and Bertagnolli 2009). Activation of the Wnt pathway leads to the suppression of the phosphorylation of the oncoprotein $\beta$-catenin, resulting in its stabilization and nuclear translocation. $\beta$-catenin then interacts with T cell factor/lymphocyte enhancer factor (TCF/LEF) to induce transcription of Wnt target proproliferative and antiapoptotic genes. In normal cells where Wnt signaling is controlled, cytoplasmic $\beta$-catenin is phosphorylated by the glycogen synthase kinase 3$\beta$ (GSK-3$\beta$) within a complex containing APC and Axin, resulting in the degradation of $\beta$-catenin through the ubiquitin proteasome pathway. APC, as component of this complex, not only contributes to the $\beta$-catenin degradation, but also inhibits its nuclear localization, thereby abrogating transcription of Wnt target genes (Buchanan and DuBois 2006).

Germline APC mutations give rise to familial adenomatous polyposis (FAP), an autosomal dominantly inherited syndrome in which patients typically develop hundreds to thousands of colorectal adenomatous polyps during their second and third decades of life. Although these are benign tumors, their large numbers virtually guarantee that some will progress to invasive lesions. Somatic mutations and deletions that inactivate both copies of APC are present in most sporadic colorectal adenomas and cancers. In a small subgroup of tumors with wild-type APC, mutations of $\beta$-catenin that render the protein resistant to its degradation promote constitutive activation of Wnt signalling (Markowitz and Bertagnolli 2009).

Animal models have played an instrumental role in demonstrating the ability of cyclooxygenase-2 (COX-2) to promote gastrointestinal (GI) tumorigenesis in the context of loss of APC. Genetic studies have demonstrated that deletion of COX-2 in $APC^{Min/+}$ and $APC^{\Delta 716}$ mouse models of intestinal tumorigenesis results in decreased small intestine and colon tumor formation (Oshima et al. 1996; Chulada et al. 2000). Furthermore, an association between increased nuclear $\beta$-catenin levels and COX-2 expression is seen in human and murine colon cancer cells and is related to defects in APC (Mei et al. 1999; Dimberg et al. 2001).

## 1.3 The Microsatellite Instability Pathway in CRC

The evidence that CRC progression occurs as a multi-step process characterized by an accumulation of genetic alterations arose from the findings that CRC patients who developed cancer from Lynch syndrome displayed tumors with a different histological profile than those with cases associated with the CIN pathway. Lynch syndrome (also termed hereditary non-polyposis CRC, or HNPCC) is the most common hereditary colon cancer syndrome, accounting for about 3 % of all CRC cases. It is an autosomal dominant disease and it is associated with a risk of CRC of about 70 % and an increased risk of a variety of other cancers, such as endometrial, ovarian, gastric, small bowel, and ureter. In Lynch syndrome, CRCs arise from adenomas but the progression of the adenoma-carcinoma sequence in this pathological setting occurs more rapidly than in the CIN pathway. However, CIN tumors have a poorer prognosis as compared to Lynch-associated CRCs. While CIN tumors are characterized by aneuploidy (abnormal number of chromosomes), multiple chromosomal rearrangements, and an accumulation of somatic mutations, Lynch-associated CRCs are typically diploid and are characterized by genetic alterations due to the inactivation of mismatch repair genes (MMR). This type of genetic alteration characterizes a well-identified aspect of genomic instability, named MSI (Ahnen 2011). Among genes identified to be affected by MSI are components of the TGF-$\beta$ signaling pathway (Markowitz et al. 1995), along with genes regulating cell proliferation, cell cycle, apoptosis, and DNA repair (Duval and Hamelin 2002). MSI is found in 15 % of CRCs, which are primarily hereditary CRCs, but it is also detected in sporadic cancers. While sporadic colorectal tumors frequently exhibit COX-2 overexpression (Wang and Dubois 2010b), up to half of MMR-deficient colorectal tumors do not show COX-2 overexpression primarily in patients with sporadic MMR-deficiencies (Castells et al. 2006) in agreement with other observations indicating reduced COX-2 protein expression in CRC with defective MMR (Karnes et al. 1998). These findings support the existence of a novel, epigenetic-based pathway that contributes to CRC disease progression and indicate potential limitations for COX-2 inhibition as chemoprevention strategy in HNPCC due to the lack functional response.

However, recent results form the first RCT of aspirin in Lynch syndrome, the colorectal adenoma/carcinoma prevention programme 2 (CAPP2), strongly support routine use of aspirin for patients with Lynch Syndrome as an adjunct to intensive cancer surveillance (Burn et al. 2011), but further RCTs with a CRC endpoint should be performed to have more definitive answers on aspirin role in the prevention of CRC in a sporadic-risk population.

## 1.4 The Epigenetic Pathway in CRC

Another mechanism of gene inactivation in CRC occurs via epigenetic-based mechanisms mainly due to aberrant DNA methylation through the introduction of a methyl group on carbon 5 of cytosine (5-methylcytosine) by DNA methylases (Kondo and Issa 2004). In the normal genome, cytosine methylation occurs in repetitive DNA sequences outside of exons, whereas in CRCs there is a global reduction of cytosine methylation and a considerable increase of aberrant cytosine methylation localized to certain gene promoter regions. These aberrant methylations associated with promoter regions can promote epigenetic silencing of genes. The two most commonly affected genes in these sporadic cases and in Lynch Syndrome are MutS homolog (hMSH)1 and hMLH2 (Issa 2004). Consistent with the MSI phenotype, hypermethylation of the COX-2 promoter has been observed in CRC samples, suggesting that the reduced expression of COX-2 may also affect sporadic forms (Toyota et al. 2000) and COX-2 gene silencing via hypermethylation was observed in approximately one-third of MMR-deficient colorectal tumors (Castells et al. 2006).

## 1.5 COX-2/mPGES-1 Pathway

Inflammation is one of the major contributors to the tumor microenvironment. In particular, chronic inflammation acts to initiate tumorigenesis and promote disease progression, and it has long been studied in relation to proinflammatory prostanoids in colon cancer (Wang and DuBois 2008). Clinical studies have shown that the use of nonsteroidal anti-inflammatory drugs (NSAIDs) [both traditional (t)NSAIDs and selective inhibitors of COX-2 (coxibs)] reduces the risk of CRC by 40–50 % (Peddareddigari et al. 2011) (for a comprehensive discussion see Chap. 4). The most plausible mechanism of the antitumorigenic effects of these drugs is through their inhibitory effect on COX-2-dependent prostanoids (Fig. 1).

NSAIDs, including aspirin, inhibit COX isozymes (COX-1 and COX-2), which catalyze the rate-limiting step in the metabolic conversion of arachidonic acid (AA) to PGs [i.e. $PGE_2$, $PGD_2$, $PGF_{2a}$, thromboxane (TX) $A_2$, and prostacyclin ($PGI_2$)] (Vane 1971). Prostanoids are second messengers which can cross the cell membrane, diffuse through the extracellular space, and interact with high-affinity G-protein coupled receptors on the same cell or in neighboring cells. The specific action of the different prostanoids in a particular type of tissue predominantly depends on the cell type-specific expression of their specific receptors and on their biosynthesis (Funk 2001) (Fig. 1).

COX-2-derived $PGE_2$ is the most abundant prostanoids found in CRC tissue, and it has been demonstrated to promote colon carcinogenesis along with other malignancies including lung, breast, and head and neck cancer (Wang and Dubois 2010a). The role of $PGE_2$ in colon cancer progression arose from studies with the $APC^{Min/+}$ mouse model of intestinal neoplasia. This genetic animal model for FAP

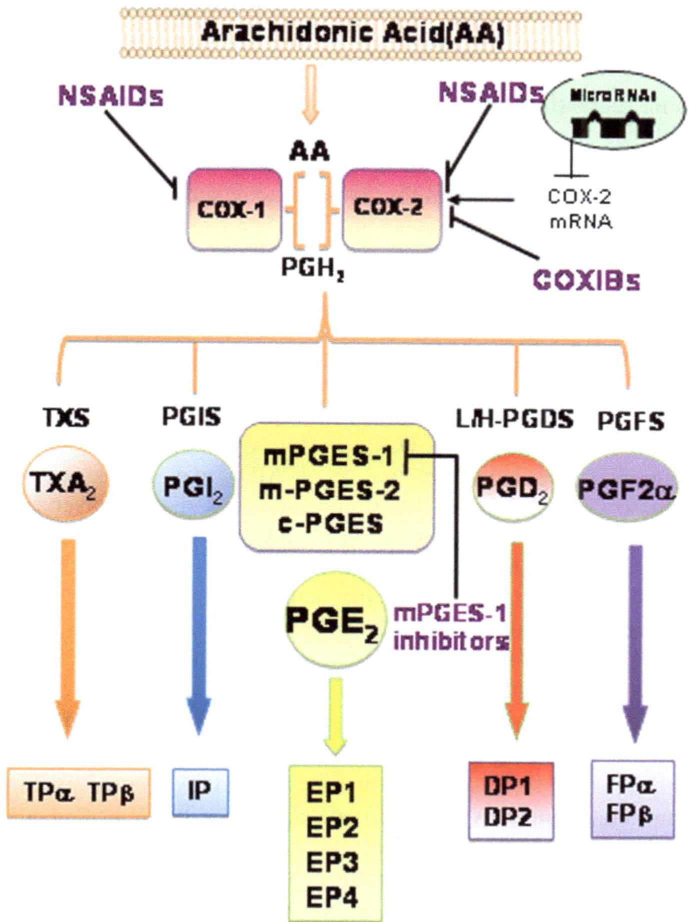


**Fig. 1** COX-2/mPGES-1 pathway. Two primary COX enzyme isoforms (COX-1 and COX-2) catalyze the rate-limiting step of PG formation: the conversion of AA into the intermediate metabolite $PGG_2$, which is further metabolized by different synthases to generate distinct PGs. The specific action of the different PGs in a particular type of tissue predominantly depends on the cell type-specific expression of their specific receptors and on their biosynthesis. NSAIDs (both traditional and COX-2 selective inhibitors, named coxibs) act by the inhibiting COX-dependent prostanoid generation. Innovative anti-inflammatory and anti-cancer strategies are based on the selective delivery of drugs affecting COX-2 activity or expression to specific tissues or by the use of selective inhibitors of mPGES-1, which by suppressing $PGE_2$ might augment the protective vascular $PGI_2$ biosynthesis. In addition, since in CRC COX-2 overexpression is controlled at post-transcriptional level through changes in its mRNA stability by miRNAs, the design of therapeutics affecting this pathway may lead to innovative therapeutic strategies in CRC. *AA* arachidonic acid, *COX* cyclooxygenase, *$PGG_2$* Prostaglandin G2, *$TXA_2$* thromboxane, *$PGI_2$* prostacyclin, *$PGD_2$* prostaglandin $D_2$, *$PGF_{2\alpha}$* prostaglandin $F_{2\alpha}$, *TXS* $TXA_2$ synthase, *PGIS* $PGI_2$ synthase, hematopoietic/lipocalin-type PGD synthase; prostaglandin F2a synthase; m(microsomal) or c(cytoplasmatic) PGES (*$PGE_2$ syntase*), TP ($TXA_2$ receptor), IP ($PGI_2$ receptor), EP1-4 ($PGE_2$ receptor), DP1-2 ($PGD_2$ receptors), FP (PGF2a receptors), *CRC* colorectal cancer

maintains inactivating mutations in the APC gene (Moser et al. 1995). Treatment of these animals with $PGE_2$ promoted a dramatic increase in small and large intestinal tumor burden (Wang et al. 2004). Moreover, studies in humans revealed that adenoma regression was more effective when $PGE_2$ tissue levels were profoundly inhibited by treatment with NSAIDs (Giardiello et al. 2004). As aforementioned, activation of the canonical Wnt pathway in the colonic epithelium is a key event in polyp formation, and this event is associated with the upregulation of several genes involved in tumor development and progression (Buchanan and DuBois 2006). Among them, overexpression of COX-2 plays a central role in intestinal tumorigenesis. In fact, elevated levels of COX-2-derived $PGE_2$ are associated with (1) resistance to apoptosis, through the upregulation of the anti-apoptotic protein Bcl-2 and the induction of nuclear factor-$\kappa$B (NF$\kappa$B) transcriptional activity (Wang and Dubois 2010a), (2) stimulation of cell proliferation, (3) simulation of cell migration, and (4) angiogenesis (Wang et al. 2004).

The well-recognized role of $PGE_2$ during tumor promotion coupled with findings demonstrating long-term use of NSAIDs may be associated with GI toxicity (Masso Gonzalez et al. 2010) and increased risk of adverse CV events (Garcia Rodriguez et al. 2008; Grosser et al. 2006), provided the rationale for the identification of novel enzymatic targets within the AA pathway, including the $PGE_2$ terminal synthases (PGES) (Wang and DuBois 2008). To date, three different gene products with PGES activity have been identified, encoding microsomal PGES-1 (mPGES-1), mPGES-2, and cytosolic PGES (cPGES), respectively (Kudo and Murakami 2005) (Fig. 1). mPGES-1 is a member of the MAPEG (membrane-associated proteins involved in eicosanoid and glutathione metabolism) superfamily, showing significant homology with other MAPEG superfamily proteins. mPGES-1 is expressed at minimal levels in most normal tissues, although abundant and constitutive expression is detected in a limited number of organs, such as the lung, kidney, and reproductive organs. mPGES-1 is also induced by cytokines and various growth factors (Samuelsson et al. 2007). The closely related mPGES-2 is expressed constitutively in a variety of human tissues, and unlike mPGES-1, it is not induced by proinflammatory signals. cPGES is expressed in a ubiquitous manner, and is thought to mediate constitutive $PGE_2$ biosynthesis based on its preferential coupling with COX-1 (Murakami et al. 2000). mPGES-1 is in general functionally coupled with COX-2 and its expression is often concomitantly induced with COX-2 overexpression, thus, contributing to the efficient generation of $PGE_2$ during inflammation (Jakobsson et al. 1999). However, studies using diverse stimuli provided evidence that COX-2 and mPGES-1 can be independently regulated (Sampey et al. 2005). This observation suggested the possibility that the pharmacological targeting of mPGES-1 may result in the suppression of $PGE_2$ production (Fig. 1) by mechanisms that circumvent the CV toxicity associated with inhibition of COX-2 activity by NSAIDs, both traditional and COX-2 selective inhibitors (named coxibs) (Bruno et al. 2010; Wang and DuBois 2008). On the basis of evidence from cell culture studies, several in vivo studies have been performed to address the impact of mPGES-1 targeting on colon tumorigenesis, but the results of these studies are conflicting (Nakanishi et al. 2010). In particular, mPGES-1 knockout mice in a mutant APC background mPGES-1 showed a significant reduction in the number and size of intestinal tumors. Interestingly, mPGES-1 deletion caused a disorganized vascular pattern within primary adenomas, implicating a novel role of $PGE_2$ in tumor angiogenesis (Nakanishi et al. 2008). In contrast, Elander et al. reported that genetic deletion of mPGES-1 resulted in accelerated intestinal tumorigenesis in $APC^{Min/+}$ mice (Elander et al. 2008). Environmental factors (i.e. Helicobacter pylori infection) may represent a possible explanation of these different responses along with genetic differences in the mouse models used. Based on these differences, the role of mPGES-1 in intestinal carcinogenesis should be further elucidated in preclinical studies prior to extended development of mPGES-1 inhibitors as novel potential chemopreventive agents (Fig. 1) (Nakanishi et al. 2010).

A different mechanism of action seems to explain the chemopreventive effect of long-term use of low-dose aspirin (Rothwell et al. 2010, 2011). In fact, several lines of clinical and experimental evidence support the notion that low-dose aspirin is an efficacious anti-thrombotic agent targeting mainly platelet COX-1 (Patrono et al. 2008; see Chap. 3). Thus, it is proposed that the same mechanism plays a role in the antitumorigenic effect of low-dose aspirin. Activated platelets may be involved in the early phase of intestinal transformation through the activation and induction of COX-2 in stromal cells (Patrono et al. 2001); these cells and their released factors may contribute to epithelial COX-2 expression in the intestinal tract, thus causing the increase of cell proliferation and the accumulation of mutations, as a consequence of inhibition of apoptosis (Cao and Prescott 2002; Prescott 2000). According with this scheme of intestinal tumorigenesis, both COX-1 and COX-2 play a role by operating sequentially, with COX-1 acting upstream of COX-2 (see Chap. 3). This is supported by experimental results showing that loss of either COX-1 or COX-2 genes blocks intestinal polyposis in mouse models of FAP by about 90 % (Chulada et al. 2000). Low-dose aspirin may affect early phase of tumorigenesis by slowing down COX-2 induction in stromal and intestinal epithelial cells, as a consequence of the inhibition of platelet activation. Differently, NSAIDs and coxibs act, as anticancer agents, in later phases of the disease by affecting the consequences of COX-2 overexpression and enhanced generation of prostanoids.

Chan et al. (2007) have shown that regular aspirin use conferred a significant reduction in the risk of CRC that overexpressed COX-2 [multivariate relative risk, 0.64; 95 % confidence interval (CI), 0.52–0.78], whereas regular aspirin use had no influence on tumors with weak or absent expression of COX-2 (multivariate relative risk, 0.96; 95 % CI, 0.73–1.26). These findings do not contradict the antiplatelet mechanism of CRC chemoprevention by aspirin but may suggest that the pathway platelet COX-1 → stromal/epithelial COX-2 overexpression occurs in the setting of genetic/epigenetic dysregulated mechanisms of COX-2 expression.

## 1.6 Prostaglandin Transporters in CRC

Intracellular $PGE_2$ can cross through the membrane by simple diffusion or via a PG efflux transporter such as MRP4, which efficiently transports $PGE_2$ in an ATP-dependent manner (Reid et al. 2003). Extracellular $PGE_2$ can be transported into the cell, where it can be inactivated or act via nuclear receptors (Zhu et al. 2006). It has been suggested that inactivation of $PGE_2$ in the tumor microenvironment occurs in two steps. First, the PG transporter (PGT) mediates the carrier-mediated membrane transport of PGs, including $PGE_2$, $PGF_{2\alpha}$, and $PGD_2$ from the extracellular milieu to the cytoplasm. Second, 15-hydroxyprostaglandin dehydrogenase (15-PGDH) catabolizes and thus inactivates $PGE_2$ (Nomura et al. 2004). It has been reported that both the expression and activity of 15-PGDH is repressed in human CRC and $APC^{Min/+}$ mouse adenomas, resulting in decreased catabolism of $PGE_2$ (Backlund et al. 2005; Myung et al. 2006; Yan et al. 2004). These findings support the role of 15-PGDH as a colon cancer suppressor gene that antagonizes the tumorigenic properties of COX-2-derived $PGE_2$. Recently, this model used to explain the increased levels of $PGE_2$ in colorectal neoplasia has been enriched by novel findings showing that other mechanisms of coordinated up- and downregulation of genes involved in $PGE_2$ transport may contribute to increase $PGE_2$ levels in tumor microenvironment. In particular, it has been shown that PGT and MRP4 mRNA levels are inversely regulated in human CRC compared to normal mucosa and in intestinal adenomas from $APC^{Min/+}$ mice, thus suggesting that $PGE_2$ transports to the cytoplasm, where it can be inactivated by 15-PGDH may be another crucial step in the regulation of $PGE_2$ levels of intestinal neoplasia (Holla et al. 2008).

## 1.7 Epidermal Growth Factor Receptor Pathway

Epidermal growth factor receptor (EGFR) mediates another important signaling involving developing colonic carcinomas. In particular, it has been shown that the early effects of COX-2-derived $PGE_2$ are in part mediated by the EGFR. The tyrosine kinase EGFR is one of four members of the HER/ErbB growth factor receptor family and its activity is increased in adenomas that occur in $APC^{Min/+}$ mice (Moran et al. 2004). Moreover, the disruption of EGFR signaling through either kinase inhibition or genetic mutation inhibits polyp formation and the growth of established tumors (Roberts et al. 2002).

As reported above, $PGE_2$ induces increased proliferation, migration, and invasiveness of colorectal carcinoma cells (Wang et al. 2004). These effects of $PGE_2$ were dependent upon the activation of the phosphatidylinositol 3-kinase/Akt pathway. $PGE_2$ also can induce activation of G proteins which classically activate PKA-mediated transcriptional activation via an increase in cAMP. This coupled activation of Akt and $G\alpha$ subunits results in the accumulation of $\beta$-catenin of the canonical Wnt pathway in the nucleus, leading to transcriptional activation of target genes. Interestingly, it has been shown that the activation of EGFR pathway by $PGE_2$ can also lead to the activation of Akt and MAPK (Buchanan and DuBois 2006). Thus, the transactivation of EGFR by $PGE_2$ is, at least in part, responsible for subsequent downstream effects including the stimulation of cell migration and invasion by COX-2-dependent $PGE_2$. In light of the CV effects associated with long-term COX-2 inhibitor use and the important role of EGFR signaling in CRC, the inhibition of both these pathways has been proposed as a novel potential therapeutic approach and has inspired several studies in animal models of CRC (Buchanan et al. 2007).

## 1.8 Peroxisome Proliferator-Activated Receptors

Growing evidence has demonstrated that peroxisome proliferator-activated receptor (PPAR) $\gamma$ serves as a tumor suppressor in CRC. PPAR$\gamma$ is one of the three different isoforms of PPARs (PPAR$\alpha$, PPAR$\beta/\delta$, and PPAR$\gamma$), which are ligand-activated transcription factors and members of the nuclear hormone receptor superfamily. They are implicated in a variety of physiologic and pathologic processes such as nutrient metabolism, energy homeostasis, inflammation, and cancer.

Evidence that PPAR$\gamma$ has an antitumor effect in CRC comes from several studies in vitro showing that PPAR$\gamma$ activation is associated with the inhibition of cell growth. This finding was corroborated in animal studies using a xenograft model of CRC in nude mice and another study using mice carrying an heterozygous deletion of PPAR$\gamma$, where an increased tendency to develop carcinogen-induced colon cancer compared with wild-type mice was observed. Importantly, the protective role of PPAR$\gamma$ is also supported by the finding that point mutations in the ligand-binding domain of one allele of the PPAR$\gamma$ gene resulted in an inability to bind ligands and control gene regulation. Interestingly, despite numerous lines of evidence supporting the role of PPAR$\gamma$ as tumor suppressor gene in CRC, different groups have reported that administration of PPAR$\gamma$ agonists, such as thiazolidinediones, enhanced colon polyp number in the $APC^{Min/+}$ mice but not in wild-type mice. These results suggest that: (1) PPAR$\gamma$ activation might be associated to a pro-tumorigenic effect when it occurs after tumor initiation, as in the $APC^{Min/+}$ mice; (2) a predisposed genetic susceptibility is necessary for the occurrence of this pro-tumorigenic effect. Thus, the assessment of the genetic predisposition may be proven useful to predict the success of PPAR$\gamma$-targeted therapy.

Although it was well established that PPAR$\gamma$ activation is associated with changes of gene expression translating into the induction of apoptosis, inhibition of cell proliferation, and angiogenesis in colon cancer cells, the molecular mechanisms of CRC suppression by PPAR$\gamma$ are complex and not completely elucidated. To date, the main mechanisms implicated in the antitumor activities of PPAR$\gamma$ ligands include the downregulation of $\beta$-catenin, the induction of caveolin-1, caveolin-2, and proline oxidase, and the upregulation of the tumor suppressor p53 (Dai and Wang 2010).

## 1.9 Tumor Microenvironment in Colorectal Carcinogenesis

The tumor microenvironment, which essentially consists of tumor-infiltrating cells, vasculature, extracellular matrix (ECM), and other matrix-associated molecules, has an important role in the multi-step process characteristic of the adenoma-carcinoma sequence in CRC. The tumor microenvironment is quite distinct from the normal tissue microenvironment and it is composed of a particular phenotype of stromal cells, including: (1) tumor-associated macrophages (TAMs), which are activated by microenvironment stimuli to a pro-tumor polarization state (called M2); (2) tumor-associated neutrophils (TANs) with a pro-tumor phenotype (called N2 neutrophils), and cancer-associated fibroblasts (CAFs). In fact, following the initiation of epithelial tumors, reciprocal interactions between transformed epithelial and stromal cells translate into a switch from a normal to a tumor microenvironment which is associated with massive infiltration of immune cells that have undergone substantial changes of their functionality. Tumor-infiltrating cells predominantly include TAMs, myeloid-derived suppressor cells (MDSCs), CD4 T-cells, CD8 T cells, CD4 regulatory T cells (Tregs), mesenchymal stem cells (MSCs), CAFs, endothelial progenitor cells (EPCs), mast cells, and platelets (Peddareddigari et al. 2011). As aforementioned, various reports demonstrate these cells can contribute to elevated prostanoid biosynthesis in the tumor microenvironment through upregulated COX-2 expression (Singer et al. 1998; Wiercinska-Drapalo et al. 1999; Prescott 2000; Cao and Prescott 2002; Dixon et al. 2006) indicating these cells are able to support tumor-associated inflammation, angiogenesis, and immune suppression, which in turn promotes tumor growth and metastasis (Peddareddigari et al. 2011).

# 2 COX-2 Gene Expression in CRC

As reported above, two primary COX enzyme isoforms have been identified to play distinct roles in physiologic and pathologic conditions. COX-1 is constitutively expressed in most cell types, and COX-1-derived PGs are necessary for protection of gastric mucosa and maintenance of vascular tone (Simmons et al. 2004). While COX-2 is normally absent in most cells, this immediate-early response gene is rapidly induced by a variety of pro-inflammatory and growth-associated stimuli, resulting in increased $PGE_2$ synthesis (Simmons et al. 2004). COX-2 has been identified to play a role in the progression of tumorigenesis, supported by various reports demonstrating that COX-2 levels are increased in premalignant and malignant tumors, and this increase in COX-2 gene expression is associated with decreased cancer patient survival (Wang and Dubois 2010a).

The relationship between COX-2 expression and CRC was first suggested by studies that demonstrated the efficacy of aspirin, NSAIDs, and coxibs to reduce colon cancer risk and also promote tumor regression in both humans and experimental animal models of colon cancer (Wang and Dubois 2010b). The molecular basis of these observations indicated that high levels of COX-2 protein were present in both human and animal colorectal tumors, whereas the normal intestinal mucosa has low-to-undetectable COX-2 expression (Wang and Dubois 2010b). COX-2 is overexpressed in approximately 80 % of colorectal adenocarcinomas and has been shown to play roles in invasiveness, apoptotic resistance, and increased tumor angiogenesis (Wang and Dubois 2010b). This association was further established in genetic studies demonstrating a significant reduction in intestinal polyposis in mice deficient for the COX-2 gene (PTGS2) (Oshima et al. 1996). These findings clearly indicate that chronic elevation of COX-2 is pathological and suggest that inhibition of COX-2 via pharmacological means or regulation of its expression can limit the development and progression of CRC.

## 2.1 Transcriptional Regulation

A variety of evidence gathered from epidemiological, experimental animal, and cellular studies indicate that unregulated COX-2 expression is an important step in CRC and it is generally well accepted that transcriptional activation of COX-2 can occur early during tumorigenesis (Fig. 2) (Dixon 2003; Wu et al. 2010). Evidence of constitutive activation of the COX-2 promoter occurring in colon cancer cells (Kutchera et al. 1996) suggested that the increased levels of COX-2 mRNA detected in colorectal adenomas and adenocarcinomas (Eberhart et al. 1994;
Kutchera et al. 1996) occur through increased transcription. Within the COX-2 promoter region lies *cis*-acting elements for the binding of several transcriptional factor complexes, such as NF$\kappa$B (Kojima et al. 2000; Schmedtje et al. 1997; Singer et al. 1998), C/EBP (Kim and Fischer 1998; Shao et al. 2000), $\beta$-catenin/TCF (Araki et al. 2003; Howe et al. 1999; Mei et al. 1999), CREB (Shao et al. 2000; Subbaramaiah et al. 2002a), NFAT (Hernandez et al. 2001), AP-1 (Miller et al. 1998; Subbaramaiah et al. 2002b), PPAR (Meade et al. 1999), and HIF$\alpha$ (Bazan and Lukiw 2002; Kaidi et al. 2006). The control of COX-2 transcription is a complex regulatory process that requires input from multiple signal transduction pathways (Dixon 2003). Due to the complexity of combined genetic alterations and inflammatory signaling occurring in the tumor microenvironment, identifying a single transcriptional pathway which plays a decisive role in promoting constitutive COX-2 expression in colon cancer has been limiting. Further efforts involving the molecular characterization of individual tumors will aid in identifying the specific cellular defects in these signaling pathways that can promote aberrant COX-2 gene transcription.

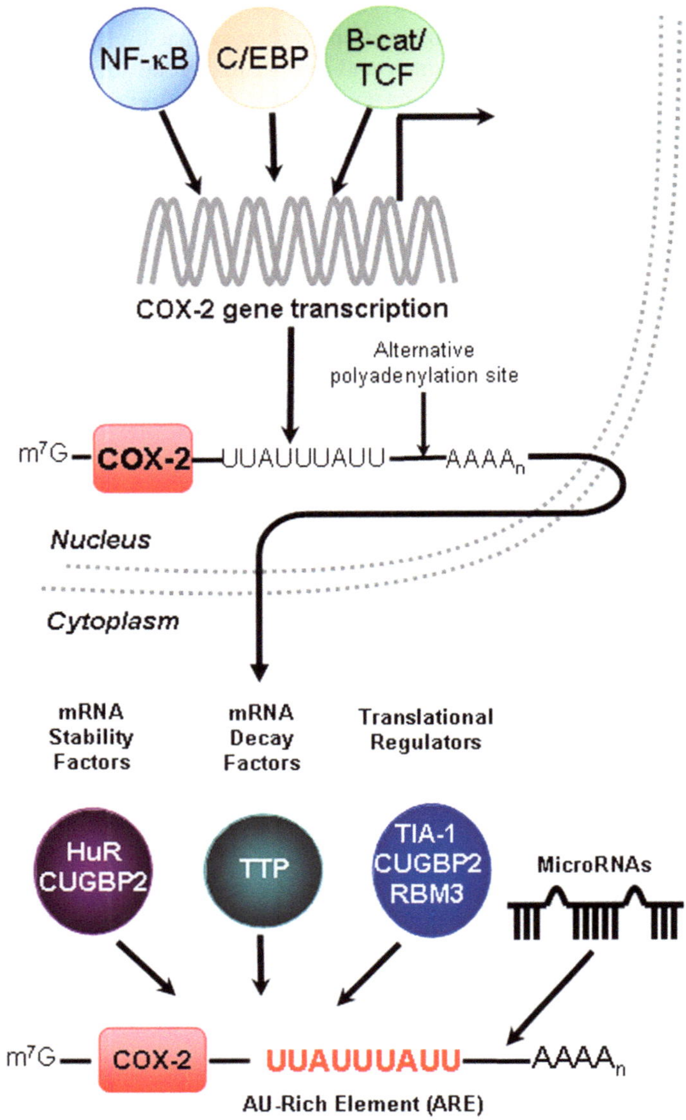


**Fig. 2** Regulation of COX-2 gene expression. Transcription of the COX-2 gene PTGS-2 can be induced by various signaling pathways to activate transcription factors NF$\kappa$B, C/EBP, and $\beta$-catenin/TCF. The primary transcript undergoes splicing, capping at the 5′ end, and polyadenylation at the 3′ end; the presence of alternative polyadenylation signals may lead to a shortened 3′UTR and subsequent loss of regulatory elements. After trafficking to the cytoplasm, COX-2 mRNA fate is mediated by sequence elements present within its 3′UTR. COX-2 expression is tightly regulated at the post-transcriptional level by RNA-binding proteins that promote mRNA stability (HuR and CUGBP2), mRNA decay (TTP), and translational inhibition (TIA-1, CUGBP2, and RMB3) through their binding of the COX-2 AU-rich element (*ARE*). Specific microRNAs have been determined to bind the COX-2 3′UTR and control COX-2 expression

## 2.2 Post-transcriptional Regulation and the 3′ Untranslated Region

An integral method in controlling gene expression is by post-transcriptional mechanisms that regulate mRNA stability and protein translation. The impact of this level of regulation is evident as microarray analysis has detected that 40–50 % of the changes in inducible gene expression occurs at the level of mRNA stability (Cheadle et al. 2005). Eukaryotic mRNAs contain two characteristic features that are integral to their function, a 5′ 7-methylguanosine cap and a 3′ poly (A) tail. In mammalian cells, the majority of mRNA decay is initiated by shortening of the poly (A) tail (deadenylation), after which degradation initiating at the 5′ end involves removal of the 5′ cap by decapping enzymes, followed by 5′ to 3′ exonucleolytic decay. Alternatively, the mRNA can be degraded by 3′ to 5′ exonucleolytic degradation through a complex of exonucleases known as the exosome (Garneau et al. 2007). These two decay pathways are not mutually exclusive and there appears to be overlap between the pathways, although the relative contribution of each mechanism is under debate (Garneau et al. 2007; Newbury et al. 2006). Many mRNAs targeted for degradation are localized to processing (P)-bodies, which are small cytoplasmic foci that contain components of both 3′ to 5′ and 5′ to 3′ decay machinery, suggesting these decay pathways converge at P-bodies (Eulalio et al. 2007; Garneau et al. 2007). An alternative fate of mRNAs observed under situations of cellular stress is their trafficking to cytoplasmic stress granules where they are translationally silenced. Current work now indicates a functional interaction between P-bodies and stress granules suggesting that mRNAs destined for decay are sorted at stress granules and delivered to P-bodies for degradation (Anderson and Kedersha 2008).

Messenger RNA regulatory elements that play a critical role in identifying specific transcripts for post-transcriptional regulation typically reside within the 3′ untranslated region (3′UTR) of the mRNA (Garneau et al. 2007). A well-established mechanism of 3′UTR-mediated post-transcriptional regulation occurs through association with various RNA-binding proteins that target select mRNAs containing adenylate- and uridylate (AU)-rich elements (AREs) within their 3′UTR (Garneau et al. 2007). More recently, small non-coding RNAs called microRNAs (miRNAs) have emerged as global mediators of post-transcriptional gene regulation through their ability to control mRNA stability and translation by imperfect base pairing to the 3′UTR of its target mRNA (Fabian et al. 2010). Currently, it is estimated that nearly one thousand miRNAs function in humans and have been predicted to regulate approximately 60 % of all protein-coding genes (Friedman et al. 2009).

Identification of multiple mRNA regulatory elements present within the COX-2 3′UTR was the first evidence suggesting that COX-2 might be regulated at a post-transcriptional level (Dixon 2003). Exon 10 of the human PTGS2 gene contains the entire 3′UTR and within this region are multiple polyadenylation signals with two signals that are primarily used to yield transcripts of ~4.6 and 2.8 kb in length (Hall-Pogar et al. 2005). Observed in most cells is the larger 4.6 kb COX-2 transcript that results from processing at a distal canonical (AAUAAA) polyadenylation site. However, a proximal non-canonical polyadenylation signal (AUUAAA) can yield transcripts with shortened 3′UTRs (Hall-Pogar et al. 2005). The significance of this alternative mRNA processing event has been shown in CRC cells as a polyadenylation variant of COX-2 mRNA lacking the distal region of the 3′UTR was selectively stabilized upon cell growth to confluence (Sawaoka et al. 2003). These findings suggest that COX-2 mRNA can escape rapid decay through alternative polyadenylation site usage resulting in deletion of potential 3′UTR regulatory elements and this phenomenon of shortening of mRNA transcripts appears to be a widespread feature occurring in cancer cells (Mayr and Bartel 2009).

## 2.3 AU-Rich Elements and ARE-Binding Proteins

A characteristic feature controlling the expression of many inflammatory cytokines, growth factors, and proto-oncogenes is their inherent ability to be targeted for rapid mRNA decay. These cancer-associated gene transcripts are unstable due to the presence of a common *cis*-acting element known as the AU-rich element (ARE) or ARE (Lopez de Silanes et al. 2007). The importance of this particular RNA element is evident, since estimates ranging from 8 to 16 % of human protein-coding genes contain an ARE sequence within their 3′UTR (Bakheet et al. 2006; Gruber et al. 2010). The functional ARE is present within the mRNA 3′UTR and is most often composed of multiple copies of an AUUUA sequence motif clustered together (Bakheet et al. 2006). Within the COX-2 3′UTR, a 116 nucleotide region containing a cluster of 6 AUUUA sequence elements located near the stop codon serves as the functional ARE (Dixon et al. 2000). post-transcriptional regulation has been shown to be dependent upon this ARE since its presence confers rapid decay of a normally stable reporter gene (Dixon et al. 2000). Furthermore, this AU-rich region is highly conserved in both sequence and location among various species of COX-2, implying that ARE function has been evolutionary conserved (Dixon 2003).

Normal cellular growth is associated with rapid decay of ARE-containing mRNAs and targeted mRNA decay is an essential way controlling their pathogenic overexpression. This aspect of COX-2 regulation is observed in non-transformed intestinal epithelial cells where rapid degradation of COX-2 mRNA occurs ($t_{1/2} \sim$ 13 min) (Sheng et al. 2000). However, a number of observations have implicated the loss of ARE-mediated post-transcriptional regulation to occur during neoplastic transformation of cells (Lopez de Silanes et al. 2007) and recent findings have demonstrated an enrichment of this subset of transcripts to occur during colon tumorigenesis. Gene expression profiling comparing adenomas to late-stage adenocarcinomas show a three- to fourfold enrichment in ARE-containing genes compared to the genome as a whole and a similar enrichment is observed as early as stage I tumors (Kanies et al. 2008), suggesting loss of ARE-mediated regulation is lost early during tumor development. With regard to COX-2 regulation, similar findings have been observed in human colon carcinoma cells (Dixon et al. 2001, 2003; Shao et al. 2000; Sheng et al. 2000). As a result of the inability of the COX-2 ARE to function properly in CRC cells, enhanced mRNA stability was detected and increased expression of a reporter gene containing the COX-2 3′UTR was also observed. Based upon the inherent genetic instability of tumor cells, it might be expected that mutations or loss of AREs might occur. However, few naturally occurring mutations in AREs have been described and the ARE region of the PTGS2 gene is intact in healthy individuals as well as in colon tumor cells (Dixon 2003). This implies that loss of ARE function in colon tumors is primarily due to altered ARE recognition by cellular *trans*-acting regulatory RNA binding proteins.

AREs mediate their regulatory function through the association of *trans*-acting RNA-binding proteins that display high affinity for AREs. The best studied ARE-binding proteins can promote rapid mRNA decay, mRNA stabilization, or translational silencing (Garneau et al. 2007). Through these mechanisms, ARE-binding proteins exhibit pleiotropic effects on gene expression, since a single ARE-binding protein can bind to multiple mRNAs and binding can occur among different classes of AREs (Barreau et al. 2005; Lopez de Silanes et al. 2007). Various cytoplasmic proteins have been detected to bind AREs and work has focused on identifying and characterizing COX-2 ARE-binding proteins. To date, 16 different RNA-binding proteins have been reported to bind the COX-2 3′UTR (Young and Dixon 2010). This chapter section will focus on well-documented RNA-binding proteins that regulate COX-2 expression and their potential impact on CRC (Fig. 2).

### 2.3.1 HuR

Hu antigen R (HuR; ELAVL1) is a ubiquitously expressed member of the ELAV (Embryonic-Lethal Abnormal Vision in *Drosophila*) family of RNA-binding proteins (Brennan and Steitz 2001). The human Hu proteins (ubiquitously expressed HuR, and neuronal-specific HuB, HuC, and HuD) were originally discovered as antigens in patients displaying paraneoplastic disorders (Voltz 2002). The cloning and characterization of HuR demonstrated that HuR contains 3 RNA recognition motifs (RRM) with high affinity and specificity for AREs and that cellular HuR overexpression stabilizes ARE-containing transcripts and promotes their translation (Brennan and Steitz 2001).

The ability of HuR to function as an ARE-stability factor appears to be linked to its subcellular localization (Keene 1999). HuR is localized predominantly in the nucleus (>90 %) and can shuttle between the nucleus and cytoplasm. It is hypothesized that the ability of HuR to promote mRNA stabilization requires its translocation to the cytoplasm, and overexpression of HuR promotes cytoplasmic localization where it binds target ARE-containing mRNAs and interferes with their rapid decay (Brennan and Steitz 2001; Keene 1999). A variety of cellular signals known to activate MAPK pathways involving p38 and ERK kinases, the

PI-3-kinase pathway, and the Wnt signaling pathway, have been shown to trigger cytoplasmic HuR localization and promote ARE-containing mRNA stabilization (Briata et al. 2003; Ming et al. 2001; Yang et al. 2004). Insight into the mechanism of HuR-mediated mRNA stabilization has been advanced with the identification of low-molecular weight inhibitors for HuR (Meisner et al. 2007). These compounds inhibit HuR cytoplasmic localization by interfering with RNA-binding (Meisner et al. 2007).

HuR has been shown to associate and post-transcriptionally regulate the expression of numerous cancer-associated transcripts bearing AREs of multiple classes (Abdelmohsen and Gorospe 2010; Lopez de Silanes et al. 2005b). Based on its ability to bind the COX-2 ARE, HuR has been identified as a *trans*-acting factor involved in regulating COX-2 expression (Dixon et al. 2001). The enhanced stabilization of COX-2 mRNA observed in colon cancer cells is, in part, due to elevated levels of HuR (Dixon et al. 2001; Young et al. 2009). Recent work evaluating HuR expression in colon cancer demonstrates that HuR is expressed at low levels and is localized to the nucleus in normal tissue, whereas HuR overexpression and cytoplasmic localization was observed in colon adenomas, adenocarcinomas, and metastases; consistent with these observations, overexpression of COX-2 co-localized with elevated HuR (Young et al. 2009). Furthermore, several studies indicate that HuR overexpression and cytoplasmic localization is a marker for elevated COX-2 that is correlated with advancing stages of malignancy and poor clinical outcome (Dixon 2003).

### 2.3.2 CUGBP2

CUG triplet repeat–binding protein 2 (CUGBP2) is an ubiquitously expressed RNA-binding protein containing 3 RRM and is a member of the CUGBP-ETR-3-like factors (CELF) family (Mukhopadhyay et al. 2003; Murmu et al. 2004). Work investigating COX-2 regulation in colon cancer cells and intestinal epithelium subjected to ionizing radiation had elucidated a novel role for CUGBP2 in regulating COX-2 expression on a post-transcriptional level (Mukhopadhyay et al. 2003; Murmu et al. 2004). CUGPB2 displays high affinity for the COX-2 ARE and radiation-induced overexpression of CUGBP2 led to COX-2 mRNA stabilization similar to the effects of HuR overexpression (Mukhopadhyay et al. 2003). In contrast to HuR, CUGBP2 repressed COX-2 translation by inhibiting ribosome loading of the COX-2 mRNA (Mukhopadhyay et al. 2003). Given that HuR enhances and CUGBP2 inhibits COX-2 protein expression indicates that these two ARE-binding proteins differ in their regulation of COX-2 expression. Although both proteins have similar affinities for the COX-2 ARE, CUGBP2 was effective in competing with HuR for ARE-binding leading to a translational block in COX-2 expression (Sureban et al. 2007). While demonstrating the ability of CUGBP2 to regulate the opposing functions of COX-2 mRNA stabilization and translational repression, these findings suggest a possible role for CUGBP2 in the early stages of tumorigenesis by counteracting the effects of HuR overexpression in order to repress COX-2 protein synthesis.

### 2.3.3 TTP

Tristetraprolin (TTP, ZFP36, TIS11) is a member of a small family of tandem Cys3His zinc finger proteins consisting of TTP, ZFP36L1, and ZFP36L2 (Sanduja et al. 2010). TTP acts on a post-transcriptional level to promote rapid decay of ARE-containing mRNAs by direct ARE binding (Carballo et al. 1998). The binding of TTP to AREs targets the transcript for rapid degradation through association with various decay enzymes (Sanduja et al. 2010). In cells, TTP localizes to P-bodies, which suggests that TTP plays a critical role in ARE-mRNA delivery to cytoplasmic sites of mRNA decay (Franks and Lykke-Andersen 2007; Kedersha et al. 2005). TTP is also a target of phosphorylation by various pathways, and this phosphorylation state likely plays a role in mediating TTP function (Sanduja et al. 2010).

Efforts to characterize the function of TTP have primarily focused on its regulation of inflammatory mediators such as TNF-$\alpha$ and GM-CSF (Carballo et al. 2000; Lai et al. 1999). The physiological consequences of TTP loss is evident, as TTP knock-out mice develop multiple inflammatory syndromes resulting from increased inflammatory factors, including COX-2, due to defects in rapid mRNA turnover (Phillips et al. 2004) and recent work has demonstrated COX-2 to be a target of TTP (Sawaoka et al. 2003; Young et al. 2009). With regard to its role in controlling COX-2 expression in colon cancer, TTP expression is low or not apparent in colon cancer cell lines, adenoma, and adenocarcinoma tissue (Young et al. 2009). This is in contrast to normal tissue where TTP was highest in normal epithelium and predominantly localized to the cytoplasm. Furthermore, adenoviral-mediated delivery of TTP to colon cancer cells resulted in downregulation of COX-2 expression coupled with a dramatic reduction in cell growth and proliferation (Young et al. 2009). These findings indicate that the presence of TTP in normal colon epithelium serves in a protective capacity by controlling expression of various inflammatory mediators including COX-2, whereas the loss of TTP expression in tumors allows for HuR to promote the stabilization and translation of COX-2 mRNA.

### 2.3.4 TIA-1

TIA-1 (T-cell intracellular antigen 1; TIA-1) was originally identified in activated T lymphocytes and is a RNA-binding protein containing 3 RRM motifs with specificity to mRNAs containing short sections of uridylate repeats (Lopez de Silanes et al. 2005a; Tian et al. 1991). Under normal cellular conditions, TIA-1 is predominantly nuclear, and in response to cellular stress translocates to the cytoplasm where it is associated with untranslated mRNAs in cytoplasmic stress granules, implicating a role in translational regulation (Anderson and Kedersha 2008; Kedersha et al. 2005). TIA-1 has been shown to bind the COX-2 ARE and regulate its expression through translational inhibition without impacting COX-2 mRNA turnover (Dixon et al. 2003). However, in colon cancer cells deficiencies in TIA-1 binding to the COX-2 ARE was observed allowing for increased polysome association with the COX-2 mRNA. In vivo, TIA-1 knockout mice maintain elevated levels of COX-2 leading to the development of arthritis (Phillips et al. 2004). These findings implicate TIA-1 as a translational silencer of COX-2 expression, and suggest that loss of TIA-1 function may be a contributing factor promoting enhanced COX-2 levels in cancer and chronic inflammation.

### 2.3.5 RBM3

RNA-binding motif protein 3 (RBM3) is a translational regulatory factor consisting of a single RRM domain and a glycine-rich region (Dresios et al. 2005). Its role in COX-2 regulation was initially identified through its binding to the AREs in the murine COX-2 3′UTR (Cok and Morrison 2001), and two hybrid screening analysis identified RBM3 to interact with HuR (Anant et al. 2010). Similar to HuR expression in cancer, RBM3 is significantly upregulated in colorectal tumors and overexpression of RBM3 in fibroblasts promoted cell transformation (Sureban et al. 2008), indicating an oncogenic capacity for this RNA-binding protein.

Consistent with its interaction with HuR, RBM3 is also a nucleocytoplasmic shuttling protein that promotes stabilization of COX-2 mRNA through binding to ARE sequences located in the first 60 nts of the COX-2 3′UTR (Sureban et al. 2008). RBM3 protein also promotes translation of COX-2 mRNA through its 3′UTR (Sureban et al. 2008); however, the mechanism underlying this effect and RBM3′s partnership with HuR to promote COX-2 mRNA translation remains to be determined. Through its ability to promote mRNA stability and translation of otherwise rapidly degraded transcripts, RBM3 is being recognized as a contributing factor promoting enhanced COX-2 expression during tumorigenesis.

## 2.4 MicroRNAs

MicroRNAs (miRNAs) are small non-coding RNAs approximately 21–24 nucleotides in length that have emerged as fundamental global regulators of gene expression via post-transcriptional mechanisms (Fabian et al. 2010). Within the genome, miRNAs can reside within gene exons or introns and can be transcribed as part of a protein-coding gene or their transcription can be regulated independently (O'Hara et al. 2009). Once transcribed, the primary miRNA transcript (pri-miRNA) is processed in the nucleus into a pre-miRNA stem-loop. The precursor miRNA (pre-miRNA) is actively transported to the cytoplasm where it is processed a second time to form a double-stranded miRNA duplex. One or both strands of the miRNA duplex generate mature miRNAs that can be loaded into the miRNA-induced silencing complex (miRISC) essential to miRNA-mediated gene targeting (Fabian et al. 2010).

MiRNAs regulate gene expression both by influencing translation and by causing degradation of target mRNAs (Fabian et al. 2010) and recent findings have implicated miRNA-mediated mRNA decay to be the predominant mechanism (Guo et al. 2010). Although similar in nature to short interfering RNAs (siRNAs) which bind target mRNA regions with 100 % complementary and promote mRNA degradation, miRNAs can bind imperfectly to the 3′UTR of targeted transcripts to attenuate target gene expression (Filipowicz et al. 2008). Based on this, a single miRNA can potentially impact expression of a large number of proteins with varying cellular functions. Due to the substantial amount of control they have over a number of putative mRNA targets, it is of considerable interest how alterations in miRNA expression in cancer can contribute to tumorigenesis. In CRC, differential expression of several miRNAs has been observed and current efforts have demonstrated that specific miRNA loss or overexpression can impact various cellular pathways associated with colon tumorigenesis (O'Hara et al. 2009; Wiemer 2007). Currently, 5 miRNAs have been reported to target COX-2 mRNA and control its expression (Fig. 2).

### 2.4.1 miR-16

The initial report implicating a role for miRNAs in cancer progression examined miR-16-1 and its function in chronic lymphocytic leukemia (CLL) (Calin et al. 2002). This miRNA is clustered with miR-15a and is located in the most commonly deleted genomic region of individuals affected by CLL who display attenuated expression of miR-16-1 and miR-15a (Calin et al. 2002; Dohner et al. 2000). It was subsequently determined that loss of miR-16-1 and miR-15a promotes cell survival, as they function to target and repress antiapoptotic factors BCL-2 and MCL1 (Cimmino et al. 2005; Sanchez-Beato et al. 2003). MiR-16-1 in particular has additionally been shown to play a role in cell cycle maintenance through regulation of several cell cycle regulatory genes (Liu et al. 2008). These results are in agreement with those showing reduced miR-16-1 levels present in the colorectal microRNAome (Cummins et al. 2006).

Based on its RNA sequence, miR-16 displays complementarity to AU-rich regions and it has been demonstrated that miR-16 can target AREs, particularly the AREs of TNF-$\alpha$, IL-6, IL-8, and COX-2 to alter their mRNA stability (Jing et al. 2005). Interestingly, these same studies determined that miR-16 works in conjunction with TTP to promote decay of ARE-containing mRNAs and this is through interactions between TTP and components of the RISC complex.

In CRC cells and tumors, miR-16 levels were observed to be decreased ~two fold and miR-16 expression in cancer cells attenuated COX-2 expression and PG synthesis (Young et al. 2011). More recent work examining miRNA-mediated regulation of COX-2 demonstrated a functional interaction between HuR and miR-16 in colon cancer cells and this interaction promoted downregulation of miR-16 (Young et al. 2011). Consistent with these observations, studies examining COX-2 regulation in response to diabetic stimuli in leukocytes has identified miR-16 to play a dynamic role in COX-2 regulation under inflammatory conditions (Shanmugam et al. 2008). These findings highlight the significance of this ARE-targeting miRNA in cancer along with demonstrating the ability of miR-16 to regulate COX-2 expression under conditions of chronic inflammation.

### 2.4.2 miR-101 and miR-199

Genomic loss of miR-101 was first detected to occur in 67 % of metastatic prostate cancer cells (Varambally et al. 2008). Since this initial report, miR-101 has further been shown to be attenuated in a variety of malignant tissues including colon, hepatocellular, and gastric cancers (Strillacci et al. 2009; Su et al. 2009; Wang et al. 2010). Initial work investigating the role of COX-2 during embryo implantation identified the murine miRNAs miR-101a and miR-199a to post-transcriptionally regulate murine COX-2 and expression of these miRNAs are inversely correlated with uterine COX-2 protein levels (Chakrabarty et al. 2007). Further work in human cells established the ability of miR-101a and miR-199a to target human COX-2 by direct binding to the 3′UTR (Chakrabarty et al. 2007; Hao et al. 2011). In the context of colon cancer, an inverse correlation between human miR-101 and COX-2 expression in colon cancer cell lines and colon tumors has been shown along with the ability of miR-101 to inhibit COX-2 translation when expressed in cells (Strillacci et al. 2009). On these same lines, COX-2 expressing colon cancer cells do not express miR-199 (Chakrabarty et al. 2007), indicating that limited expression of these miRNAs in colon cancer can contribute to observed COX-2 overexpression.

### 2.4.3 miR-143

MiR-143 is located on Chr 5q32 and is thought to originate from the same pri-miRNA transcript as miR-145; however, some studies have suggested tissue-specific transcriptional regulation may account for their independent regulation (Akao et al. 2007; Cordes et al. 2009; Wu et al. 2011). Expression of miR-143 is attenuated at the adenoma and carcinoma stages of CRC (Michael et al. 2003), and is consistently attenuated in colorectal tumors and cell lines (Akao et al. 2006; Bandres et al. 2006; Slaby et al. 2007). Furthermore, reintroduction of miR-143 into GI cancer cells has been shown to repress abnormal cell growth and proliferation (Akao et al. 2006; Chen et al. 2009; Takagi et al. 2009). More recently, miR-143 has been found to promote COX-2 down regulation in a bladder carcinoma cellular model, resulting in reduced cell proliferation and mobility (Song et al. 2011).

### 2.4.4 miR-542-3p

Various examples of dysregulated miRNA expression have been shown to contribute to the pathogenesis most cancers (Croce 2009) and more recently, genetic polymorphisms in components of miRNA networks and their targets are being recognized as contributing factors in disease etiology (Ryan et al. 2010). Several studies have identified a common single nucleotide polymorphism (SNP) in the COX-2 gene at position 8473 (T8473C; rs5275) that is associated with increased risk and/or NSAID responsiveness in a number of cancers where COX-2 overexpression is a contributing factor (Ali et al. 2005; Campa et al. 2004; Ferguson et al. 2008; Gong et al. 2009; Langsenlehner et al. 2006; Ozhan et al. 2010; Shen et al. 2006; Siezen et al. 2005; Vogel et al. 2008). The T8473C SNP is located in exon 10 which encodes the COX-2 3′UTR suggesting a potential role in post-transcriptional regulation. Recent findings have demonstrated that this SNP lies within a region that targets COX-2 mRNA for degradation by miR-542-3p (Moore et al. 2011). This miRNA was identified to bind transcripts derived from the 8473T allele and promote mRNA decay, whereas the cancer-associated variant 8473C allele interfered with miR-542-3p binding allowing for mRNA stabilization. Colon cancer cells and tissue displayed COX-2 expression levels that were dependent on T8473C allele dosage and allelic-specific expression of COX-2 was observed to be a contributing factor promoting COX-2 overexpression (Moore et al. 2011). These findings provide a novel molecular explanation underlying cancer susceptibility associated with COX-2 T8473C SNP and identify it as a potential marker for identifying cancer patients best served through selective COX-2 inhibition.

## 3 Conclusions

Numerous evidences sustain a key role of COX-2 overexpression in the development of cancers, in particular CRC (Prescott 2000; Cha and Dubois 2007, Harper and Tyson-Capper 2008; Young et al. 2009). A proof of concept of the role of COX-2 in human tumorigenesis is evidenced by the efficacy of selective COX-2 inhibitors (such as celecoxib) to decrease the risk of colorectal adenoma recurrence (Bertagnolli et al. 2006; Steinbach et al. 2000). However, the use of selective COX-2 inhibitors seems to be inappropriate due to the interference with CV homeostasis by the coincident inhibition of vascular COX-2-dependent $PGI_2$ (Grosser et al. 2006). The challenge of the next years will be to improve the management of CRC by using a double approach based on the development of innovative prevention-based strategies and anticancer therapies. Although important strides have been made through the understanding of the genetic mechanisms associated with the adenoma-carcinoma sequence, thus allowing for the development of improved strategies to identify patients at high risk to develop CRC, biomarkers of early detection and of safe and effective chemopreventive agents are still lacking. Furthermore, the reduced capacity of colorectal screening programs in detecting proximal colon cancers represents another important limitation in prevention of CRC. In the future, mechanistic studies should be performed to clarify the molecular pathways of the chemopreventive effects of low-dose aspirin in CRC (Rothwell et al. 2010, 2011) and the results of these studies may open the way to a new promising strategy for the primary prevention of CRC, based on the use of low-dose aspirin as chemopreventive agent.

On the other hand, the use of selective inhibitors of mPGES-1, which are under development (Samuelsson et al. 2007), may represent a very promising therapeutic approach to overcome the limits of COX-2 inhibitors due to the CV hazard (Grosser et al. 2006). In fact, mPGES-1 inhibitors cause a selective inhibition of $PGE_2$ by affecting a $PGE_2$ synthase downstream of COX-2 and thus, they do not affect, or even can augment, the biosynthesis of the vasoprotective $PGI_2$ (Wang et al. 2008). However, the knowledge that in cancer, COX-2 overexpression is controlled at the post-transcriptional level through changes in its mRNA stability by miRNAs open the way to innovative strategies for design of therapeutics affecting this pathway involved in colon tumorigenesis (Fig. 2). In this perspective, the development of tissue-specific delivery system for specific miRNAs is just beginning and it looks promising.

**Acknowledgments** This work was supported by the National Institutes of Health (R01 CA134609 to D.A. Dixon) and American Cancer Society (RSG-06-122-01-CNE to D.A. Dixon). We apologize to our colleagues for not being able to reference all primary work due to space limitations.

## References

Abdelmohsen K, Gorospe M (2010) Post-transcriptional regulation of cancer traits by HuR. Wiley Interdisc Rev RNA 1:214–229
Ahnen DJ (2011) The American college of gastroenterology emily couric lecture–the adenoma-carcinoma sequence revisited: Has the era of genetic tailoring finally arrived? Am J Gastroenterol 106:190–198
Akao Y, Nakagawa Y, Naoe T (2006) MicroRNAs 143 and 145 are possible common onco-microRNAs in human cancers. Oncol Rep 16:845–850
Akao Y, Nakagawa Y, Naoe T (2007) MicroRNA-143 and -145 in colon cancer. DNA Cell Biol 26:311–320
Ali IU, Luke BT, Dean M et al (2005) Allellic variants in regulatory regions of cyclooxygenase-2: association with advanced colorectal adenoma. Br J Cancer 93:953–959
Anant S, Houchen CW, Pawar V et al (2010) Role of RNA-binding proteins in colorectal carcinogenesis. Curr Colorectal Cancer Rep 6:68–73
Anderson P, Kedersha N (2008) Stress granules: the tao of RNA triage. Trends Biochem Sci 33:141–150
Araki Y, Okamura S, Hussain SP et al (2003) Regulation of cyclooxygenase-2 expression by the wnt and ras pathways. Cancer Res 63:728–734
Atkin WS, Edwards R, Kralj-Hans I et al (2010) Once-only flexible sigmoidoscopy screening in prevention of colorectal cancer: a multicentre randomised controlled trial. Lancet 375:1624–1633
Backlund MG, Mann JR, Holla VR et al (2005) 15-hydroxyprostaglandin dehydrogenase is down-regulated in colorectal cancer. J Biol Chem 280:3217–3223
Bakheet T, Williams BR, Khabar KS (2006) ARED 3.0: the large and diverse AU-rich transcriptome. Nucleic Acids Res 34:D111–D114
Bandres E, Cubedo E, Agirre X et al (2006) Identification by real-time PCR of 13 mature microRNAs differentially expressed in colorectal cancer and non-tumoral tissues. Mol Cancer 5:29
Barreau C, Paillard L, Osborne HB (2005) AU-rich elements and associated factors: Are there unifying principles? Nucleic Acids Res 33:7138–7150
Bazan NG, Lukiw WJ (2002) Cyclooxygenase-2 and presenilin-1 gene expression induced by interleukin-1beta and amyloid beta 42 peptide is potentiated by hypoxia in primary human neural cells. J Biol Chem 277:30359–30367
Bertagnolli MM, Eagle CJ, Zauber AG et al (2006) Celecoxib for the prevention of sporadic colorectal adenomas. N Engl J Med 355:873–884
Brennan CM, Steitz JA (2001) HuR and mRNA stability. Cell Mol Life Sci 58:266–277

Briata P, Ilengo C, Corte G et al (2003) The wnt/beta-catenin → pitx2 pathway controls the turnover of pitx2 and other unstable mrnas. Mol Cell 12:1201–1211
Bruno A, Di Francesco L, Coletta I et al (2010) Effects of af3442 [n-(9-ethyl-9 h-carbazol-3-yl)-2-(trifluoromethyl)benzamide], a novel inhibitor of human microsomal prostaglandin e synthase-1, on prostanoid biosynthesis in human monocytes in vitro. Biochem Pharmacol 79:974–981
Buchanan FG, DuBois RN (2006) Connecting COX-2 and wnt in cancer. Cancer Cell 9:6–8
Buchanan FG, Holla V, Katkuri S et al (2007) Targeting cyclooxygenase-2 and the epidermal growth factor receptor for the prevention and treatment of intestinal cancer. Cancer Res 67:9380–9388
Burn J, Bishop DT, Chapman PD et al (2011) A randomized placebo-controlled prevention trial of aspirin and/or resistant starch in young people with familial adenomatous polyposis. Cancer Prev Res 4:655–665
Calin GA, Dumitru CD, Shimizu M et al (2002) Frequent deletions and down-regulation of micro-RNA genes mir15 and mir16 at 13q14 in chronic lymphocytic leukemia. Proc Nat Acad Sci USA 99:15524–15529
Campa D, Zienolddiny S, Maggini V et al (2004) Association of a common polymorphism in the cyclooxygenase 2 gene with risk of non-small cell lung cancer. Carcinogenesis 25:229–235
Cao Y, Prescott SM (2002) Many actions of cyclooxygenase-2 in cellular dynamics and in cancer. J Cell Physiol 90:279–286
Carballo E, Lai WS, Blackshear PJ (1998) Feedback inhibition of macrophage tumor necrosis factor-a production by tristetraprolin. Science 281:1001–1005
Carballo E, Lai WS, Blackshear PJ (2000) Evidence that tristetraprolin is a physiological regulator of granulocyte-macrophage colony-stimulating factor messenger RNA deadenylation and stability. Blood 95:1891–1899
Castells A, Paya A, Alenda C et al (2006) Cyclooxygenase 2 expression in colorectal cancer with DNA mismatch repair deficiency. Clin Cancer Res 12:1686–1692
Cha YI, DuBois RN (2007) NSAIDs and cancer prevention: targets downstream of COX-2. Annu Rev Med 58:239–252
Chakrabarty A, Tranguch S, Daikoku T et al (2007) MicroRNA regulation of cyclooxygenase-2 during embryo implantation. Proc Nat Acad Sci USA 104:15144–15149
Chan AT, Ogino S, Fuchs CS (2007) Aspirin and the risk of colorectal cancer in relation to the expression of COX-2. N Engl J Med 356:2131–2142
Cheadle C, Fan J, Cho-Chung YS et al (2005) Control of gene expression during t cell activation: alternate regulation of mRNA transcription and mRNA stability. BMC Genomics 6:75
Chen X, Guo X, Zhang H et al (2009) Role of miR-143 targeting kras in colorectal tumorigenesis. Oncogene 28:1385–1392
Chulada PC, Thompson MB, Mahler JF et al (2000) Genetic disruption of ptgs-1, as well as ptgs-2, reduces intestinal tumorigenesis in min mice. Cancer Res 60:4705–4708
Cimmino A, Calin GA, Fabbri M et al (2005) MiR-15 and miR-16 induce apoptosis by targeting bcl2. Proc Nat Acad Sci USA 102:13944–13949
Cok SJ, Morrison AR (2001) The 3′-untranslated region of murine cyclooxygenase-2 contains multiple regulatory elements that alter message stability and translational efficiency. J Biol Chem 276:23179–23185
Cordes KR, Sheehy NT, White MP et al (2009) MiR-145 and miR-143 regulate smooth muscle cell fate and plasticity. Nature 460:705–710
Croce CM (2009) Causes and consequences of microRNA dysregulation in cancer. Nat Rev Genet 10:704–714
Cummins JM, He Y, Leary RJ et al (2006) The colorectal micrornaome. Proc Nat Acad Sci USA 103:3687–3692
Dai Y, Wang WH (2010) Peroxisome proliferator-activated receptor gamma and colorectal cancer. World J Gastrointest Oncol 2:159–164

Dimberg J, Hugander A, Sirsjo A et al (2001) Enhanced expression of cyclooxygenase-2 and nuclear beta-catenin are related to mutations in the APC gene in human colorectal cancer. Anticancer Res 21:911–915
Dixon DA (2003) Regulation of COX-2 expression in human cancer. Prog Exp Tumor Res 37:52–71
Dixon DA, Balch GC, Kedersha N et al (2003) Regulation of cyclooxygenase-2 expression by the translational silencer TIA-1. J Exp Med 198:475–481
Dixon DA, Kaplan CD, McIntyre TM et al (2000) Post-transcriptional control of cyclooxygenase-2 gene expression. The role of the 3′-untranslated region. J Biol Chem 275:11750–11757
Dixon DA, Tolley ND, King PH et al (2001) Altered expression of the mRNA stability factor HuR promotes cyclooxygenase-2 expression in colon cancer cells. J Clin Invest 108:1657–1665
Dixon DA, Tolley ND, Bemis-Standoli K et al (2006) Expression of COX-2 in platelet-monocyte interactions occurs via combinatorial regulation involving adhesion and cytokine signaling. J Clin Invest 116:2727–2738
Dohner H, Stilgenbauer S, Benner A et al (2000) Genomic aberrations and survival in chronic lymphocytic leukemia. N Engl J Med 343:1910–1916
Dresios J, Aschrafi A, Owens GC et al (2005) Cold stress-induced protein RBM3 binds 60s ribosomal subunits, alters microRNA levels, and enhances global protein synthesis. Proc Nat Acad Sci USA 102:1865–1870
Duval A, Hamelin R (2002) Mutations at coding repeat sequences in mismatch repair-deficient human cancers: toward a new concept of target genes for instability. Cancer Res 62:2447–2454
Eberhart CE, Coffey RJ, Radhika A et al (1994) Up-regulation of cyclooxygenase 2 gene expression in human colorectal adenomas and adenocarcinomas. Gastroenterology 107:1183–1188
Elander N, Ungerback J, Olsson H et al (2008) Genetic deletion of mPGES-1 accelerates intestinal tumorigenesis in apc(min/+) mice. Biochem Biophys Res Commun 372:249–253
Eulalio A, Behm-Ansmant I, Izaurralde E (2007) P bodies: at the crossroads of post-transcriptional pathways. Nat Rev Mol Cell Biol 8:9–22
Fabian MR, Sonenberg N, Filipowicz W (2010) Regulation of mRNA translation and stability by microRNAs. Annu Rev Biochem 79:351–379
Ferguson HR, Wild CP, Anderson LA et al (2008) Cyclooxygenase-2 and inducible nitric oxide synthase gene polymorphisms and risk of reflux esophagitis, barrett's esophagus, and esophageal adenocarcinoma. Cancer Epidemiol Biomarkers Prev 17:727–731
Filipowicz W, Bhattacharyya SN, Sonenberg N (2008) Mechanisms of post-transcriptional regulation by microRNAs: Are the answers in sight? Nat Rev Genet 9:102–114
Franks TM, Lykke-Andersen J (2007) TTP and BRF proteins nucleate processing body formation to silence mRNAs with AU-rich elements. Genes Dev 21:719–735
Friedman RC, Farh KK, Burge CB et al (2009) Most mammalian mRNAs are conserved targets of microRNAs. Genome Res 19:92–105
Funk CD (2001) Prostaglandins and leukotrienes: advances in eicosanoid biology. Science 294:1871–1875
Garcia Rodriguez LA, Tacconelli S, Patrignani P (2008) Role of dose potency in the prediction of risk of myocardial infarction associated with nonsteroidal anti-inflammatory drugs in the general population. J Am Coll Cardiol 52:1628–1636
Garneau NL, Wilusz J, Wilusz CJ (2007) The highways and byways of mRNA decay. Nat Rev Mol Cell Biol 8:113–126
Giardiello FM, Casero RA Jr, Hamilton SR et al (2004) Prostanoids, ornithine decarboxylase, and polyamines in primary chemoprevention of familial adenomatous polyposis. Gastroenterology 126:425–431
Gong Z, Bostick RM, Xie D et al (2009) Genetic polymorphisms in the cyclooxygenase-1 and cyclooxygenase-2 genes and risk of colorectal adenoma. Int J Colorectal Dis 24:647–654

Grady WM, Carethers JM (2008) Genomic and epigenetic instability in colorectal cancer pathogenesis. Gastroenterology 135:1079–1099
Grosser T, Fries S, FitzGerald GA (2006) Biological basis for the cardiovascular consequences of COX-2 inhibition: therapeutic challenges and opportunities. J Clin Invest 116:4–15
Gruber AR, Fallmann J, Kratochvill F et al (2010) Aresite: a database for the comprehensive investigation of AU-rich elements. Nucleic Acids Res 39:D66–D69
Guo H, Ingolia NT, Weissman JS et al (2010) Mammalian microRNAs predominantly act to decrease target mRNA levels. Nature 466:835–840
Hall-Pogar T, Zhang H, Tian B et al (2005) Alternative polyadenylation of cyclooxygenase-2. Nucleic Acids Res 33:2565–2579
Hao Y, Gu X, Zhao Y et al (2011) Enforced expression of miR-101 inhibits prostate cancer cell growth by modulating the COX-2 pathway in vivo. Cancer Prev Res (Phila) 4:1073–1083
Harper KA, Tyson-Capper AJ (2008) Complexity of COX-2 gene regulation. Biochem Soc Trans 36:543–545
Hernandez GL, Volpert OV, Iniguez MA et al (2001) Selective inhibition of vascular endothelial growth factor-mediated angiogenesis by cyclosporin a: roles of the nuclear factor of activated t cells and cyclooxygenase 2. J Exp Med 193:607–620
Holla VR, Backlund MG, Yang P et al (2008) Regulation of prostaglandin transporters in colorectal neoplasia. Cancer Prev Res 1:93–99
Howe LR, Subbaramaiah K, Chung WJ et al (1999) Transcriptional activation of cyclooxygenase-2 in wnt-1-transformed mouse mammary epithelial cells. Cancer Res 59:1572–1577
Issa JP (2004) CpG island methylator phenotype in cancer. Nat Rev Cancer 4:988–993
Jakobsson PJ, Thoren S, Morgenstern R et al (1999) Identification of human prostaglandin E synthase: a microsomal, glutathione-dependent, inducible enzyme, constituting a potential novel drug target. Proc Nat Acad Sci USA 96:7220–7225
Jemal A, Bray F, Center MM et al (2011) Global cancer statistics. CA Cancer J Clin 61:69–90
Jing Q, Huang S, Guth S et al (2005) Involvement of microRNA in AU-rich element-mediated mRNA instability. Cell 120:623–634
Kaidi A, Qualtrough D, Williams AC et al (2006) Direct transcriptional up-regulation of cyclooxygenase-2 by hypoxia-inducible factor (HIF)-1 promotes colorectal tumor cell survival and enhances HIF-1 transcriptional activity during hypoxia. Cancer Res 66:6683–6691
Kanies CL, Smith JJ, Kis C et al (2008) Oncogenic ras and transforming growth factor-beta synergistically regulate AU-rich element-containing mRNAs during epithelial to mesenchymal transition. Mol Cancer Res 6:1124–1136
Karnes WE, Shattuck-Brandt R, Burgart LJ et al (1998) Reduced COX-2 protein in colorectal cancer with defective mismatch repair. Cancer Res 58:5473–5477
Kedersha N, Stoecklin G, Ayodele M et al (2005) Stress granules and processing bodies are dynamically linked sites of mRNP remodeling. J Cell Biol 169:871–884
Keene J (1999) Why is Hu where? Shuttling of early-response messenger RNA subsets. Proc Nat Acad Sci USA 96:5–7
Kim Y, Fischer SM (1998) Transcriptional regulation of cyclooxygenase-2 in mouse skin carcinoma cells. Regulatory role of ccaat/enhancer-binding proteins in the differential expression of cyclooxygenase-2 in normal and neoplastic tissues. J Biol Chem 273:27686–27694
Kojima M, Morisaki T, Izuhara K et al (2000) Lipopolysaccharide increases cyclo-oxygenase-2 expression in a colon carcinoma cell line through nuclear factor-kappa B activation. Oncogene 19:1225–1231
Kondo Y, Issa JP (2004) Epigenetic changes in colorectal cancer. Cancer Metastasis Rev 23:29–39
Kudo I, Murakami M (2005) Prostaglandin e synthase, a terminal enzyme for prostaglandin E2 biosynthesis. J Biochem Mol Biol 38:633–638

Kulendran M, Stebbing JF, Marks CG et al (2011) Predictive and prognostic factors in colorectal cancer: a personalized approach. Cancers 3:1622–1638

Kutchera W, Jones DA, Matsunami N et al (1996) Prostaglandin synthase 2 is abnormally expressed in human colon cancer: evidence for a transcriptional effect. Proc Nat Acad Sci USA 93:4816–4820

Lai WS, Carballo E, Strum JR et al (1999) Evidence that tristetraprolin binds to AU-rich elements and promotes the deadenylation and destabilization of tumor necrosis factor alpha mRNA. Mol Cell Biol 19:4311–4323

Langsenlehner U, Yazdani-Biuki B, Eder T et al (2006) The cyclooxygenase-2 (PTGS2) 8473T > C polymorphism is associated with breast cancer risk. Clin Cancer Res 12:1392–1394

Liu Q, Fu H, Sun F et al (2008) Mir-16 family induces cell cycle arrest by regulating multiple cell cycle genes. Nucleic Acids Res 36:5391–5404

Lopez de Silanes I, Galban S, Martindale JL et al (2005a) Identification and functional outcome of mRNAs associated with RNA-binding protein tia-1. Mol Cell Biol 25:9520–9531

Lopez de Silanes I, Lal A, Gorospe M (2005b) HuR: post-transcriptional paths to malignancy. RNA Biol 2:11–13

Lopez de Silanes I, Quesada MP, Esteller M (2007) Aberrant regulation of messenger RNA 3′-untranslated region in human cancer. Cell Oncol 29:1–17

Markowitz SD, Bertagnolli MM (2009) Molecular origins of cancer: molecular basis of colorectal cancer. N Engl J Med 361:2449–2460

Markowitz S, Wang J, Myeroff L et al (1995) Inactivation of the type II TGF-beta receptor in colon cancer cells with microsatellite instability. Science 268:1336–1338

Masso Gonzalez EL, Patrignani P, Tacconelli S et al (2010) Variability among nonsteroidal antiinflammatory drugs in risk of upper gastrointestinal bleeding. Arthritis Rheum 62:1592–1601

Mayr C, Bartel DP (2009) Widespread shortening of 3′UTRs by alternative cleavage and polyadenylation activates oncogenes in cancer cells. Cell 138:673–684

Meade EA, McIntyre TM, Zimmerman GA et al (1999) Peroxisome proliferators enhance cyclooxygenase-2 expression in epithelial cells. J Biol Chem 274:8328–8334

Mei JM, Hord NG, Winterstein DF et al (1999) Differential expression of prostaglandin endoperoxide H synthase-2 and formation of activated beta-catenin-lef-1 transcription complex in mouse colonic epithelial cells contrasting in APC. Carcinogenesis 20:737–740

Meisner NC, Hintersteiner M, Mueller K et al (2007) Identification and mechanistic characterization of low-molecular-weight inhibitors for HuR. Nat Chem Biol 3:508–515

Michael MZ, OC SM, van Holst Pellekaan NG et al (2003) Reduced accumulation of specific microRNAs in colorectal neoplasia. Mol Cancer Res 1:882–891

Miller C, Zhang M, He Y et al (1998) Transcriptional induction of cyclooxygenase-2 gene by okadaic acid inhibition of phosphatase activity in human chondrocytes: co-stimulation of AP-1 and cre nuclear binding proteins. J Cell Biochem 69:392–413

Ming XF, Stoecklin G, Lu M et al (2001) Parallel and independent regulation of interleukin-3 mRNA turnover by phosphatidylinositol 3-kinase and p38 mitogen-activated protein kinase. Mol Cell Biol 21:5778–5789

Moore AE, Young LE, Dixon DA (2011) A common single-nucleotide polymorphism in cyclooxygenase-2 disrupts microRNA-mediated regulation. Oncogene (in press)

Moran AE, Hunt DH, Javid SH et al (2004) APC deficiency is associated with increased EGFR activity in the intestinal enterocytes and adenomas of C57Bl/6j-Min/+ mice. J Biol Chem 279:43261–43272

Moser AR, Luongo C, Gould KA et al (1995) APCmin: a mouse model for intestinal and mammary tumorigenesis. Eur J Cancer 31A:1061–1064

Mukhopadhyay D, Houchen CW, Kennedy S et al (2003) Coupled mRNA stabilization and translational silencing of cyclooxygenase-2 by a novel RNA binding protein, CUGBP2. Mol Cell 11:113–126

Murakami M, Naraba H, Tanioka T et al (2000) Regulation of prostaglandin E2 biosynthesis by inducible membrane-associated prostaglandin E2 synthase that acts in concert with cyclooxygenase-2. J Biol Chem 275:32783–32792

Murmu N, Jung J, Mukhopadhyay D et al (2004) Dynamic antagonism between RNA-binding protein cugbp2 and cyclooxygenase-2-mediated prostaglandin E2 in radiation damage. Proc Nat Acad Sci USA 101:13873–13878

Myung SJ, Rerko RM, Yan M et al (2006) 15-hydroxyprostaglandin dehydrogenase is an in vivo suppressor of colon tumorigenesis. Proc Nat Acad Sci USA 103:12098–12102

Nakanishi M, Gokhale V, Meuillet EJ et al (2010) mPGES-1 as a target for cancer suppression: a comprehensive invited review "phospholipase A2 and lipid mediators". Biochimie 92:660–664

Nakanishi M, Montrose DC, Clark P et al (2008) Genetic deletion of mPGES-1 suppresses intestinal tumorigenesis. Cancer Res 68:3251–3259

Newbury SF, Muhlemann O, Stoecklin G (2006) Turnover in the alps: an mRNA perspective. Workshops on mechanisms and regulation of mRNA turnover. EMBO Rep 7:143–148

Nomura T, Lu R, Pucci ML et al (2004) The two-step model of prostaglandin signal termination: in vitro reconstitution with the prostaglandin transporter and prostaglandin 15 dehydrogenase. Mol Pharmacol 65:973–978

O'Hara SP, Mott JL, Splinter PL et al (2009) MicroRNAs: key modulators of post-transcriptional gene expression. Gastroenterology 136:17–25

Oshima M, Dinchuk JE, Kargman SL et al (1996) Suppression of intestinal polyposis in APCΔ716 knockout mice by inhibition of cyclooxygenase 2 (COX-2). Cell 87:803–809

Ozhan G, Yanar TH, Ertekin C et al (2010) The effect of genetic polymorphisms of cyclooxygenase 2 on acute pancreatitis in Turkey. Pancreas 39:371–376

Patrono C, Patrignani P, García Rodríguez LA (2001) Cyclooxygenase-selective inhibition of prostanoid formation: transducing biochemical selectivity into clinical read-outs. J Clin Invest 108:7–13

Patrono C, Baigent C, Hirsh J et al (2008) Antiplatelet drugs: American college of chest physicians evidence-based clinical practice guidelines. Chest 133:199S–233S (8th edn)

Peddareddigari VG, Wang D, Dubois RN (2011) The tumor microenvironment in colorectal carcinogenesis. Cancer Microenviron 3:149–166

Phillips K, Kedersha N, Shen L et al (2004) Arthritis suppressor genes TIA-1 and TTP dampen the expression of tumor necrosis factor alpha, cyclooxygenase 2, and inflammatory arthritis. Proc Nat Acad Sci USA 101:2011–2016

Prescott SM (2000) Is cyclooxygenase-2 the alpha and the omega in cancer? J Clin Invest 105:1511–1513

Reid G, Wielinga P, Zelcer N et al (2003) The human multidrug resistance protein MRP4 functions as a prostaglandin efflux transporter and is inhibited by nonsteroidal antiinflammatory drugs. Proc Nat Acad Sci USA 100:9244–9249

Roberts RB, Min L, Washington MK et al (2002) Importance of epidermal growth factor receptor signaling in establishment of adenomas and maintenance of carcinomas during intestinal tumorigenesis. Proc Nat Acad Sci USA 99:1521–1526

Rothwell PM, Fowkes FG, Belch JF et al (2011) Effect of daily aspirin on long-term risk of death due to cancer: analysis of individual patient data from randomised trials. Lancet 377:31–41

Rothwell PM, Wilson M, Elwin CE et al (2010) Long-term effect of aspirin on colorectal cancer incidence and mortality: 20-year follow-up of five randomised trials. Lancet 376:1741–1750

Ryan BM, Robles AI, Harris CC (2010) Genetic variation in microRNA networks: the implications for cancer research. Nat Rev Cancer 10:389–402

Sampey AV, Monrad S, Crofford LJ (2005) Microsomal prostaglandin E synthase-1: the inducible synthase for prostaglandin E2. Arthritis Res Ther 7:114–117

Samuelsson B, Morgenstern R, Jakobsson PJ (2007) Membrane prostaglandin E synthase-1: a novel therapeutic target. Pharmacol Rev 59:207–224

Sanchez-Beato M, Sanchez-Aguilera A, Piris MA (2003) Cell cycle deregulation in B-cell lymphomas. Blood 101:1220–1235

Sanduja S, Blanco FF, Dixon DA (2010) The roles of TTP and BRF proteins in regulated mRNA decay. Wiley Interdisc Rev RNA 2:42–57

Sawaoka H, Dixon DA, Oates JA et al (2003) Tristetrapolin binds to the 3′ untranslated region of cyclooxygenase-2 mRNA: a polyadenylation variant in a cancer cell line lacks the binding site. J Biol Chem 278:13928–13935

Schmedtje JF Jr, Ji YS, Liu WL et al (1997) Hypoxia induces cyclooxygenase-2 via the NF-kappaB p65 transcription factor in human vascular endothelial cells. J Biol Chem 272:601–608

Shanmugam N, Reddy MA, Natarajan R (2008) Distinct roles of heterogeneous nuclear ribonuclear protein K and microRNA-16 in cyclooxygenase-2 RNA stability induced by s100b, a ligand of the receptor for advanced glycation end products. J Biol Chem 283:36221–36233

Shao J, Sheng H, Inoue H et al (2000) Regulation of constitutive cyclooxygenase-2 expression in colon carcinoma cells. J Biol Chem 275:33951–33956

Shen J, Gammon MD, Terry MB et al (2006) Genetic polymorphisms in the cyclooxygenase-2 gene, use of nonsteroidal anti-inflammatory drugs, and breast cancer risk. Breast Cancer Res 8:R71–R80

Sheng H, Shao J, Dixon DA et al (2000) Transforming growth factor-beta1 enhances Ha-ras-induced expression of cyclooxygenase-2 in intestinal epithelial cells via stabilization of mRNA. J Biol Chem 275:6628–6635

Siezen CL, van Leeuwen AI, Kram NR et al (2005) Colorectal adenoma risk is modified by the interplay between polymorphisms in arachidonic acid pathway genes and fish consumption. Carcinogenesis 26:449–457

Simmons DL, Botting RM, Hla T (2004) Cyclooxygenase isozymes: the biology of prostaglandin synthesis and inhibition. Pharmacol Rev 56:387–437

Singer II, Kawka DW, Schloemann S et al (1998) Cyclooxygenase 2 is induced in colonic epithelial cells in inflammatory bowel disease. Gastroenterology 115:297–306

Slaby O, Svoboda M, Fabian P et al (2007) Altered expression of miR-21, miR-31, miR-143 and miR-145 is related to clinicopathologic features of colorectal cancer. Oncology 72:397–402

Song T, Zhang X, Wang C et al (2011) Expression of miR-143 reduces growth and migration of human bladder carcinoma cells by targeting cyclooxygenase-2. Asian Pac J Cancer Prev 12:929–933

Steinbach G, Lynch PM, Phillips RK et al (2000) The effect of celecoxib, a cyclooxygenase-2 inhibitor, in familial adenomatous polyposis. N Engl J Med 342:1946–1952

Strillacci A, Griffoni C, Sansone P et al (2009) Mir-101 downregulation is involved in cyclooxygenase-2 overexpression in human colon cancer cells. Exp Cell Res 315:1439–1447

Su H, Yang JR, Xu T et al (2009) MicroRNA-101, down-regulated in hepatocellular carcinoma, promotes apoptosis and suppresses tumorigenicity. Cancer Res 69:1135–1142

Subbaramaiah K, Cole PA, Dannenberg AJ (2002a) Retinoids and carnosol suppress cyclooxygenase-2 transcription by creb-binding protein/p300-dependent and -independent mechanisms. Cancer Res 62:2522–2530

Subbaramaiah K, Norton L, Gerald W et al (2002b) Cyclooxygenase-2 is overexpressed in HER-2/neu-positive breast cancer. Evidence for involvement of AP-1 and PEA3. J Biol Chem 277:18649–18657

Sureban SM, Murmu N, Rodriguez P et al (2007) Functional antagonism between RNA binding proteins HuR and CUGBP2 determines the fate of COX-2 mRNA translation. Gastroenterology 132:1055–1065

Sureban SM, Ramalingam S, Natarajan G et al (2008) Translation regulatory factor RBM3 is a proto-oncogene that prevents mitotic catastrophe. Oncogene 27:4544–4556

Takagi T, Iio A, Nakagawa Y et al (2009) Decreased expression of microRNA-143 and -145 in human gastric cancers. Oncology 77:12–21

Tian Q, Streuli M, Saito H et al (1991) A polyadenylate binding protein localized to the granules of cytolytic lymphocytes induces DNA fragmentation in target cells. Cell 67:629–639
Toyota M, Shen L, Ohe-Toyota M et al (2000) Aberrant methylation of the cyclooxygenase 2 CpG island in colorectal tumors. Cancer Res 60:4044–4048
Vane JR (1971) Inhibition of prostaglandin synthesis as a mechanism of action for aspirin-like drugs. Nat New Biol 231:232–523
Varambally S, Cao Q, Mani RS et al (2008) Genomic loss of microRNA-101 leads to overexpression of histone methyltransferase EZH2 in cancer. Science 322:1695–1699
Vogel U, Christensen J, Wallin H et al (2008) Polymorphisms in genes involved in the inflammatory response and interaction with NSAID use or smoking in relation to lung cancer risk in a prospective study. Mutat Res 639:89–100
Voltz R (2002) Paraneoplastic neurological syndromes: an update on diagnosis, pathogenesis, and therapy. Lancet Neurol 1:294–305
Wang D, DuBois RN (2008) Pro-inflammatory prostaglandins and progression of colorectal cancer. Cancer Lett 267:197–203
Wang D, Dubois RN (2010a) Eicosanoids and cancer. Nat Rev Cancer 10:181–193
Wang D, Dubois RN (2010b) The role of COX-2 in intestinal inflammation and colorectal cancer. Oncogene 29:781–788
Wang HJ, Ruan HJ, He XJ et al (2010) MicroRNA-101 is down-regulated in gastric cancer and involved in cell migration and invasion. Eur J Cancer 46:2295–2303
Wang M, Song WL, Cheng Y et al (2008) Microsomal prostaglandin E synthase-1 inhibition in cardiovascular inflammatory disease. J Intern Med 263:500–505
Wang D, Wang H, Shi Q et al (2004) Prostaglandin E(2) promotes colorectal adenoma growth via transactivation of the nuclear peroxisome proliferator-activated receptor delta. Cancer Cell 6:285–295
Wiemer EA (2007) The role of microRNAs in cancer: no small matter. Eur J Cancer 43:1529–1544
Wiercinska-Drapalo A, Flisiak R, Prokopowicz D (1999) Effects of ulcerative colitis activity on plasma and mucosal prostaglandin E2 concentration. Prostaglandins Other Lipid Mediat 58:159–165
Wu BL, Xu LY, Du ZP et al (2011) MiRNA profile in esophageal squamous cell carcinoma: downregulation of miR-143 and miR-145. World J Gastroenterol 17:79–88
Wu WK, Sung JJ, Lee CW et al (2010) Cyclooxygenase-2 in tumorigenesis of gastrointestinal cancers: an update on the molecular mechanisms. Cancer Lett 295:7–16
Yan M, Rerko RM, Platzer P et al (2004) 15-hydroxyprostaglandin dehydrogenase, a COX-2 oncogene antagonist, is a tgf-beta-induced suppressor of human gastrointestinal cancers. Proc Nat Acad Sci USA 101:17468–17473
Yang X, Wang W, Fan J et al (2004) Prostaglandin a2-mediated stabilization of p21 mRNA through an erk-dependent pathway requiring the RNA-binding protein HuR. J Biol Chem 279:49298–49306
Young LE, Dixon DA (2010) Post-transcriptional regulation of cyclooxygenase 2 expression in colorectal cancer. Curr Colorectal Cancer Rep 6:60–67
Young LE, Moore AE, Sokol L et al. (2011) The mRNA stability factor HuR inhibits microRNA-16 targeting of cyclooxygenase-2. Mol Cancer Res (in press)
Young LE, Sanduja S, Bemis-Standoli K et al (2009) The mRNA binding proteins HuR and tristetraprolin regulate cyclooxygenase 2 expression during colon carcinogenesis. Gastroenterology 136:1669–1679
Zhu T, Gobeil F, Vazquez-Tello A et al (2006) Intracrine signaling through lipid mediators and their cognate nuclear G-protein-coupled receptors: a paradigm based on PGE2, PAF, and LPA1 receptors. Can J Physiol Pharmacol 84:377–391

# Mode of Action of Aspirin as a Chemopreventive Agent

Melania Dovizio, Annalisa Bruno, Stefania Tacconelli and Paola Patrignani

**Abstract**

Aspirin taken for several years at doses of at least 75 mg daily reduced long-term incidence and mortality due to colorectal cancer. The finding of aspirin benefit at low-doses given once daily, used for cardioprevention, locates the antiplatelet effect of aspirin at the center of its antitumor efficacy. In fact, at low-doses, aspirin acts mainly by an irreversible inactivation of platelet cyclooxygenase (COX)-1 in the presystemic circulation, which translates into a long-lasting inhibition of platelet function. Given the short half-life of aspirin in the human circulation(approximately 20 min) and the capacity of nucleated cells to resynthesize the acetylated COX-isozyme(s), it seems unlikely that a nucleated cell could be the target of aspirin chemoprevention. These findings convincingly suggest that colorectal cancer and atherothrombosis may share a common mechanism of disease, i.e. platelet activation in response to epithelial(in tumorigenesis) and endothelial(in tumorigenesis and atherothrombosis) injury. Activated platelets may also enhance the metastatic potential of cancer cells (through a direct interaction and/or the release of soluble mediators or exosomes) at least in part by inducing the overexpression of COX-2. COX-independent mechanisms of aspirin, such as the inhibition of NF-kB signaling and Wnt/$\beta$-catenin signaling and the acetylation of extra-COX proteins, have

M. Dovizio · S. Tacconelli · P. Patrignani (✉)
Center of Excellence on Aging (CeSI) and Department of Neuroscience and Imaging,
G. d'Annunzio University, School of Medicine, Via dei Vestini 31, 66100 Chieti, Italy
e-mail: ppatrignani@unich.it

A. Bruno
Center of Excellence on Aging (CeSI) and Department of Medicine and Aging,
G. d'Annunzio University, School of Medicine,
Via dei Vestini 31, 66100 Chieti, Italy

A. T. Chan and E. Detering (eds.), *Prospects for Chemoprevention of Colorectal Neoplasia*, Recent Results in Cancer Research 191, DOI: 10.1007/978-3-642-30331-9_3, 

been suggested to play a role in its chemopreventive effects. However, their relevance remains to be demonstrated in vivo at clinical doses.

## Abbreviations

| | |
|---|---|
| 15R-HETE | 15R-hydroxyeicosapentaenoic acid |
| 5-LOX | 5-lipoxygenase |
| ADP | Adenosine diphosphate |
| apaf-1 | Apoptotic protease activating factor-1 |
| AA | Arachidonic acid |
| CRC | Colorectal cancer |
| COX | Cyclooxygenase |
| EGFR | Epidermal growth factor receptor |
| ERK | Extracellular signal-regulated kinase |
| FAP | Familial adenomatous polyposis |
| FGF | Fibroblast growth factor |
| IGF | Insulin-like growth factor |
| IL | Interleukin |
| LPS | Bacterial endotoxin |
| MPs | Microparticles |
| mPGES-1 | Microsomal $PGE_2$ synthase-1 |
| NK | Natural killer |
| NSAID | Nonsteroidal anti-inflammatory drug |
| NF-kB | Nuclear factor kappa B |
| PDGF | Platelet-derived growth factor |
| PDGF | Platelet-derived growth factor |
| $PGI_2$ | Prostacyclin |
| PG | Prostaglandin |
| PKC | Protein kinase C |
| Ser | Serine |
| S1P | Sphingosine-1-phosphate |
| Lef | T-cell factor (Tcf)/lymphoid enhancer factor |
| TX | Thromboxane |
| TIMP | Tissue inhibitor of metalloproteinases |
| TCIPA | Tumor cell-induced platelet aggregation |
| TXAS | $TXA_2$ synthase |
| VEGF | Vascular endothelial growth factor |

## Contents



## 1 Introduction

Most clinical evidence of a chemopreventive effect of aspirin in colorectal cancer (CRC) derives from epidemiological studies (Thun et al. 2002; Cuzick et al. 2009). Indeed, the vast majority of them reported an inverse association between the use of aspirin (acetyl salicylic acid, ASA) and incidence of CRC and also CRC mortality. Only one cohort study reported a positive association (Paganini-Hill et al. 1989). It is noteworthy to point out that in this study, an increase in cardiovascular events was detected in the aspirin group. A recent study has followed-up five randomised trials of aspirin versus control in primary and secondary prevention of vascular events and established the effect of aspirin on risk of CRC over 20 years during and after the trials (Rothwell et al. 2010). In this study, aspirin taken at doses of at least 75 mg daily (recommended for the prevention against cardiovascular disease) reduced the incidence and mortality of CRC. Also, randomised controlled trials (RCTs) and epidemiological studies have reported a risk reduction of the incidence or recurrence of adenomatous polyps with aspirin. Several RCTs have demonstrated that aspirin (81–325 mg daily) reduces colorectal adenoma risk in average/high-risk population (Baron et al. 2003; Sandler et al. 2003; Benamouzig et al. 2003).

Interestingly, one of the cardiovascular RCTs (Meade et al. 1998) in which the cancer chemopreventive effect of ASA was detected on long-term follow-up (Rothwell et al. 2010), involved the administration of a controlled-release formulation of ASA (75 mg) with negligible systemic bioavailability (Charman et al. 1993) translating into a selective inhibition of platelet COX-1 pathway (Clarke et al. 1991). This finding sustains the hypothesis that the antiplatelet effect of aspirin plays a central role in its antitumor efficacy (Patrono et al. 2001).

In this chapter we will develop the theme of CRC and atherothrombosis sharing a common mechanism of disease, i.e. platelet activation in response to epithelial (in tumorigeneis) and endothelial (in tumorigenesis and atherothrombosis) injury. While some lipid products of platelet metabolism and release [e.g. thromboxane (TX)$A_2$] would act primarily through their specific receptors on other platelets and smooth muscle cells to evoke platelet aggregation and vasoconstriction in a major arterial (e.g. coronary) vessel at sites of plaque rupture (Davì and Patrono 2007), other platelet protein products stored and released from $\alpha$-granules [such as platelet-derived growth factor (PDGF)] (Italiano et al. 2008) or generated and released (such as interleukin(IL)-1$\beta$] (Dixon et al. 2006) would act primarily on adjacent (e.g. stromal) cells to evoke cyclooxygenase (COX)-2 induction, an event involved in adenoma development and growth (Prescott 2000; Patrono et al. 2001; Cha and Dubois 2007). We propose that platelet activation is involved in the early stages of colorectal carcinogenesis in man and by the induction of a COX-2-mediated paracrine signaling between stromal cells and epithelial cells within adenomas (Fig. 1).

The finding that aspirin benefit was greatest for cancers of the proximal colon (Rothwell et al. 2010) may suggest that platelet-induced tumorigenesis is the mechanism involved in the initiation and/or progression of proximal colon carcinoma. Previous data provide strong support for the hypothesis that proximal and distal colon carcinoma might differ in mechanisms of their initiation and/or progression possibly because the proximal and the distal colon have different embryonic origins and a different vascular supply (Delattre et al. 1989; Iacopetta 2002).

Finally, in this chapter we will discuss COX-independent mechanisms possibly involved in aspirin chemoprevention and we will verify their clinical relevance by considering the available information of pharmacokinetic and pharmacodynamic of aspirin at clinical doses.

## 2 Mechanisms of Action of Aspirin

### 2.1 Historical Overview of Aspirin and its Mechanism of Action (Box. 1)

Salicylates, in the form of willow bark, were used as an analgesic during the time of Hippocrates, and their antipyretic effects have been recognized for more than 200 years (Stone 1763). Acetyl salicilyc acid (ASA, aspirin), was introduced in the late 1890s (Dreser 1899) and has been used to treat a variety of inflammatory conditions; however, the antiplatelet activity of this agent was not recognized until almost 70 years later (Weiss and Aledort 1967). Insight into the molecular mechanism of action of aspirin was provided by Gerry Roth and Phil Majerus who used aspirin labeled with $^3$H at the acetyl group to demonstrate acetylation of

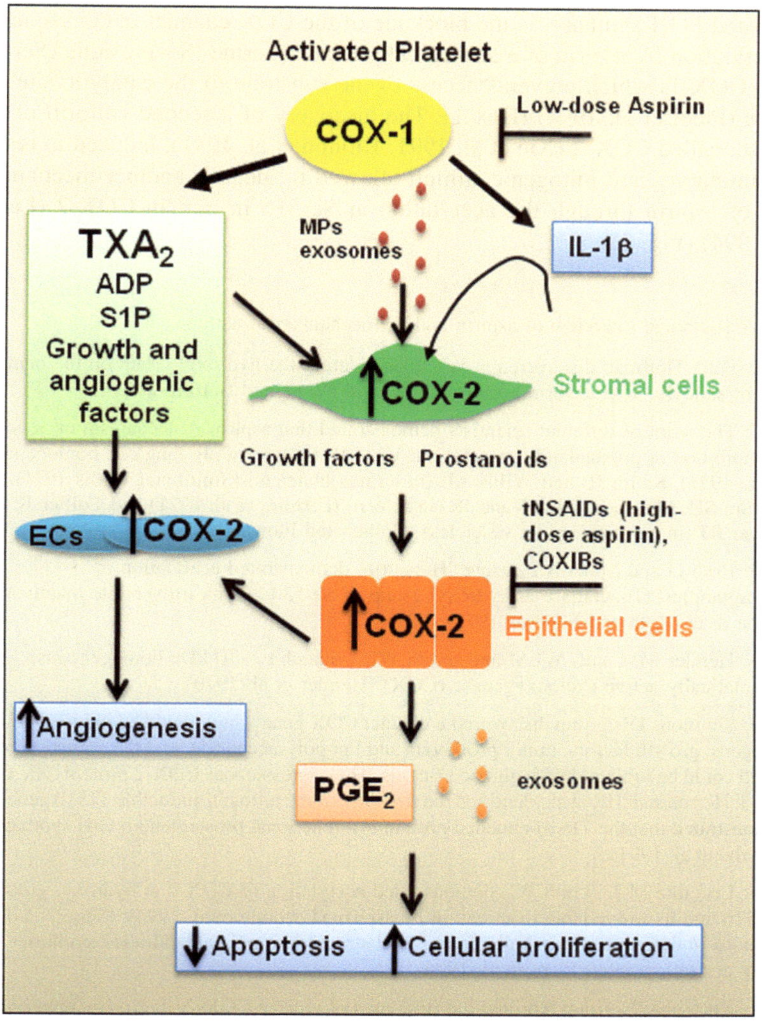


**Fig. 1** Platelet COX-1 mechanism of colon tumorigenesis. Platelets may play an early role in colon tumorigenesis through the release of soluble factors and/or microparticles and exosomes), which can activate stromal cells (macrophages and fibroblasts) translating into an over-expression of COX-2 and the release of prostanoids and growth factors. They may induce intestinal epithelial cell transformation, in part as a consequence of COX-2 expression. Later, in tumor progression there will be the induction of COX-2 also in endothelial cells and this will contribute to a proangiogenic response. Abbreviations: microparticle (*MP*), endothelial cells (*EC*), sphingosine-1-phosphate (*S1P*)

prostaglandin (PG) H-synthase (also known as COX) and its irreversible inactivation by the drug (Roth and Majerus 1975; Roth et al. 1975). Importantly, the structural basis of the enzyme inactivation, inferred from the crystal structure of inactivated PGH-synthase, is the blockade of the COX channel in consequence of the acetylation by aspirin of a strategically located serine (Ser) residue (Ser529 in human COX-1) which prevents access of the substrate to the catalytic site of the enzyme (Picot et al. 1994) (Box 1). The discovery of a second isoform of PGH-synthase, called COX-2 (Xie et al. 1991; Kujubu et al. 1991), induced in response to inflammatory and mitogenic stimuli allowed to identify another mechanism of action of aspirin through the acetylation at Ser516 in human COX-2 (Lecomte et al. 1994) (Fig. 2).

Box 1 Historical overview of aspirin and its mechanism of action

1890: Felix Hoffman discovered a way to acetylating the hydroxyl group on the benzene ring of salicylic acid to form acetylsalicylic acid (Vane and Botting 2003).

1971: The work of different scientists demonstrated that aspirin's mechanism of action is the inhibition of prostaglandin generation: Vane JR (in guinea pig lung cell homogenates) (Vane 1971), Smith JB and Willis AL (in human platelets) (Smith and Willis 1971), Ferreira SH, Moncada S and Vane JR (in spleen) (Ferreira et al. 1971) and Collier JC and Flower RJ (in human seminal vescicles) (Collier and Flower 1971).

1975: Roth G and Majerus P, using $^{3}$H-aspirin, demonstrated acetylation of prostaglandin(PG)-synthase at hydroxyl group of Ser530 and its irreversible inactivation by the drug (Roth and Majerus 1975).

1976: Hemler M, Lands WEM and Smith WL isolated a ~70 kDa homogeneous, enzymatically active cyclooxygenase (COX) (Hemler et al. 1976).

1991: Simmons D's group discovered a distinct COX gene which could be induced with mitogens, growth factors, tumor promoters and lipopolysaccharide, and the induction of which could be inhibited with glucocorticoids. This gene encodes COX-2 protein (Xie et al. 1991); Herschman HR et al. identified the structure of the mitogen-inducible TIS10 gene and demonstrated that the TIS10-encoded protein is a functional prostaglandin G/H synthase (Kujubu et al. 1991).

1994: Lecomte M & Smith WL demonstrated acetylation of COX-2 at hydroxyl group of Ser 516 and its irreversible inactivation by aspirin (Lecomte et al. 1994); Picot D, Loll P, Garavito M determined the three-dimensional structure of prostaglandin H2 synthase-1 by X-ray crystallography (Picot et al. 1994).

1996: Kurumbail's group reported the structures of murine COX-2; these structures explained the structural basis for the selective inhibition of COX-2 (Kurumbail et al. 1996).

## 2.2 Insights into the Mechanism of Inhibition of COXs by Aspirin

Aspirin is the only nonsteroidal anti-inflammatory drug (NSAID) which causes an irreversible inactivation of COX-1 and COX-2 by acetylation of a specific serine moiety (Ser529 of COX-1 and Ser516 of COX-2) (Loll et al. 1995; Picot et al. 1994; Lecomte et al. 1994) (Fig. 2).

Both COX-1 and COX-2 catalyze the conversion of arachidonic acid (AA) to prostanoids [prostaglandin (PG)$E_2$, $PGF_{2\alpha}$, $PGD_2$, prostacyclin($PGI_2$), and

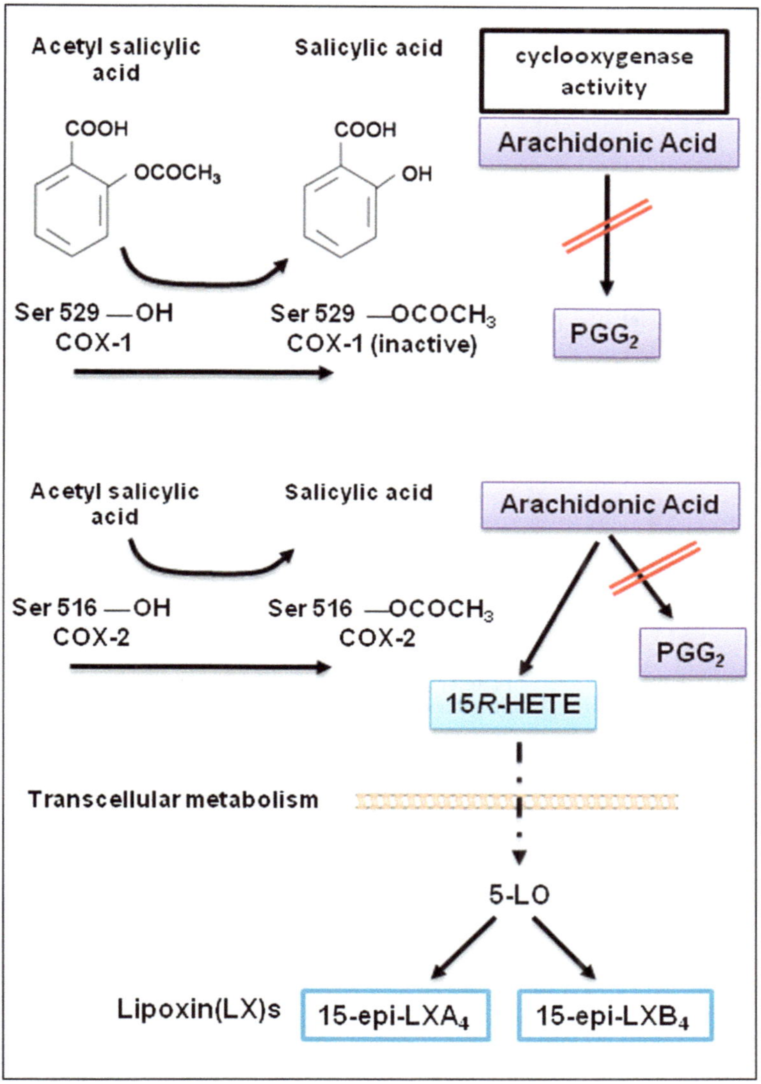


**Fig. 2** The molecular mechanism of irreversible inactivation of the cyclooxygenase activity of COX-1 and COX-2 by aspirin through the acetylation of a strategically located serine residue (i.e, Ser529 in the human COX-1 and Ser516 in the human COX-2). In COX-2 expressing cells (such as endothelial cells, leukocytes and epithelial cells), the acetylation of the enzyme by aspirin inhibits its cyclooxygenase activity (preventing the generation of $PGG_2$) but arachidonic acid can be metabolized to 15(*R*)-hydroxyeicosatetraenoic acid (*HETE*). 15(R)-HETE can be transformed to 15(*R*)-epilipoxin(*LX*)$A_4$ and 15epi-$LXB_4$ in leukocytes via 5-lipoxygenase (*5-LO*)

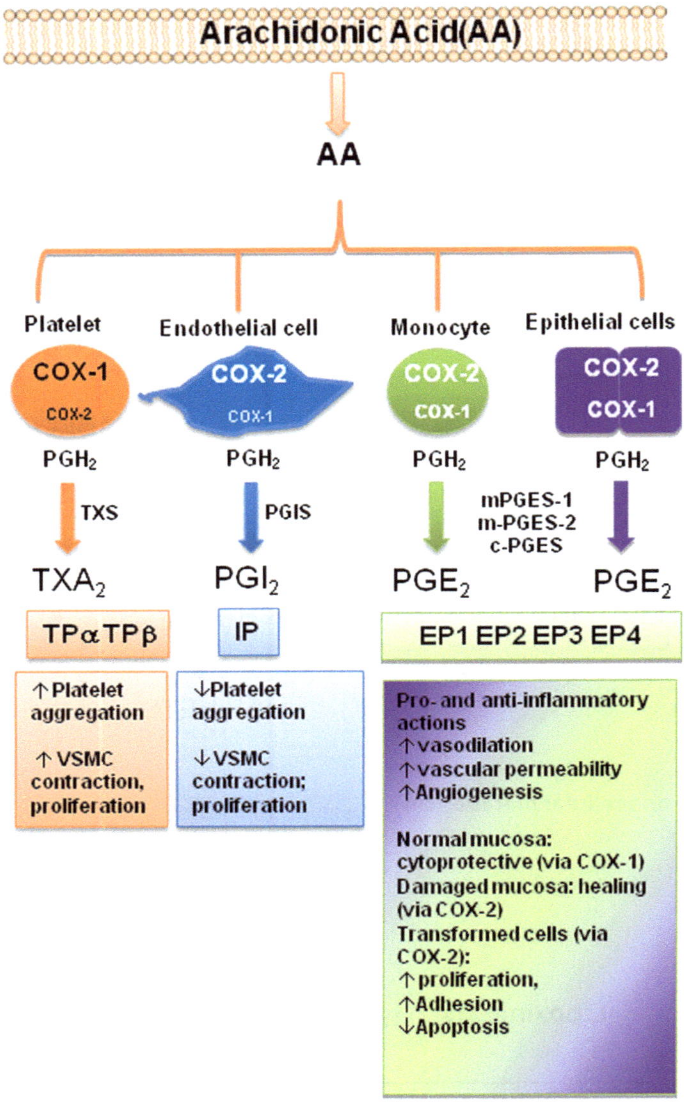


**Fig. 3** The product of cyclooxygenase activity of COX-1 and COX-2, $PGH_2$ is metabolized to different prostanoids by tissue-specific synthases. Released prostanoids regulate different functions by the interaction with G-protein coupled receptors. Abbreviations: COX cyclooxygenase; $TXA_2$ synthase (*TXS*), $PGI_2$ synthase (*PGIS*), microsomal (*m*) or cytoplasmatic (*c*), $PGE_2$ synthase (*PGES*), $TXA_2$ receptor (*TP*), $PGI_2$ receptor (*IP*), EP1-4 ($PGE_2$ receptor)

thromboxane(TX)$A_2$] (FitzGerald 2003) (Fig. 3). COX-1 gene is considered a "housekeeping gene" and it is highly expressed in platelets and gastric epithelial cells where it plays a role in causing platelet activation, via the generation of

$TXA_2$, and gastric cytoprotection, via the generation mainly of $PGE_2$, respectively (Patrono et al. 2001; Capone et al. 2007; Smyth et al. 2009). Differently, the gene for COX-2 is a primary response gene with many regulatory sites (Kang et al. 2007). However, COX-2 is constitutively expressed in some cells in physiologic conditions, such as endothelial cells (Topper et al. 1996), where COX-2-dependent-$PGI_2$ induces an antithrombtic and vasoprotective signaling (Grosser et al. 2006; Di Francesco et al. 2009), and in pathological conditions, such as cancer cells where the major product is $PGE_2$ (Dixon et al. 2001). COX-2 overexpression, in cancer cells, occurs through post-transcriptional mechanisms, in part due to altered expression of trans-acting factors that bind to AREs (AU-rich) elements and regulate the status of mRNA stability (Harper and Tyson-Capper 2008) (see Chap. 2 for a detailed description by Dixon et al.).

Both the COX-isozymes have two catalytic activities (Fig. 4): (1) a COX activity responsible for oxygenating AA to $PGG_2$; and (2) a peroxidase (POX) activity that catalyzes a two-electron reduction of $PGG_2$ to $PGH_2$.

COX-1 and COX-2 are homodimers that exhibit half of sites with COX activity, with AA as the substrate (Yuan et al. 2006; Sidhu et al. 2010) (Fig. 5): only one monomer is able to catalyze a reaction at a given time. The noncatalytic monomer functions as an allosteric regulator of the catalytic monomer (Kulmacz and Lands 1985; Yuan et al. 2006, 2009). This is of potential importance in vivo, where certain fatty acids can function as allosteric regulators of COXs, inhibiting COX-1 and stimulating COX-2 (Yuan et al. 2009).

Aspirin binds to one monomer of COX-1 and -2 by the interaction with Arg120 residue and modifies covalently COX isoenzymes by the acetylation of Ser529 and Ser516 on COX-1 and COX-2, respectively; the acetylated monomer becomes the allosteric subunit, and the partner monomer becomes the catalytic monomer. Acetylation of the allosteric subunit of COX-1 causes an irreversible inactivation of the COX activity of the enzyme which translates into the inhibition of the generation of $PGG_2$ from AA (Fig. 2). In other words, aspirin acts as negative allosteric effector by binding to one monomer of COX-1, thus markedly reducing or even eliminating the activity of the partner monomer (Rimon et al. 2010).

Aspirin inhibits COX-2 activity, in a concentration-dependent fashion, through the acetylation of a single monomer of the enzyme (Sharma et al. 2010) (Fig. 2). However, the outcome is somewhat more complex than that seen with COX-1. The acetylated COX-2 has a significantly compromised ability to form $PGG_2$ but produces an alternative product, 15R-hydroxyeicosapentaenoic acid (15R-HETE) from AA (Lecomte et al. 1994). Sophisticated experiments performed by Smith's group (Sharma et al. 2010) showed that aspirin acetylation of the regulatory monomer of COX-2 is associated with an irreversible inhibition of the catalytic monomer to form $PGG_2$. In contrast, the acetylated monomer forms primarily 15R-HETE from AA (Fig. 2). Thus, the effect of aspirin on COX-2 is an incomplete allosteric inhibitory effect compared with that seen with COX-1 (Sharma et al. 2010).

Several studies in vitro have shown that 15R-HETE is then metabolized to the epi-lipoxins (LXs) in monocytes and leukocytes through the action of 5-lipoxygenase (5-LOX) (Fig. 2) (Gilroy 2005; Serhan 2005), the enzyme also responsible

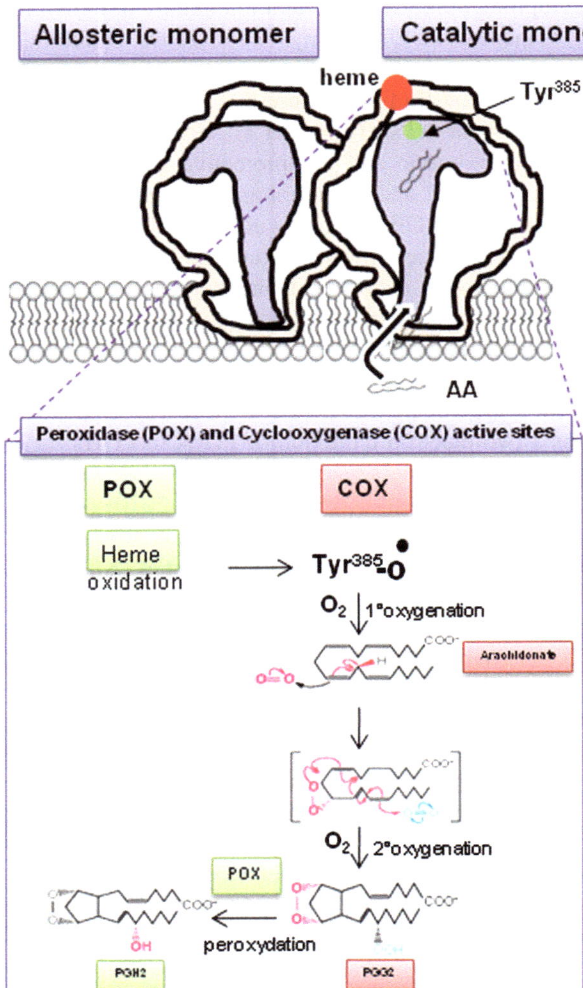


**Fig. 4** Mechanism of $PGH_2$ generation by COX-1 and COX-2. Both COX-1 and COX-2 possess peroxydase (*POX*) and cyclooxygenase (*COX*) activities. Thus, COX-isozymes generate the same product $PGH_2$. The first step is the oxidation of the heme group at the POX active site, which causes the formation of a tyrosyl radical at Tyr385 in COX active site. The Tyr385 radical stereospecifically abstracts a hydrogen atom from carbon13 of arachidonic acid (*AA*)(1st oxygenation), then the carbon radical induces the formation of an oxane ring. The addition of a second $O_2$ molecule at carbon 15 ultimately produces $PGG_2$ (2nd oxygenation). $PGG_2$ is the substrate of POX activity which converts peroxide group of $PGG_2$ to hydroxyl forming $PGH_2$

for initiation of leukotriene synthesis. The epi-LXs may cause antiproliferative and anti-inflammatory actions (Serhan 2005; Fierro et al. 2002; Romano 2010). However, convincing evidences that these lipid mediators triggered by aspirin are

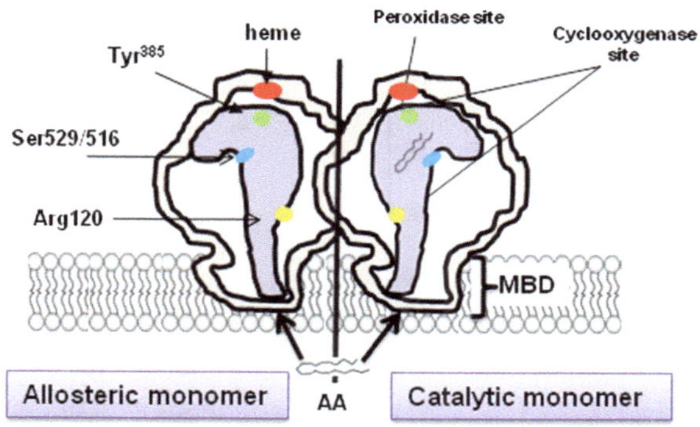


**Fig. 5** Dimeric structure of COXs. COX-1 and -2 are homodimers composed of 2 monomers (about 72 kDa) that are tightly bonded to one another. Each monomer is anchored to the cellular membrane through a membrane binding domain (MBD) and contains both cyclooxygenase (*COX*) and peroxidare (*POX*) sites

generated in vivo in humans are lacking. In particular, the analytical assays (mainly immunoassays) (Romano 2006) used to measure their levels in urinary collections were not rigorously validated by comparison with mass-spectrometry analysis.

# 3 Pharmacology/Pharmacokinetic of Aspirin

## 3.1 COX-Isozyme Selectivity in Vitro

The inhibitory effect of aspirin on platelet COX-1 activity is evaluated by assessing $TXB_2$ generated during whole blood clotting for 1 h at 37 °C (serum $TXB_2$) (Patrono et al. 1980). As shown in Fig. 6a, aspirin affects platelet COX-1 activity with an $IC_{50}$ value (concentration which inhibits by 50 % the activity of COXs) of 18 μM. In heparinized human whole blood incubated for 24 h with bacterial endotoxin LPS (which causes a time-dependent induction of COX-2 mainly in monoctyes) (Patrignani et al. 1994), aspirin inhibits $PGE_2$ generation with an $IC_{50}$ value of approximately 5 mM (Fig. 6a). Under these experimental conditions, salicylic acid (the hydrolysis product of aspirin) affects platelet COX-1 and monocyte COX-2 activities with comparable $IC_{50}$ values of approximately 1 mM (Fig. 6b). This may suggest the contribution of salicylic acid to the inhibition of COX-2 in whole blood by aspirin, assessed at 24 h of incubation. In fact, aspirin is unstable in blood and it can be deacetylated to salicilic acid by the activity of plasma esterases. We have shown that in human whole blood, aspirin loses its capacity to inhibit platelet COX-1, in a time-dependent fashion, with a $t_{1/2}$ of approximately 2 h (Fig. 7) (Cipollone et al. 1997). In order to avoid the influence of aspirin metabolism in plasma to its potency to affect COX-isozymes, we assessed aspirin inhibitory effects in washed human platelets (expressing only COX-1) and isolated human monocytes (expressing COX-2 after overnight incubation with LPS), incubated at 37 °C for 60 min with a low concentration of AA, i.e. 0.5 μM. Under these experimental conditions, aspirin results 60-fold more potent to inhibit platelet COX-1 than monocyte COX-2 (Fig. 8).

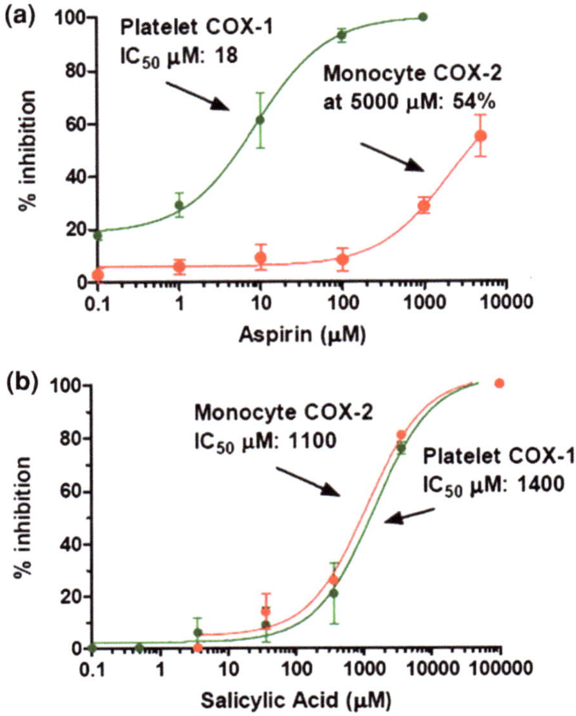


**Fig. 6** Inhibitory effects of Aspirin and Salicylic Acid on platelet COX-1- and monocyte COX-2-dependent prostanoid biosynthesis in human whole blood. **a** Increasing concentrations of Aspirin (0.1–5,000 µM) were used and concentration–response curves for inhibition of platelet COX-1 activity (in *green*; assessed by measuring $TXB_2$ levels in an aliquot of human whole blood allowed to clot for 1 h at 37 °C) and of monocyte COX-2 activity (in *red*, assessed by measuring of $PGE_2$ in LPS-stimulated human whole blood for 24 h) were depicted. **b** Concentration–response curves for inhibition of platelet COX-1 and monocyte COX-2 by increasing concentration of Salicylic acid (0.1–5,000 µM). $IC_{50}$ values were reported for all curves with the exception of the inhibition curve of monocyte COX-2 by Aspirin in which the maximun inhibition value reached with 5,000 µM of aspirin was 54 %. Concentration–response curves were fitted, and $IC_{50}$ values were analysed with PRISM (GraphPad, San Diego, CA, USA)

## 3.2 Pharmacokinetic

Aspirin is rapidly absorbed in the stomach and primarily in the upper intestine. Peak plasma levels occur 30–40 min after aspirin ingestion. In contrast, it can take up to 3–4 h to reach peak plasma levels after administration of enteric-coated aspirin (Patrono et al. 2008). The inhibition of platelet COX-1 activity (assessing serum $TXB_2$) ex vivo (after oral dosing) is detectable before aspirin reaches the systemic circulation which is consistent with the inhibition of platelet COX-1 in the presystemic (portal) circulation (Pedersen and FitzGerald 1984). This is further sustained by the fact that the administration of low-dose aspirin (75–100 mg)

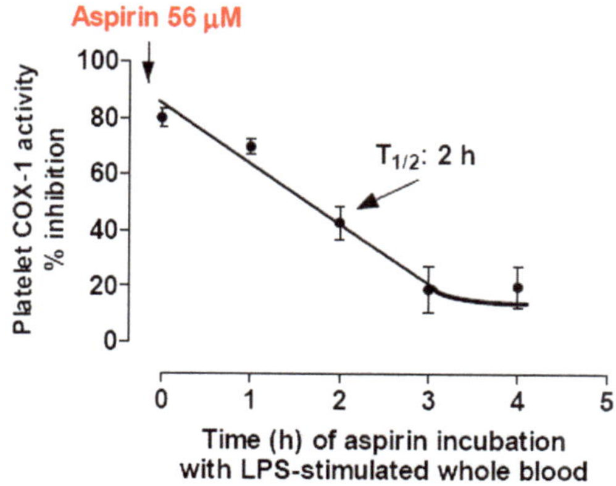


**Fig. 7** Time-dependent deacetylation of aspirin in blood. Aspirin was incubated with 1-mL aliquots of heparinized blood samples for 0, 1, 2, 3 and 4 h at 37 °C in the presence of LPS (10 μg/mL). At the end of each incubation, plasma was separated by centrifugation and an aliquot of plasma (corresponding to 56 μM of aspirin) were immediately added to 1-mL samples of whole blood that were allowed to clot at 37 °C for 60 min; serum $TXB_2$ levels were then measured. The half-life of the loss of inhibitory capacity of platelet COX-1 activity was reported

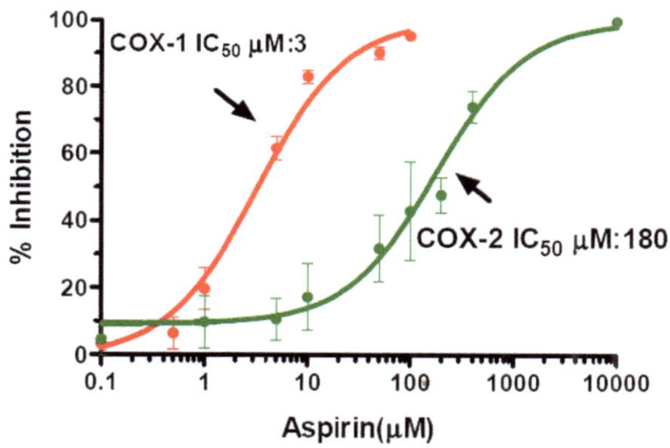


**Fig. 8** Effects of Aspirin on prostanoid biosynthesis by washed human platelets (expressing COX-1) and isolated monocytes (expressing COX-2). Concentration–response curves for inhibition of platelet COX-1 and monocyte COX-2 were obtained by the treatment of washed human platelets (expressing only COX-1) and isolated human monocytes (previously incubated overnight with LPS to induce COX-2) with increasing concentrations of Aspirin (0.1–5,000 μM) and AA (0.5 mM) for 60 min at 37 °C. The inhibition of platelet COX-1 activity was assessed by measuring $TXB_2$ levels, while monocyte COX-2 activity was assessed by measuring $PGE_2$ levels. Concentration–response curves were fitted, and $IC_{50}$ values were analysed with PRISM (GraphPad, San Diego, CA, USA)

causes an almost complete suppression of serum $TXB_2$ ($\geq$95 %) (Patrignani et al. 1982) which cannot be explained by circulating plasma concentrations of aspirin (approximately 7 μM; Table 1) (Charman et al. 1993). In fact, as shown in Fig. 6a,

**Table 1** Peak plasma concentrations ($C_{max}$) of aspirin and salicylic acid after the administration of different doses of aspirin

| Aspirin doses | Aspirin $C_{max}$ | Salicylic acid $C_{max}$ |
|---|---|---|
| Antiplatelet dose, 75 mg/day | | |
| Solution | 7.31 μM[a] | 15 μM |
| Controlled release | 0.29–0.54 μM[a] | 4 μM |
| Analgesic doses, 325–600 mg/4–6 h | 28–80 μM[b,c] | 500 μM[d] (1 g single dose) |
| Anti-inflammatory dose, 1.2 g/4–6 h | 142 μM[c] | 1500–2500 μM[d,e] |

[a] Charman et al. Br J Clin Pharm 1993;36:470–473
[b] Pedersen et al. N Engl J Med 1984;311:1206–1211
[c] Seymour et al. J Clin Pharm 1982;13:807–810
[d] Smyth et al. J Pharm Pharmacol 1971;23:729–744
[e] Rumble et al. Br J Clin Pharm 1980;9:41–45

an almost complete inhibition of platelet COX-1 can be obtained by adding 100 μM of aspirin to whole blood aliquots. The inhibition of platelet function is evident by 1 h after oral dosing with aspirin (Patrono et al. 1985).

The plasma half-life of aspirin is only 20 min; however, because platelets have a limited capacity to generate COX-1 de novo (Evangelista et al. 2006), the irreversible inhibition on platelet COX-1 by aspirin lasts for the duration of the life of the platelet (i.e. 10 days) (Patrignani et al. 1982). For all these reasons, the oral administration of aspirin at low-doses, once daily, causes an almost complete suppression of platelet COX-1 which persists throughout dosing interval (Patrignani et al. 1982). This is a fundamental requisite to obtain an antithrombotic effect (Patrono et al. 2008). In fact, even tiny concentrations of $TXA_2$ can activate platelets and they can synergize with low-concentrations of other agonists to cause a complete platelet aggregation (Minuz et al. 2006).

The oral bioavailability of regular aspirin tablets is approximately 40–50 % over a wide range of doses (Pedersen and FitzGerald 1984). A considerably lower bioavailability has been reported for enteric-coated tablets and sustained-release, microencapsulated preparations (Charman et al. 1993; Clarke et al. 1991). Because platelet COX-1 is acetylated in the presystemic circulation, the antiplatelet effect of aspirin is largely independent of systemic bioavailability (Pedersen and FitzGerald 1984).

### 3.3 Determinants of Achieved COX-Isozyme Selectivity by Clinical Doses of Aspirin

The administration of low-dose aspirin is associated with a preferential inhibition of platelet COX-1 ex vivo (Patrignani et al. 1982; Patrono et al. 1985). In fact, the levels of aspirin (approximately 7 μM) detectable in the systemic circulation (Charman et al. 1993) can cause only a trivial (Figs. 6a and 8) and reversible inhibition of COX-2 expressed in nucleated cells (for de novo synthesis of the acetylated protein). In contrast, platelet COX-1 is completely and irreversibly inhibited in the presystemic circulation and this effect persists for the interval between doses because platelets are anucleated cell fragments. This platelet COX-1 selectivity can be enhanced by the slow administration of low-dose aspirin. In fact, a controlled-release formulation of aspirin 75 mg with negligible systemic bioavailability (Charman et al. 1993; Table 1) has been shown to achieve selective inhibition of platelet $TXA_2$ production without suppressing systemic $PGI_2$ synthesis (Clarke et al. 1991), which is mainly derived from vascular COX-2 (Grosser et al. 2006), and presumably other prostanoids generated in other nucleated cell types.

Aspirin administered at analgesic (325–600 mg every 4–6 h) and anti-inflammatory (1.2 g every 4–6 h) doses is associated with circulating concentrations in the range of 30–150 μM (Pedersen and FitzGerald 1984; Seymour and Rawlins 1982; Table 1) that may affect COX-2 activity in a dose-dependent fashion (Figs. 6a and 8). Circulating concentrations of aspirin hydrolysis product, i.e. salicylic acid, might contribute to affect COX-2 activity or expression when aspirin is administered at very high doses (>1000 mg) (Smyth and Dawkins 1971; Rumble et al. 1980; Table 1).

### 3.3.1 Dose-Dependence of Gastrointestinal Toxicity

Observational studies (García Rodríguez et al. 2001, 2011) and a meta-analysis of randomized clinical trials in high-risk patients (Baigent and Collaboration 2002) have demonstrated that long-term therapy with low-dose aspirin approximately doubles the risk of major extracranial (mostly, upper gastrointestinal) bleeding (Patrono et al. 2005). It is likely that these complications are related to inhibition of platelet COX-1 (Patrono et al. 2001). However, the risk of upper gastrointestinal bleeding increases at higher doses of aspirin (García Rodríguez et al. 2001) and this is plausibly due to the contribution of the inhibition of gastrointestinal COX-1 (Fig. 3) by systemic plasma concentrations of aspirin.

## 4 Role of Platelets in Tumorigenesis

### 4.1 Platelet-Mediated Mechanisms in Tumorigenesis and Metastasis

Platelets represent an important linkage between tissue damage/dysfunction and the inflammatory response initially acting to repair the damage but, if platelet activation is uncontrolled, this translates into a wide spectrum of pathological conditions, such as atherothrombosis and cancer. Moreover, the role of platelets has been recognized from a long time in the process of spreading of neoplastic cells to other organs or to lymph nodes far from the primary tumor (called metastatic disease) (Gay and Felding-Habermann 2011). Interestingly, Folkman and associates showed that platelets sequester angiogenesis regulatory proteins and that the analysis of the "platelet angiogenesis proteome" could be used for ultra-early detection of recurrent cancer years before it is symptomatic or can be anatomically located (Cervi et al. 2008).

Platelets store and release, after activation, various angiogenic-regulating factors, such as vascular endothelial growth factor (VEGF), PDGF, fibroblast growth factor (FGF), insulin-like growth factor (IGF), endostatin, thrombospondin-1, tissue inhibitor of metalloproteinases (TIMP). These products are present in different sets of $\alpha$-granules suggesting a differential release of pro- and anti-angiogenic factors in different districts (Italiano et al. 2008). In addition, platelets can synthesize and release cytokines, such as IL-1$\beta$ (Dixon et al. 2006). Platelet-derived IL-1$\beta$, generated by the interaction of platelets with monocytes, has been shown to contribute to monocytic COX-2 induction through a post-transcriptional mechanism which stabilizes COX-2 mRNA (Dixon et al. 2006).

Activated platelets may play a role in tumor progression and metastasis also by the release of microparticles (MPs) and exosomes (Janowska-Wieczorek et al. 2005). These platelet-derived MPs are approximately 0.1–1.0 μm in diameter in humans and express P-selectin (CD62P) and GP IIb-IIIa. They adhere to a variety of cells, can activate endothelial cells, leukocytes and other platelets, and deliver signals through chemokines (Mause and Weber 2010). Exosomes, range in size from 0.04 to 0.1 μm, arise from the internal membrane vesicles of multivesicular bodies and platelets $\alpha$-granules. Unlike MPs, exosomes do not share a similar surface phenotype of activated platelets. However, both MPs and exosomes are known to carry and deliver cellular signals, suggesting a potential role in platelet-derived signaling.

Another mechanism by which platelets influence tumorigenesis is through the generation of $TXA_2$, a major product of platelet COX-1, which promotes platelet aggregation and vasoconstriction (Grosser et al. 2006). $TXA_2$ has been reported to be involved in angiogenesis and development of tumor metastasis (Honn 1983). Interestingly, it has been shown that enhanced $TXA_2$ generation by the introduction of the downstream $TXA_2$ synthase (TXAS) into murine colon-26 adenocarcinoma cell line (C26) enhanced tumor growth in vivo through the stimulation of tumor angiogenesis (Pradono et al. 2002). Similarly, $TXA_2$ promotes the interaction between metastasizing tumor cells and the host hemostatic system (Pradono et al. 2002). Thus, pharmacological inhibition of $TXA_2$ synthase (TXAS) has been shown significantly to inhibit tumor cell growth, invasion, metastasis and angiogenesis in a range of experimental models (Honn 1983). However, the recent finding that aspirin reduces the incidence and mortality of CRC, at doses of at least 75 mg daily (Rothwell et al. 2010), recommended for the prevention against heart disease (Patrono et al. 2005), strongly suggests a role of $TXA_2$, derived mainly from platelets, in tumorigenesis (Patrono et al. 2001) (Fig. 1).

Recent findings have shown that platelets generate and store high amounts of sphingosine-1-phosphate (S1P) which is released upon stimulation with activators of protein kinase C (PKC), such as thrombin, but also with a $TXA_2$ mimetic (Ulrych et al. 2011). Once released, S1P may regulate processes such as inflammation, neovascularization, cell growth and survival (Pyne and Pyne 2010). Interestingly, it was found that oral ASA (500 mg single dose or 100 mg over 3 days) attenuated S1P release from platelets in healthy volunteers ex vivo and it was proposed that the inhibition of $TXA_2$ by aspirin might play a role in the depression of S1P release (Ulrych et al. 2011). Aspirin added in vitro to washed human platelets caused a concentration-dependent reduction of S1P release which however, it was not complete even at 300 μM (Ulrych et al. 2011). Thus, aspirin is more potent to inhibit $TXB_2$ than S1P, both ex vivo and in vitro. Further studies should be performed to address whether the partial depression of platelet S1P release ex vivo might contribute to aspirin chemoprevention of CRC.

Enhanced platelet activation has been detected in humans, in coloreactal cancer and familial adenomatous polyposis (FAP) (Sciulli et al. 2005; Dovizio et al. 2012). A plausible mechanism explaining platelet activation in colon tumorigenesis is that tumor cell-derived products may cause endothelial dysfunction and increase vascular permeability (Padua et al. 2008). This phenomenon may facilitate the interaction of platelets with tumor constituents which are capable of inducing platelet aggregation (Jurasz et al. 2004). In this scenario, vascular $PGI_2$ might play an important role by curbing platelet activation and the release of α-granules, which segregate angiogenesis-regulatory proteins (Menter et al. 1987). Inhibition of COX-2-dependent $PGI_2$, without affecting platelet COX-1 activity by selective COX-2 inhibitors (coxibs), might limit their chemopreventive efficacy. It is noteworthy that low-dose aspirin has a reverse impact on vascular COX-2 and platelet COX-1: it affects only marginally vascular $PGI_2$ while almost completely suppresses platelet $TXA_2$ (Capone et al. 2004).

Activated platelets may release several mediators, such as $TXA_2$, S1P, growth and angiogenic factors and cytokines that may play a role in the upregulation of COX-2 in different cell types (Fig. 1), and this seems a central phenomenon in colon tumorigenesis.

In CRC, COX-2 expression is induced early in stromal cells, and subsequently at high levels in epithelial cells (Prescott 2000), where it correlates with advanced tumor invasion and poor clinical outcomes (Sheehan et al. 1999). Finally, it has been suggested that COX-2 overexpression and associated prostanoid synthesis mitigates immunologic self-tolerance, and antitumor immune responses (Sharma et al. 2005). The role of COX-2 in human tumorigenesis is evidenced by the efficacy of selective COX-2 inhibitors (such as celecoxib) to decrease the risk of colorectal adenoma recurrence (Bertagnolli et al. 2006; Steinbach et al. 2000). However, the use of selective COX-2 inhibitors seems to be inappropriate due to the interference with cardiovascular homeostasis by the coincident inhibition of vascular COX-2-dependent $PGI_2$ (Grosser et al. 2006, see also Chap. 4).

$PGE_2$ is a key prostanoid in tumorigenesis generated through the activity of coordinate expression of COX-2 and mPGES-1 (microsomal $PGE_2$ synthase-1), an enzyme downstream of COX-2 (Wang and DuBois 2010). $PGE_2$ exerts its autocrine/paracrine effects on target cells by coupling to four subtypes of G-protein-coupled receptors classified as EP1, EP2, EP3, and EP4 (E-series prostanoid receptors) (Fig. 3). Recently, it has been shown that EP2 stimulation causes transactivation of the epidermal growth factor receptor (EGFR) signaling pathway to promote tumor cell proliferation and invasion (Donnini et al. 2007).

As shown in Fig. 1, platelets may play an early role in tumorigenesis (Patrono et al. 2001) through the activation of stromal cells, which are the earliest cells to over-express COX-2 during colon carcinogenesis. The stromal COX-2 expression may result in the release of higher levels of prostanoids and growth factors. This step may contribute to epithelial COX-2 expression in the intestinal tract which may cause the increase of cell proliferation and the accumulation of mutations, as a consequence of inhibition of apoptosis (Cao and Prescott 2002; Prescott 2000). Later in tumor progression there will be the induction of COX-2 also in endothelial cells and this will contribute to a proangiogenic response. In this scheme of intestinal tumorigenesis (Fig. 1), both COX-1 and COX-2 play a role but the two COX pathways operate sequentially. This is supported by experimental studies showing that loss of either COX-1 or COX-2 genes blocks intestinal polyposis in mouse models of FAP by about 90 % (Chulada et al. 2000).

Extensive experimental evidence shows that platelets support tumour metastasis (Gay and Felding-Habermann 2011). The activation of platelets and the coagulation system have a crucial role in the progression of cancer. During metastatization, tumor cells acquire the capacity to invade locally and to spread to distant district though the systemic circulation. Thus, tumor cells may interact with platelets and cause their aggregation, a phenomenon known as tumor cell-induced platelet aggregation (TCIPA) (Jurasz et al. 2004). During tumor-platelet interaction, cancer cells have the ability to stimulate the release of platelet granules leading to the release of potent proaggregatory mediators, such as adenosine diphosphate (ADP), an element of platelet dense granules, and $TXA_2$ (Jurasz et al. 2004; Needleman et al. 1976). Platelets-tumor cells interactions confer a number of advantages to the survival of the tumor cells in the vasculature and in its successful metastasis. In fact, platelets provide a physical barrier to natural killer (NK) cell contact, and exert paracrine suppression of NK-mediated cytolytic activity (Nieswandt et al. 1999).

## 4.2 Role of Platelet COX-1 in Aspirin Chemoprevention

Several lines of evidence are consistent with the inhibitory effect of platelet COX-1 by aspirin playing a key role in cancer chemoprevention:

1. Apparent saturability of the chemopreventive effect of aspirin at low-doses given once daily found both in long term analyses of cardiovascular RCTs (Rothwell et al. 2010; Rothwell et al. 2011) and RCTs of adenoma recurrence (Baron et al. 2003; Sandler et al. 2003) as well as in the vast majority of observational studies performed in different settings and with different methodology (Cuzick et al. 2009). A remarkably similar saturability of the cardioprotective effect of aspirin at low-doses given once daily is explained by the irreversible nature of COX-1 inactivation in platelets (Patrignani et al. 1982; Patrono et al. 2008), and limited capacity of human platelets of de novo protein synthesis (Evangelista et al. 2006).
2. It seems unlikely that a nucleated cell can be the target of the chemopreventive effect obtained by one daily administration of low-dose aspirin; in fact, (1) aspirin has a short half-life in human circulation (approximately 20 min), (2) circulating

levels of aspirin, at anti-thrombotic and analgesic doses (Table 1), are below the $IC_{50}$ values for inhibition of COX-2 [$IC_{50}$ value of 180 μM, in the absence of plasma proteins (Fig. 8); in the presence of plasma proteins, it can be approximately 400 μM, considering an aspirin plasma protein binding of 50 %], (3) rapid recovery of acetylated COX-2 in a nucleated cells.

3. One of the cardiovascular RCTs (Meade et al. 1998) in which the chemopreventive effect of aspirin was detected on long term follow-up (Rothwell et al. 2010) involved the administration of a controlled-release formulation of aspirin (75 mg) with negligible systemic bioavailability (Clarke et al. 1991; Charman et al. 1993).
4. Enhanced platelet activation and $TXA_2$ generation in vivo have been demonstrated in patients with CRC and it was cumulatively inhibited by aspirin 50 mg daily (Sciulli et al. 2005).

## 5 COX-Independent Mechanisms of Aspirin Chemoprevention

Several evidences have shown that some NSAIDs, including aspirin, are able to inhibit the proliferation and to induce apoptosis of colon cancer cells in vitro independently from their inhibitory effect on COX-dependent prostanoid biosynthesis (Hanif et al. 1996). We will describe some of the major molecular mechanisms affected by aspirin which may play a role in its antiproliferative and proapototic effects: (1) the interruption of nuclear factor kappa B (NF-kB) signaling (Kopp and Ghosh 1994; Yin et al. 1998; Stark et al. 2001), (2) the interruption of extracellular signal-regulated kinases (ERK) (Pan et al. 2008), (3) the induction of various apoptotic pathways (Jana 2008), (4) the inhibition of Wnt/$\beta$-catenin signaling (Bos et al. 2006). These findings are of interest for the development of novel therapeutics to curb tumorigenesis. However, it seems unlikely that they may play a relevant role in the clinical efficacy of aspirin, as cancer chemopreventive agent. In fact, the different molecular and cellular effects were mainly detected in vitro at very high concentrations of aspirin, often in the millimor range that are not reached in vivo, in the systemic circulation, even when aspirin is administered at high anti-inflammatory doses. Finally, the possible capacity of aspirin to acetylate extra-COX proteins is discussed.

### 5.1 Inhibition of NF-kB

NF-kB is a transcription factor involved in the regulation of antiapoptotic gene expression (Bours et al. 2000); it is sequestered in the cytoplasm of cells by inhibitory proteins, such as IkB. In response to extracellular signals, IkB is phosphorylated by a cellular kinase complex known as IKK (constituted by two subunit IKK$\alpha$ and IKK$\beta$) and it is then degraded by the ubiquitin–proteasome machinery (Chen et al. 1995), thus allowing NF-kB to translocate to the nucleus and to regulate the expression of several genes. It has been demonstrated that aspirin and sodium salicylate inhibit IKK-$\beta$ activity in vitro at millimolar

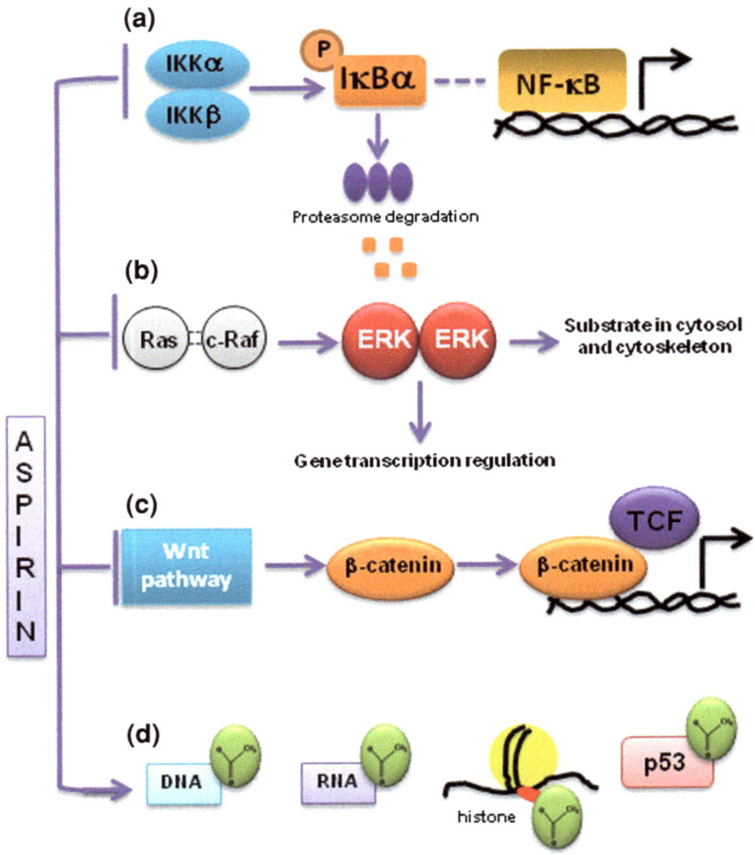


**Fig. 9** COX-independent mechanisms of aspirin action. Aspirin is able to alter intestinal tumor growth rates and modulate carcinogenesis by a variety of COX-independent mechanisms: **a** the inhibition of IKK$\beta$, thereby preventing the activation by NF-kB and its capacity to regulate the expression of several genes that cause suppression of the apoptotic response in cancer cells; **b** the inhibition of the binding of c-Raf with Ras, leading to the inhibition of ERK signaling, involved in the regulation of diverse cellular processes, such as proliferation, survival, differentiation and migration; **c** the inhibition of the Wnt/$\beta$-catenin pathway which plays a role in the expression of genes involved in tumorigenesis; **d** the acetylation of key proteins, such as the tumor suppressor p53 which increased its DNA binding activity

concentration (Yin et al. 1998). The mechanism of aspirin and sodium salicylate for this inhibition is due to their binding to IKK-$\beta$, thus, competing with ATP for the binding to the kinase, an event necessary to phosphorylate IKB (Kopp and Ghosh 1994; Grilli et al. 1996) Fig. 9.

### 5.2 Interruption of Extracellular Signal-Regulated Kinases

Another tumorigenic pathway affected by NSAIDs, including aspirin, is the extracellular signal-regulated kinase (ERK) signaling (Pan et al. 2008). The ERK signaling pathway has been found to be a major controller in the regulation of diverse cellular processes such as proliferation, survival, differentiation and migration (Geest and Coffer 2009). Aberrant activation of signaling molecules, such as activating mutations of tyrosine kinase receptors, causes the binding of Ras oncogene and c-Raf kinase that leads to constitutive activation of ERK and tumorigenesis. Recently, it has been shown that aspirin (at 500 μM) in vitro inhibits the binding of c-Raf with Ras, leading to the inhibition of ERK signaling (Pan et al. 2008).

### 5.3 Induction of Apoptosis by Caspase Activation

Aspirin at millimolar concentrations was found to induce apoptosis through mitochondrial pathways, i.e. cytochrome c release and activation of caspase-9 (Zimmermann et al. 2000), and extrinsic pathways, i.e. activation of caspase-8 (Gu et al. 2005). Cytochrome c released into the cytosol can bind to the apoptotic protease activating factor-1 (apaf-1) and forms the apoptosome complex, which in turn leads to the sequential activation of caspase-9 and caspase-3. Caspases are members of the cysteine protease family, which plays a crucial role in apoptotic pathways by cleaving a variety of key cellular proteins (Creagh et al. 2003).

### 5.4 Inhibition of Wnt/β-Catenin Pathway

Wnt/β-catenin pathway is the most essential oncogenic pathway in colon cancer; the essential feature is an increase in the levels of free cytoplasmic β-catenin (Miller et al. 1999). Subsequently, β-catenin translocates into the nucleus where it binds with members of the T-cell factor (Tcf)/lymphoid enhancer factor (Lef) family of transcription factors, and activates the transcription of Wnt target gene expression such as cyclin D, COX-2 and Myc (Mann et al. 1999).

It has been found that aspirin at millimolar concentrations caused a concentration-dependent inhibiton of the Wnt/β-catenin pathway by stimulating the phosphorylation and breakdown of β-catenin, in vitro (Bos et al. 2006).

## 6 Aspirin-Mediated Acetylation of Extra-COX Proteins

Aspirin has been shown to acetylate proteins and biomolecules in addition to COX-isozymes, such as hemoglobin, DNA, RNA and histones, as well as several plasma constituents, including hormones and enzymes, in vitro at higher concentrations than those reached in the systemic circulation after dosing with low-dose aspirin (Alfonso et al. 2009a).

It was demonstrated that aspirin at 100 μM, a concentration which is reached in the systemic circulation after dosing with anti-inflammatory doses but not after low-dose aspirin (Seymour and Rawlins 1982; Pedersen et al. 1984; Table 1) acetylates the tumor suppressor protein p53 (Alfonso et al. 2009a). Increased acetylation of p53 by aspirin was correlated with increased p53 DNA binding activity and the expression of two of its target genes, $p21^{CIP1}$, a protein involved in cell cycle arrest, and Bax, a mitochondrial pro-apoptotic protein.

These findings should arouse the interest to perform further studies to verify the spectrum of proteins and nucleic acids acetylated by the oral administration of aspirin, in blood cells and epithelial cells of the gastrointestinal tract.

## 7 Conclusions

CRC is the second most common cancer in developed countries. In contrast to cardiovascular and infectious diseases, whose prevention has had a substantial impact on their associated morbidity and mortality, gains in cancer prevention have been limited. The main reasons for this can be due to the lack of biomarkers of early detection and of safe and effective chemopreventive agents. A recent clinical study showed that after 5 years of taking aspirin, death rates were 54 % less for gastrointestinal cancers (Rothwell et al. 2011). The finding of aspirin benefit at low-doses, used for cardioprevention, to reduce long-term incidence and mortality due to CRC (Rothwell et al. 2010) locates the antiplatelet effect of aspirin at the center of its antitumor efficacy. At low-doses, aspirin acts mainly by a preferential and irreversible inactivation of platelet COX-1 thus causing a profound and persistent inhibition of platelet function (Patrignani et al. 1982; Davì and Patrono 2007).

All these pieces of evidence suggest that arterial occlusion and adenoma formation represent different phenotypes of the same abnormal repair process mediated by platelet activation at distinct sites of injury. These extreme phenotypes of a physiologic repair process might result from unfavourable genetic and/or environmental influences on the nature of the lesion, the extent and duration of platelet activation in response to injury and/or the downstream events triggered by platelet-derived lipid and protein mediators.

The study of the successful paradigm of CRC chemoprevention by aspirin may allow the characterization of novel mechanisms of disease and the development of biomarkers for early diagnosis and individualized prevention.

**Acknowledgements** This work was supported by research funding from the Associazione Italiana per la Ricerca sul Cancro (AIRC) to Paola Patrignani. We would like to thank, for fruitful discussions and suggestions, Dr Carlo Patrono (Catholic University, Rome, Italy), Luis A Garcia Rodriguez (CEIFE, Madrid, Spain) and Angel Lanas (University of Zaragoza, Spain). We apologize to our colleagues for not being able to reference all primary work due to space limitations.

## References

Alfonso LF, Srivenugopal KS, Arumugam TV et al (2009a) Aspirin inhibits camptothecin-induced p21CI P1 levels and potentiates apoptosis in human breast cancer cells. Int J Oncol 34:597–608
Alfonso LF, Srivenugopal KS, Bhat GJ (2009b) Does aspirin acetylate multiple cellular proteins? Mol Med Report 2:533–537
Archer SY, Hodint RA (1999) Histone acetylation and cancer. Curr Opin Genet Dev 9:171–174
Baigent C and Antithrombotic Trialists' Collaboration (2002) Collaborative meta-analysis of randomised trials of antiplatelet therapy for prevention of death, myocardial infarction, and stroke in high-risk patients. BMJ 324:71–86
Baron JA, Cole BF, Sandler RS et al (2003) A randomized trial of aspirin to prevent colorectal adenomas. N Engl J Med 348:891–899
Bastida E, Escolar G, Ordinas A et al (1986) Morphometric evaluation of thrombogenesis by microvesicles from human tumor cell lines with thrombin-dependent (U87MG) and adenosine diphosphate-dependent (SKNMC) platelet-activating mechanisms. J Lab Clin Med 108:622–627
Benamouzig R, Deyra J, Martin A et al (2003) Daily soluble aspirin and prevention of colorectal adenoma recurrence: one-year results of the APACC trial. Gastroenterology 125:328–336
Bertagnolli MM, Eagle CJ, Zauber AG et al (2006) Celecoxib for the prevention of sporadic colorectal adenomas. N Engl J Med 355:873–884
Bos CL, Kodach LL, van den Brink GR et al (2006) Effect of aspirin on the Wnt/beta-catenin pathway is mediated via protein phosphatase 2A. Oncogene 25:6447–6456
Bours V, Bentires-Alj M, Hellin AC et al (2000) Nuclear factor-kappa B, cancer, and apoptosis. Biochem Pharmacol 60:1085–1089
Cao Y, Prescott SM (2002) Many actions of cyclooxygenase-2 in cellular dynamics and in cancer. J Cell Physiol 90:279–286
Capone ML, Tacconelli S, Di Francesco L et al (2007) Pharmacodynamic of cyclooxygenase inhibitors in humans. Prostaglandins Other Lipid Mediat 82:85–94
Capone ML, Tacconelli S, Sciulli MG et al (2004) Clinical pharmacology of platelet, monocyte, and vascular cyclooxygenase inhibition by naproxen and low-dose aspirin in healthy subjects. Circulation 109:1468–1471
Cervi D, Yip TT, Bhattacharya N et al (2008) Platelet-associated PF-4 as a biomarker of early tumor growth. Blood 111:1201–1207
Cha YI, DuBois RN (2007) NSAIDs and cancer prevention: targets downstream of COX-2. Annu Rev Med 58:239–252
Charman WN, Charman SA, Monkhouse DC et al (1993) Biopharmaceutical characterisation of a low-dose (75 mg) controlled-release aspirin formulation. Br J Clin Pharmac 36:470–473
Chen Z, Hagler J, Palombella VJ et al (1995) Signal-induced site-specific phosphorylation targets I kappa B alpha to the ubiquitin-proteasome pathway. Genes Dev 9:1586–1597
Chulada PC, Thompson MB, Mahler JF et al (2000) Genetic disruption of Ptgs-1, as well as Ptgs-2, reduces intestinal tumorigenesis in Min mice. Cancer Res 60:4705–4708
Cipollone F, Patrignani P, Greco A et al (1997) Differential suppression of thromboxane biosynthesis by indobufen and aspirin in patients with unstable angina. Circulation 96:1109–1116
Clarke RJ, Mayo G, Price P et al (1991) Suppression of thromboxane A2 but not of systemic prostacyclin by controlled-release aspirin. N Engl J Med 325:1137–1141
Collier JC, Flower RJ (1971) Effect of Aspirin on human seminal prostaglandins. Lancet ii:852–853
Creagh EM, Conroy H, Martin SJ (2003) Caspase-activation pathways in apoptosis and immunity. Immunol Rev 193:10–21
Cuzick J, Otto F, Baron JA et al (2009) Aspirin and non-steroidal anti-inflammatory drugs for cancer prevention: an international consensus statement. Lancet Oncol 10:501–507
Davì G, Patrono C (2007) Platelet activation and atherothrombosis. N Engl J Med 357:2482–2494
Delattre O, Olschwang S, Law DJ et al (1989) Multiple genetic alterations in distal and proximal colorectal cancer. Lancet 2:353–356

Di Francesco L, Totani L, Dovizio M et al (2009) Induction of prostacyclin by steady laminar shear stress suppresses tumor necrosis factor-alpha biosynthesis via heme oxygenase-1 in human endothelial cells. Circ Res 104:506–513
Dixon DA, Tolley ND, Bemis-Standoli K et al (2006) Expression of COX-2 in platelet-monocyte interactions occurs via combinatorial regulation involving adhesion and cytokine signaling. J Clin Invest 116:2727–2738
Dixon DA, Tolley ND, King PH et al (2001) Altered expression of the mRNA stability factor HuR promotes cyclooxygenase-2 expression in colon cancer cells. J Clin Invest 2108:1657–1665
Donnini S, Finetti F, Solito R et al (2007) EP2 prostanoid receptor promotes squamous cell carcinoma growth through epidermal growth factor receptor transactivation and iNOS and ERK1/2 pathways. FASEB J 21:2418–2430
Dovizio M, Tacconelli S, Ricciotti E et al (2012) Effects of celecoxib on prostanoid biosynthesis and circulating angiogenesis proteins in familial adenomatous polyposis. J Pharmacol Exp Ther 341:242–250
Dreser H (1899) Pharmakologisches über aspirin (acetylsalicylsäure). Pfluger's Arch 76:306–318
Evangelista V, Manarini S, Di Santo A et al (2006) De novo synthesis of cyclooxygenase-1 counteracts the suppression of platelet thromboxane biosynthesis by aspirin. Circ Res 98:593–595
Ferreira SH, Moncada S, Vane JR (1971) Indomethacin and Aspirin abolish prostaglandin release from spleen. Nature 231:237–239
Fierro IM, Kutok JL, Serhan CN (2002) Novel lipid mediator regulators of endothelial cell proliferation and migration: aspirin-triggered-15R-lipoxin A(4) and lipoxin A(4). J Pharmacol Exp Ther 300:385–392
FitzGerald GA (2003) COX-2 and beyond: Approaches to prostaglandin inhibition in human disease. Nat Rev Drug Discov 2:879–890
García Rodríguez LA, Hernández-Díaz S, de Abajo FJ (2001) Association between aspirin and upper gastrointestinal complications: systematic review of epidemiologic studies. Br J Clin Pharmacol 52:563–571
García Rodríguez LA, Lin KJ, Hernández-Díaz S et al (2011) Risk of upper gastrointestinal bleeding with low-dose acetylsalicylic acid alone and in combination with clopidogrel and other medications. Circulation 2011(123):1108–1115
Gay LJ, Felding-Habermann B (2011) Contribution of platelets to tumour metastasis. Nat Rev Cancer 11:123–134
Geest CR, Coffer PJ (2009) MAPK signaling pathways in the regulation of hematopoiesis. J Leukoc Biol 86:237–250
Gilroy DW (2005) The role of aspirin-triggered lipoxins in the mechanism of action of aspirin. Prostaglandins Leukot Essent Fatty Acids 73:203–210
Grilli M, Pizzi M, Memo M et al (1996) Neuroprotection by aspirin and sodium salicylate through blockade of NF-kB activation. Science 274:1383–1385
Grosser T, Fries S, FitzGerald GA (2006) Biological basis for the cardiovascular consequences of COX-2 inhibition: therapeutic challenges and opportunities. J Clin Invest 116:4–15
Gu Q, Wang JD, Xia HH et al (2005) Activation of the caspase-8/Bid and Bax pathways in aspirin-induced apoptosis in gastric cancer. Carcinogenesis 26:541–546
Hanif R, Pittas A, Feng Y et al (1996) Effects of nonsteroidal anti-inflammatory drugs on proliferation and on induction of apoptosis in colon cancer cells by a prostaglandin-independent pathway. Biochem Pharmacol 52:237–245
Harper KA, Tyson-Capper AJ (2008) Complexity of COX-2 gene regulation. Biochem Soc Trans 36:543–545
Hemler M, Lands WEM, Smith WL (1976) Purification of the cyclooxygenase that forms prostaglandins: demonstration of two forms of iron in the holoenzyme. J Biol Chem 251:5575–5579
Honn K (1983) Inhibition of tumor cell metastasis by modulation of the vascular prostacyclin/thromboxane A2 system. Clin Exp Metastasis 1:103–114
Iacopetta B (2002) Are there two sides to colorectal cancer? Int J Cancer 101:403–408

Italiano JE Jr, Richardson JL, Patel-Hett S et al (2008) Angiogenesis is regulated by a novel mechanism: pro- and antiangiogenic proteins are organized into separate platelet alpha granules and differentially released. Blood 111:1227–1233
Jana NR (2008) NSAIDs and apoptosis. Cell Mol Life Sci 65:1295–1301
Janowska-Wieczorek A, Wysoczynski M, Kijowski J et al (2005) Microvesicles derived from activated platelets induce metastasis and angiogenesis in lung cancer. Int J Cancer 113:752–760
Jurasz P, Alonso-Escolano D, Radomski MW (2004) Platelet–cancer interactions: mechanisms and pharmacology of tumour cell-induced platelet aggregation. Br J Pharmacol 143:819–826
Kang YJ, Mbonye UR, DeLong CJ et al (2007) Regulation of intracellular cyclooxygenase levels by gene transcription and protein degradation. Prog Lipid Res 46:108–125
Kopp E, Ghosh S (1994) Inhibition of NF-kappa B by sodium salicylate and aspirin. Science 265:956–959
Kujubu DA, Fletcher BS, Varnum BC (1991) TIS10, a phorbol ester tumor promoter-inducible mRNA from Swiss 3T3 cells, encodes a novel prostaglandin synthase/cyclooxygenase homologue. J Biol Chem 266:12866–12872
Kulmacz RJ, Lands WE (1985) Stoichiometry and kinetics of the interaction of prostaglandin H synthase with anti-inflammatory agents. J Biol Chem 260:12572–12578
Kurumbail RG, Stevens AM, Gierse JK et al (1996) Structural basis for selective inhibition of cyclooxygenase-2 by anti-inflammatory agents. Nature 384:644–648
Lecomte M, Laneuville O, Ji C et al (1994) Acetylation of human prostaglandin endoperoxide synthase-2 (cyclooxygenase-2) by aspirin. J Biol Chem 269:13207–13215
Loll PJ, Picot D, Garavito RM (1995) The structural basis of aspirin activity inferred from the crystal structure of inactivated prostaglandin H2 synthase. Nat Struct Biol 2:637–643
Mann B, Gelos M, Siedow A et al (1999) Target genes of beta-catenin-T cell-factor/lymphoid-enhancer-factor signaling in human colorectal carcinomas. Proc Natl Acad Sci U S A 96:1603–1608
Mause SF, Weber C (2010) Microparticles: protagonists of a novel communication network for intercellular information exchange. Circ Res 107:1047–1057
Meade TW, Framework The Medical Research Council's General Practice Research (1998) Thrombosis prevention trial: randomised trial of low-intensity oral anticoagulation with warfarin and low-dose aspirin in the primary prevention of ischaemic heart disease in men at increased risk. Lancet 351:233–241
Menter DG, Onoda JM, Moilanen D et al (1987) Inhibition by prostacyclin of the tumor cell-induced platelet release reaction and platelet aggregation. J Natl Cancer Inst 78:961–969
Miller JR, Hocking AM, Brown JD et al (1999) Mechanism and function of signal transduction by the Wnt/beta-catenin and Wnt/$Ca^{2+}$ pathways. Oncogene 18:7860–7872
Minuz P, Fumagalli L, Gaino S et al (2006) Rapid stimulation of tyrosine phosphorylation signals downstream of Gprotein- coupled receptors for thromboxane A2 in human platelets. Biochem J. 400:127–134
Needleman P, Moncada S, Bunting S et al (1976) Identification of an enzyme in platelet microsomes which generates thromboxane A2 from prostaglandin endoperoxides. Nature 261:558–560
Nieswandt B, Hafner M, Echtenacher B et al (1999) Lysis of tumor cells by natural killer cells in mice is impeded by platelets. Cancer Res 59:1295–1300
Okajima F (2002) Plasma lipoproteins behave as carriers of extracellular sphingosine 1-phosphate: is this an atherogenic mediator or an anti-atherogenic mediator? Biochim Biophys Acta 1582:132–137
Pacienza N, Pozner RG, Bianco GA et al (2008) The immunoregulatory glycan-binding protein galectin-1 triggers human platelet activation. FASEB J 22:1113–1123
Padua D, Zhang XH, Wang Q et al (2008) TGFbeta primes breast tumors for lung metastasis seeding through angiopoietin-like 4. Cell 133:66–77
Paganini-Hill A, Chao A, Ross RK et al (1989) Aspirin use and chronic diseases: a cohort study of the elderly. BMJ 299:1247–1250

Pan MR, Chang HC, Hung WC (2008) Non-steroidal anti-inflammatory drugs suppress the ERK signaling pathway via block of Ras/c-Raf interaction and activation of MAP kinase phosphatases. Cell Signal 20:1134–1141
Patrignani P, Filabozzi P, Patrono C (1982) Selective cumulative inhibition of platelet thromboxane production by low-dose aspirin in healthy subjects. J Clin Invest 69:1366–1372
Patrignani P, Panara MR, Greco A et al (1994) Biochemical and pharmacological characterization of the cyclooxygenase activity of human blood prostaglandin endoperoxide synthases. J Pharmacol Exp Ther 271:1705–1712
Patrono C, Baigent C, Hirsh J et al (2008) Antiplatelet drugs: American college of chest physicians evidence-based clinical practice guidelines. Chest 133:199S–233S 8th edn
Patrono C, Ciabattoni G, Patrignani P et al (1985) Clinical pharmacology of platelet cyclooxygenase inhibition. Circulation 72:1177–1184
Patrono C, Ciabattoni G, Pinca E et al (1980) Low dose aspirin and inhibition of thromboxane B2 production in healthy subjects. Thromb Res 17:317–327
Patrono C, García Rodríguez LA, Landolfi R et al (2005) Low-dose aspirin for the prevention of atherothrombosis. N Engl J Med 353:2373–2383
Patrono C, Patrignani P, García Rodríguez LA (2001) Cyclooxygenase-selective inhibition of prostanoid formation: transducing biochemical selectivity into clinical read-outs. J Clin Invest 108:7–13
Pedersen AK, FitzGerald GA (1984) Dose-related kinetics of aspirin: presystemic acetylation of platelet cyclo-oxygenase. N Engl J Med 311:1206–1211
Picot D, Loll PJ, Garavito RM (1994) The X-ray crystal structure of the membrane protein prostaglandin H2 synthase-1. Nature 367:243–249
Pradono P, Tazawa R, Maemondo M et al (2002) Gene transfer of thromboxane A(2) synthase and prostaglandin I(2) synthase antithetically altered tumor angiogenesis and tumor growth. Cancer Res 62:63–66
Prescott SM (2000) Is cyclooxygenase-2 the alpha and the omega in cancer? J Clin Invest 105:1511–1513
Pyne NJ (2010) Pyne S (2010) Sphingosine 1-phosphate and cancer. Nat Rev Cancer 10:489–503
Rimon G, Sidhu RS, Lauver DA et al (2010) Coxibs interfere with the action of aspirin by binding tightly to one monomer of cyclooxygenase-1. Proc Natl Acad Sci USA 107:28–33
Romano M (2006) Lipid mediators: lipoxin and aspirin-triggered 15-epi-lipoxins. Inflamm Allergy Drug Targets 5:81–90
Romano M (2010) Lipoxin and aspirin-triggered lipoxins. Sci World J 10:1048–1064
Roth GJ, Majerus PW (1975) The mechanism of the effect of aspirin on human platelets: 1 acetylation of a particulate fraction protein. J Clin Invest 56:624–632
Roth GJ, Stanford N, Majerus PW (1975) Acetylation of prostaglandin synthase by aspirin. Proc Natl Acad Sci U S A 72:3073–3076
Rothwell PM, Fowkes FG, Belch JF et al (2011) Effect of daily aspirin on long-term risk of death due to cancer: analysis of individual patient data from randomised trials. Lancet 377:31–41
Rothwell PM, Wilson M, Elwin CE et al (2010) Long-term effect of aspirin on colorectal cancer incidence and mortality: 20 year follow-up of five randomised trials. Lancet 376:1741–1750
Rumble RH, Brooks PM, Roberts MS (1980) Metabolism of salicylate during chronic aspirin therapy. Br J Clin Pharmac 9:41–45
Sandler RS, Halabi S, Baron JA et al (2003) A randomized trial of aspirin to prevent colorectal adenomas in patients with previous colorectal cancer. N Engl J Med 348:883–890
Sciulli MG, Filabozzi P, Tacconelli S et al (2005) Platelet activation in patients with colorectal cancer. Prostaglandins Leukot Essent Fatty Acids 72:79–83
Serhan CN (2005) Lipoxins and aspirin-triggered 15-epi-lipoxins are the first lipid mediators of endogenous anti-inflammation and resolution. Prostaglandins Leukot Essent Fatty Acids 73:141–162
Seymour RA, Rawlins MD (1982) Efficacy and pharmacokinetics of aspirin in post-operative dental pain. J. Clin. Pharmac. 13:807–810

Sharma NP, Dong L, Yuan C et al (2010) Asymmetric acetylation of the cyclooxygenase-2 homodimer by aspirin and its effects on the oxygenation of arachidonic, eicosapentaenoic, and docosahexaenoic acids. Mol Pharmacol 77:979–986

Sharma S, Yang SC, Zhu L et al (2005) Tumor cyclooxygenase-2/prostaglandin E2-dependent promotion of FOXP3 expression and $CD^{4+}$ $CD^{25+}$ T regulatory cell activities in lung cancer. Cancer Res 65:5211–5220

Sheehan KM, Sheahan K, O'Donoghue DP et al (1999) The relationship between cyclooxygenase-2 expression and colorectal cancer. JAMA 282:1254–1257

Sidhu RS, Lee JY, Yuan C et al (2010) Comparison of cyclooxygenase-1 crystal structures: cross-talk between monomers comprising cyclooxygenase-1 homodimers. Biochemistry 49:7069–7079

Smith JB, Willis AL (1971) Aspirin selectively inhibits prostaglandin production in human platelets. Nature 231:235–237

Smyth EM, Grosser T, Wang M et al (2009) Prostanoids in health and disease. J Lipid Res 50:S423–S428

Smyth MJH, Dawkins PD (1971) Salicylates and enzyme. J Pharm Pharmacol 23:729–744

Stark LA, Din FV, Zwacka RM et al (2001) Aspirin-induced activation of the NF-kappaB signaling pathway: a novel mechanism for aspirin-mediated apoptosis in colon cancer cells. FASEB J 15:1273–1275

Steinbach G, Lynch PM, Phillips RK et al (2000) The effect of celecoxib, a cyclooxygenase-2 inhibitor, in familial adenomatous polyposis. N Engl J Med 342:1946–1952

Stone E (1763) An account of the success of the bark of the willow tree in the cure of agues. Philos Trans R Soc Lond. 53:195–200

Tani M, Sano T, Ito M et al (2005) Mechanisms of sphingosine and sphingosine 1-phosphate generation in human platelets. J Lipid Res 46:2458–2467

Thun MJ, Henley SJ, Patrono C (2002) Nonsteroidal anti-inflammatory drugs as anticancer agents: mechanistic. Pharmacologic, Clin Issues J Natl Cancer Inst 94:252–266

Topper JN, Cai J, Falb D et al (1996) Identification of vascular endothelial genes differentially responsive to fluid mechanical stimuli: cyclooxygenase-2, manganese superoxide dismutase, and endothelial cell nitric oxide synthase are selectively up-regulated by steady laminar shear stress. PNAS 93:10417–10422

Ulrych T, Böhm A, Polzin et al (2011) Release of sphingosine-1-phosphate from human platelets is dependent on thromboxane formation. J Thromb Haemost 9:790–798

Vane JR (1971) Inhibition of prostaglandin synthesis as a mechanism of action for Aspirin-like drugs. Nat New Biol 231:232–235

Vane JR, Botting RM (2003) The mechanism of action of aspirin. Thromb Res 110:255–258

Wang D, Dubois RN (2010) Eicosanoids and cancer. Nat Rev Cancer 10:181–193

Weiss HJ, Aledort LM (1967) Impaired platelet-connective-tissue reaction in man after aspirin ingestion. Lancet 2:495–497

Xie W, Chipman JG, Robertson DL et al (1991) Expression of a mitogen-responsive gene encoding prostaglandin synthase is regulated by mRNA splicing. Proc Natl Acad Sci U S A 88:2692–2696

Yin MJ, Yamamoto Y, Gaynor RB (1998) The anti-inflammatory agents aspirin and salicylate inhibit the activity of I(kappa)B kinase-beta. Nature 396:77–80

Yuan C, Rieke CJ, Rimon G et al (2006) Partnering between monomers of cyclooxygenase-2 homodimers. Proc Natl Acad Sci U S A. 103:6142–6147

Yuan C, Sidhu RS, Kuklev DV et al (2009) Cyclooxygenase Allosterism, Fatty Acid-mediated Cross-talk between Monomers of Cyclooxygenase Homodimers. J Biol Chem 284:10046–10055

Zimmermann KC, Waterhouse NJ, Goldstein JC et al (2000) Aspirin induces apoptosis through release of cytochrome c from mitochondria. Neoplasia 2:505–513

# Coxibs: Pharmacology, Toxicity and Efficacy in Cancer Clinical Trials

Luis A. Garcia Rodriguez, Lucia Cea-Soriano, Stefania Tacconelli and Paola Patrignani

**Abstract**

This chapter briefly summarizes the current knowledge about the role of nonsteroidal anti-inflammatory drugs (NSAIDs), specially focusing on those selective for cyclooxygenase (COX)-2 (coxibs), on colorectal cancer (CRC) onset, and progression. Both epidemiological and experimental studies have reported that these drugs reduce the risk of developing colonic tumors. However, the promising use of coxibs in chemoprevention was halted abruptly due to the detection on enhanced cardiovascular (CV) risks. Thus, we discuss the clinical data and plausible mechanisms of CV hazards associated with traditional NSAIDs and coxibs. The extent of inhibition of COX-2-dependent prostacyclin, an important vasoprotective and anti-thrombotic pathway, in the absence of a complete suppression of COX-1-dependent platelet function, at common doses of NSAIDs, might play a role in CV toxicity. Coxibs might still be reserved for younger patients with familial adenomatous polyposis (FAP). However, it should be taken into consideration that recent findings of enhanced thromboxane (TX)$A_2$ biosynthesis in colon tumorigenesis, detected in humans. In this context, the use of low-dose aspirin (which mainly acts by inhibiting platelet COX-1-dependent $TXA_2$) may have a place for chemoprevention of CRCs (see also Chap. 3). The possible use of coxibs to prevent CRC will depend mainly on research progresses in biomarkers able to identify the

L. A. Garcia Rodriguez (✉) · L. Cea-Soriano
Centro Español de Investigacion Farmacoepidemiologica (CEIFE),
2 Almirante 28, 28004 Madrid, Spain
e-mail: lagarcia@ceife.es

S. Tacconelli · P. Patrignani (✉)
Center of Excellence On Aging (CeSI) and Department of Neuroscience and Imaging,
G. d'Annunzio University, School of Medicine, Via dei Vestini 31, 66100 Chieti CH, Italy
e-mail: ppatrignani@unich.it

A. T. Chan and E. Detering (eds.), *Prospects for Chemoprevention of Colorectal Neoplasia*,
Recent Results in Cancer Research 191, DOI: 10.1007/978-3-642-30331-9_4, 

patients uniquely susceptible to developing thrombotic events by inhibition of COX-2.

## Abbreviations

| | |
|---|---|
| AMI | Acute myocardial infarction |
| ASA | Aspirin |
| CV | Cardiovascular |
| CNS | Central nervous system |
| CRC | Colorectal cancer |
| COX | Cyclooxygenase |
| EMA | European medicine agency |
| EU | European union |
| FAP | Familial adenomatous polyposis |
| FDA | Food and drug administration |
| GI | Gastrointestinal |
| $PGI_2$ | Prostacyclin |
| PG | Prostaglandin |
| RCT | Randomized clinical trial |
| RR | Relative risk |
| RA | Rheumatoid arthritis |
| $TXA_2$ | Thromboxane |
| tNSAID | Traditional nonsteroidal anti-inflammatory drug |
| US | United States |

## Contents

# 1 Introduction

Colorectal cancer (CRC) is the second cancer-related death in the world and it is one of the most preventable. Incidence and mortality from CRC appears similar in both men and women (Parkin et al. 1999). Data from the World Health Organization (WHO) indicate that CRC has reached the highest incidence of all malignancies in Europe (Weir et al. 2003). Survival is directly linked to the stage of the disease at the time of diagnosis. New progress in surgery, such as mesorectal resection, minimal manipulation, and resection of metastasis has decreased the mortality in those patients (Choti et al. 2002; Headrick et al. 2001).

CRC is preventable in up to 80–90 % of the cases. A large body of evidence indicates that genetic mutations, epigenetic changes, diet, lifestyle as smoking habits and alcohol consumption, insulin and insulin growth factor, diabetes, and chronic inflammation are risk factors for CRC (Wang and Dubois 2010a; Garcia Rodriguez et al. 2000; Willett et al. 1990; Larsson et al. 2005; Cheng et al. 2011).

Some of the most significant lifestyle habits are periodic physical activity, abstinence from smoking, and a healthy diet. It has been suggested that having a diet low in calories high in fruit and vegetables, low in red meat and animal (saturated) fat, and rich in antioxidants and other micronutrients may have a protecting effect against CRC (Boursi and Arber 2007).

Subjects with type two diabetes have consistently been shown to be at increased risk of CRC (Larsson et al. 2005; Jiang et al. 2011). In a meta-analysis of 15 case control and cohort studies involving 2,593,935 participants, diabetic individuals had 30 % increased risk of CRC (RR = 1.30, 95 % confidence interval (CI) 1.20–1.40) (Larsson et al. 2005). The mechanist explanation of this association is not completely understood. It has been proposed that insulin and insulin-like growth factor (IGF-1), in diabetes, may activate different signaling leading to tumor cell transformation, such as Wnt-$\beta$-catenin pathway (Giouleme et al. 2011), which triggers the expression of different genes involved in cell proliferation; among them it is, noteworthy, the possible overexpression of COX-2 (Buchanan and Dubois 2006; see Chap. 2). It has been recently shown that four single nucleotide polymorphisms (SNPs), identified by genome-wide association studies (GWAS) as susceptibility locus for type two diabetes, i.e THADA, JAZF1, KCNJ11 and TSPAN8, also impact the risk of CRC (Cheng et al. 2011). However, further studies would be performed to confirm these findings before they could be used as predictor biomarkers of susceptibility of CRC development.

Some factors described above might play a major etiologic role and so that they are preventive strategies of CRC. It is pointed out that calcium intake could have an inhibitory effect on tumors with *ras* mutations (Janne and Mayer 2000; Bautista et al. 1997; Lipkin and Newmark 1985). Analysis from the Nurses' Health Study and the Health Professionals Follow-Up Study found that consumption of calcium reduced the risk of distal colon cancer but not of proximal cancer (Wu et al. 2002). However, the results from Women's Health Initiative (WHI) did not observe effect for daily calcium with vitamin D intake on the incidence of CRC among postmenopausal women (Wactawski-Wende et al. 2006). In addition, epidemiological studies found that individuals with the highest dietary folate intake had a lower incidence of CRC, whereas individuals with diets that are low in folate appear to have an increased risk of CRC (Boursi and Arber 2007). Antioxidants as vitamin C, D and carotenes have been thought to protect the mucosa as they neutralize the free radicals, but data did not lead enough evidence to support a recommendation that individuals obtaining supplementary sources of antioxidants to reduce their risk of CRC (Greenberg et al. 1994; Hennekens et al. 1996). Meta-analysis conducted by Trock et al. and meta-analysis of several case-control studies observed that a high fiber intake was associated with an approximately 40 % reduction in CRC risk but not for adenomas (Trock et al. 1990; Fuchs et al. 1999; Lev-Ari et al. 2006). Physical activity is a protective factor independent from other lifestyle habits that may be related to CRC risk (Campos et al. 2005; Giovannucci 2002). In spite of these alternatives to reduce the risk of cancer onset to that date there was no progress in eliminating these risk factors.

One of the promising prevention strategies consists in drug intervention also known as chemoprevention (Hong et al. 1990; King et al. 2001). Chemoprevention involves long-term use of a variety of oral drugs that can delay, prevent or even reverse the development of adenomas in the large bowel, and interfere with the progression from adenoma to carcinoma. The ideal chemopreventive agent should meet the following criteria: to be effective, have a convenient dosing schedule, be easily administered, have low cost, and most importantly, it should have a very low side effect profile in the target population.

Long-term use of nonsteroidal anti-inflammatory drugs (NSAIDs), particularly aspirin (ASA) (described in detail in Chaps. 3 and 7) and selective cyclooxygenase (COX)-2 inhibitors (coxibs, Fig. 1) have been one of the most studied class of drugs in CRC chemoprevention, since both epidemiological and experimental studies have reported that these drugs reduce the risk of developing colonic tumors.

NSAIDs, one of the most frequently used therapeutic family of drugs worldwide, are a heterogenous group of compounds often chemically unrelated (although most of them are organic acids) (Burke et al. 2006), which act by inhibiting the synthesis of prostanoids, a family of biologically active mediators generated by the activity of COXs (FitzGerald and Patrono 2001; Simmons et al. 2004). NSAIDs are grouped on the basis of pharmacodynamic features, i.e. COX-1/COX-2 selectivity (Capone et al. 2007). This is assessed in vitro and ex vivo (after dosing) using the human whole blood assays (Patrignani et al. 1994; Patrono et al. 1980) which evaluate the effects of drugs on platelet COX-1 and monocyte COX-2 (Fig. 2). Traditional tNSAIDs are a group of drugs which inhibit both COX-1 and COX-2 at therapeutic doses (also called nonselective NSAIDs), while coxibs are selective inhibitors of COX-2.

tNSAIDs use was its gastrointestinal (GI) safety (Fig. 3). NSAIDs have been repeatedly shown to induce GI events ranging from dyspepsia/gastric intolerance to serious (mainly upper) GI bleeding (Brun and Jones 2001; Hernandez-Diaz and Garcia Rodrìguez 2000). Apart from ASA and NSAID therapy, other factors as

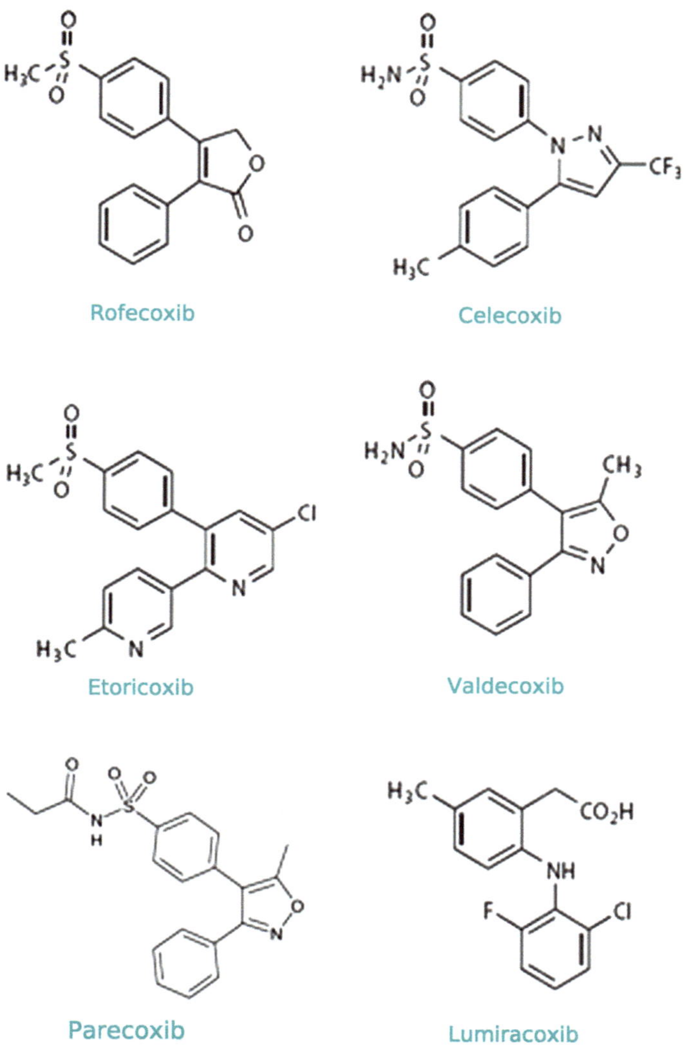


**Fig. 1** Chemical structures of coxibs. Rofecoxib and etoricoxib, celecoxib, and valdecoxib are diaryleterocyclic derivatives containing a phenylsulphone and a phenylsulphonamide moiety, respectively. Parecoxib is the water soluble and injectable prodrug of valdecoxib. Differently from the other coxibs, lumiracoxib is a phenyl acetic acid derivative of diclofenac

advanced age, history of peptic ulcer and comedication with corticosteroids, or anticoagulants have been associated with an increased risk of upper GI disorders (Laine 2001; Lanas and Scheiman 2007). Different prevention strategies to overcome/minimize GI problems have been developed in the last decades. The discovery of *Helicobacter pylori* contribution to the atrophy of the gastric mucosa and

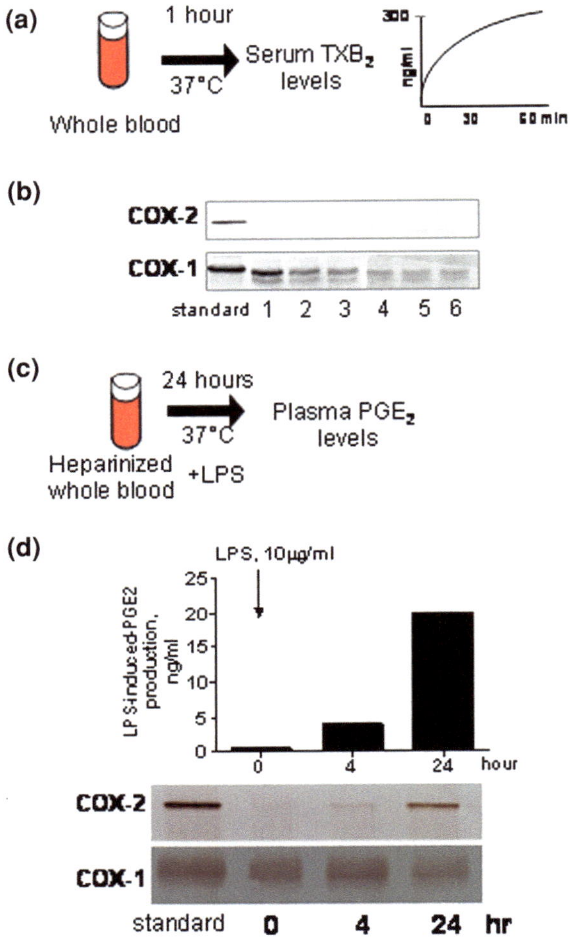


**Fig. 2** Whole blood assays to evaluate the effects of COX inhibitors on platelet COX-1 and monocyte COX-2 activities. **a** The measurement of $TXB_2$ production during whole blood clotting is used as an index of platelet COX-1 activity (Patrono et al. 1980). In panel **b**, western blot shows that COX-1 but not COX-2 is detected in platelets of healthy subjects (adapted from Patrignani et al. 1999). **c** The measurement of $PGE_2$ production in response to bacterial endotoxin (*LPS*) added to heparinized blood samples reflects the time-dependent induction of COX-2 in circulating monocytes (Patrignani et al. 1994). In panel **d**, the time course of COX-1, COX-2, and $PGE_2$ biosynthesis in monocytes stimulated with *LPS* is shown. The Western blot of COX-1 and COX-2 in isolated monocytes stimulated (or not) with *LPS* has been adapted from Sciulli et al. (2003)

subsequently peptic ulcer and gastric cancer onset, together with its eradication therapy have contributed to a better knowledge and control. Some randomized controlled trials (RCTs) and observational studies have found that proton pump inhibitors (PPIs) reduce the risk of upper GI bleeding in patients under antiplatelet and NSAID treatment. Study performed by Lai et al. found that, among ASA users, lansoprazole therapy was associated with a reduced recurrence of ulcer complications when compared with placebo (1.6 vs. 14.8 %) (Lai et al. 2002). Chan et al. showed that among users of NSAIDs other than ASA, omeprazole therapy was associated with a reduced rate of recurrent bleeding compared with *Helicobacter pylori* eradication therapy (4.4 vs. 18.8 %) (Chan et al. 2001). A recent observational study by Lin et al. observed how PPI use was associated with a lower risk of upper GI bleeding in the general population as well as in patients on antithrombotic or anti-inflammatory therapy (Lin et al. 2011).

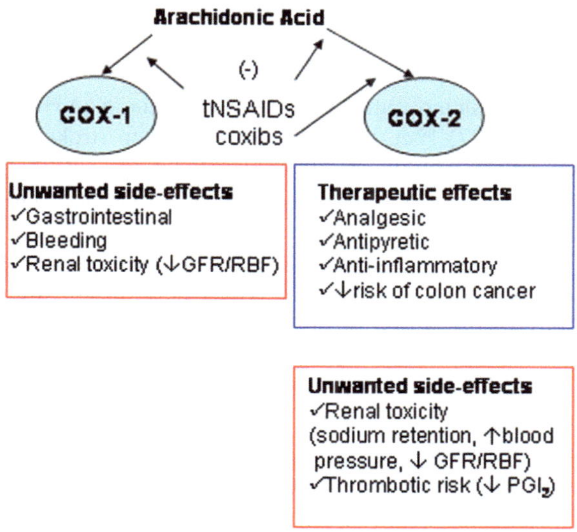


**Fig. 3** Pharmacological effects of COX-1 and COX-2 inhibition by traditional (t)NSAIDs and selective COX-2 inhibitors (coxibs). *GFR* glomerular filtration rate; *RBF* renal blood flow

Thus, according with the ACCF/ACG/AHA 2008 expert consensus guideline concurrent therapy of PPIs is now the standard therapy for patients receiving ASA and NSAIDs (Bhatt et al. 2008).

Although adverse upper GI events appear to be a class effect, not all tNSAIDs exhibit the same degree of GI toxicity at therapeutic doses. A large body of evidence comparing the GI safety profile across most individual tNSAIDs has been reported in detail (Massó González et al. 2010) and clinicians may now make better-informed clinical and therapeutical decisions on which NSAID to use. With this background of increased risk of GI events observed with all tNSAIDs, the research community together with the industry started to work on the appealing notion of attaining the same analgesic and anti-inflammatory effect, but limiting the undesirable GI effects leading to the development of a novel class of NSAIDs (FitzGerald and Patrono 2001). Inhibition of COX-2 was thought to transduce all the beneficial effects of NSAIDs, while inhibiton of COX-1 was considered to be responsible for all the unintended adverse effects on the GI mucosa (Fig. 3). The introduction of coxibs (Fig. 1) in the 1990s was a major breakthrough thought by many to solve all the GI safety problems once and forever (Box 1). Actually, coxibs demonstrated to be as effective as tNSAIDs and presented an improved GI safety profile though they still carried a small increased risk of serious cardiovascular (CV) events (Grosser et al. 2006). Yet, soon after the market introduction of coxibs which was a huge success, some data started to emerge questioning their effect on CV homeostasis, in particular whether they could increase the risk of acute myocardial infarction (AMI), which led to the withdrawn from the United States (US) and European Union (EU) of two coxibs, rofecoxib and valdecoxib, in 2004, and 2005, respectively. Lumiracoxib was approved in the EU in 2006, but was withdrawn from the market in several countries the following year because of liver toxicity.

An increased risk of hemorrhagic stroke associated with NSAIDs has been also reported in a recent statement by the American Heart Association (AHA) (Antman et al. 2007). Yet, the association between stroke and use of NSAID still remains controversial with several studies yielding conflicting results. A number of studies investigating this relationship have not demonstrated any significant association (Thrift et al. 1999; Bak et al. 2003; Johnsen et al. 2003; Choi et al. 2008). Other authors reported an increased risk of subarachnoid hemorrhage associated with the use of NSAIDs and coxibs (Haag et al. 2008; Roumie et al. 2008; Chang et al. 2010). Use of low-dose ASA has been associated with a small increased risk of intracranial hemorrhage: Antithrombotic Trialists' (ATT) Collaboration reported a nonsignificant increase (between 30 and 60 %) in hemorrhagic stroke (Baigent et al. 2009). This existing controversy around a true association between NSAIDs and hemorrhagic stroke denotes the necessity of further large-scale studies, especially in target populations as elderly or in a population with multiple potential risk factors for CV events.

This chapter briefly summarizes the current knowledge of chemopreventive role of NSAIDs specially focusing on coxibs on colon cancer onset and progression. Finally, we performed an overview of the different aspects of NSAID-related CV toxicity such as the observed heterogeneity between different individual NSAIDs and its determinants, the time course of the effect, and the potential interaction between ASA and NSAIDs.

**Box 1**

Marketing authorzation was granted for rofecoxib and celecoxib as first representatives of this new pharmacological class in 1999 in the EU and US with the indication for osteoarthritis (OA) and Rheumatoid Arthritis (RA). In 2000, rofecoxib received the marketing authorzation for treatment of acute pain and pain associated with primary dysmenorrhoea in the EU.

During the following years, a number of second generation of coxibs obtained the marketing authorization in the EU and US.

Etoricoxib received the marketing authorization for rheumatic diseases, including gouty arthritis in some EU member states. Valdecoxib was granted the marketing authorization via the EMA central procedure for treatment of RA and OA and pain associated with primary dysmenorrhoea. Parecoxib, the prodrug of valdecoxib, received the marketing authorzation via the central EMA procedure for short-term treatment of post-surgical pain, when used intravenously or intramuscularly. Finally, lumiracoxib received the marketing authorization for symptomatic treatment of OA and acute pain associated with dental and orthopedic surgery and primary dysmenorrhoea. In addition, celecoxib obtained the marketing authorization for an orphan drug indication (FAP) via the EMA central procedure.

From a regulatory point of view, the VIGOR study (Bombardier et al. 2000), together with epidemiological data, which also raised concerns about the CV safety of coxibs, constituted the starting point for a reconsideration of the benefit/risk balance of the coxibs approved at that point of time (celecoxib, etoricoxib, parecoxib, rofecoxib, valdecoxib) with respect to adverse CV and GI effects, in 2002. In addition, serious hypersensitivity and serious skin reactions have been observed with valdecoxib, some in patients with a history of allergic-type reactions to sulphonamides. Thus, an assessment of serious hypersensitivity reactions (e.g. anaphylaxis and angioedema) and serious adverse skin reactions (including Stevens-Johnson syndrome, toxic epidermal necrolysis, erythema multiforme, and exfoliative dermatitis) was added in October 2002, based on concerns raised by epidemiological data. As a result of this first EU coxib-referral, the European Commission concluded in April 2004 that the benefit/risk balance of the coxibs remained favorable; however, that additional warnings should be added to the product informations concerning CV safety (mainly concerning the risk of MI), GI safety (mainly concerning the association with ASA), and observed or potential serious skin effects and hypersensitivity reactions and that the sections on undesirable effects and pharmacodynamic properties should be updated accordingly.

The CV hazard associated with the use of rofecoxib and valdecoxib led to the voluntary withdrawal from the US and EU markets of them, in 2004, and 2005 respectively.

In 2005, FDA has decided to allow celecoxib to remain in the market and has asked Pfizer to revise its label in order to include a boxed warning containing the class NSAID warnings and contraindication about CV and GI risk, plus specific information on the controlled clinical trial data that demonstrate an increased risk of adverse CV events for celecoxib and to encourage practitioners to use the lowest effective dose for the shortest duration consistent with individual patient treatment goals.

Actually, etoricoxib is approved in more than 70 countries worldwide but not in the US, where FDA have required additional safety and efficacy data. Current therapeutic indications are: treatment of RA, psoriatic arthritis, osteoarthritis, ankylosing spondylitis, chronic low back pain, acute pain, and gout. However, the approved indications differ by country.

Valdecoxib was approved by the FDA on 2001 and was available by prescription in tablet form until 2005, when it was removed from the market due to its CV hazard.

Parecoxib is currently available in Europe and is indicated for short-term treatment of postoperative pain, while it has not been approved in US by FDA.

Lumiracoxib is currently marketed in few countries, including Mexico, Ecuador, and the Dominican Republic. In EU, its marketing was approved in 2006, but was withdrawn from the market in several countries the following year because of liver toxicity. It has never been approved for use in the US.

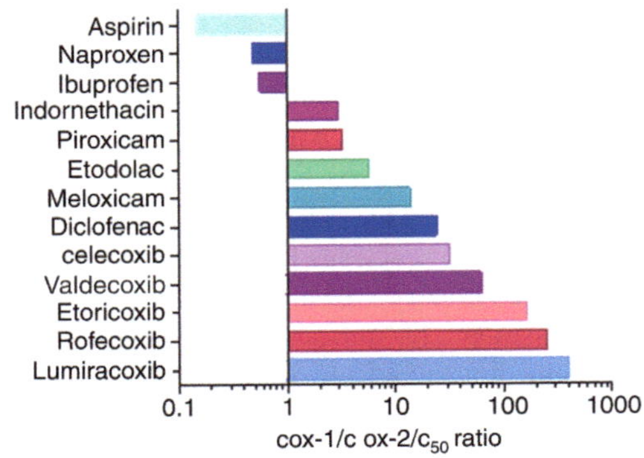


**Fig. 4** Biochemical selectivity, assessed as COX-1/COX-2 $IC_{50}$ values of some COX inhibitors. The value 1 mirrors an equivalent potency to inhibit both COX-isozymes. Higher values (>1) mirror higher selectivity versus COX-2. Lower values (<1) mirror higher selectivity for COX-1

## 2 Pharmacology of tNSAIDs and Coxibs

Although NSAIDs have been used for centuries, the exact mechanism of action and pathways of these drugs was not unveiled until 1970s (Vane 1971; Simmons et al. 2004). It was discovered that an enzyme called COX is responsible for the crucial step of prostanoid biosynthesis. This enzyme catalyzes the conversion of arachidonic acid into prostaglandin (PG)$H_2$, an intermediate which is converted by different tissue-specific synthases into prostanoids, such as prostacyclin ($PGI_2$), thromboxane (TX)$A_2$, $PGE_2$, $PGF_{2\alpha}$, $PGD_2$, each with a broad spectrum of biological activities (Simmons et al. 2004; Smyth et al. 2009). There are two isoforms of COX, named COX-1 and COX-2. COX-1 is expressed constitutively in many tissues and it plays a central role in platelet aggregation and gastric cytoprotection (FitzGerald and Patrono 2001), while COX-2 is induced during inflammation, wound healing, and neoplasia. However, COX-2 gene is constitutively expressed in endothelial cells and central nervous system (CNS) (Smyth et al. 2009). As shown in Fig. 3, inhibition of COX-2 by tNSAIDs and coxibs mediates their therapeutic actions (i.e analgesia, antiinflammatory and antitumorigenic effects) but also some unwanted side effects for the CV system. In fact, in endothelial cells of macrocirculation, COX-2 is the major source of $PGI_2$, even in physiological conditions (Grosser et al. 2006; Capone et al. 2007). $PGI_2$ inhibits aggregation of platelets induced by all recognized agonists, vascular smooth muscle cell proliferation and vascular tone, leucocyte-endothelial cell interactions, and cholesteryl ester hydrolase (Grosser et al. 2006). Recently, an antioxidant role for $PGI_2$, through the induction of hemoxygenase-1, has been reported (Grosser et al. 2006; Di Francesco et al. 2009). For all these biological actions, $PGI_2$ has the distinctive features of a cardioprotective mediator. Animal models that were genetically modified for COX-2 or the receptor for $PGI_2$ or $TXA_2$ (named IP and TP, respectively) convincingly showed that reduction of COX-2-dependent $PGI_2$ translates into a hazardous phenotype for the CV system by leaving unconstrained the intricate network of stimuli, such as $TXA_2$, thus predisposing to thrombosis, atherogenesis, and hypertension (Grosser et al. 2006).

Using the human whole blood assays (Fig. 2) which evaluate the effects of drugs on platelet COX-1 and monocyte COX-2 in vitro, the selectivity towards COX-2 by tNSAIDs, and coxibs was characterized (Capone et al. 2007; Patrignani et al. 2008a). In Fig. 4, the COX-2/COX-1 selectivity of the most used NSAIDs is shown. ASA, naproxen and ibuprofen were more potent inhibitors of COX-1 than COX-2, while the majority of NSAIDs (traditional and coxibs) resulted more selective for COX-2 (Capone et al. 2007; Patrignani et al. 2008a). The most selective COX-2 inhibitors are the coxibs rofecoxib, etoricoxib and lumiracoxib, which display COX-1/COX-2 $IC_{50}$ ratios >100 ($IC_{50}$: concentration required to inhibit the activity of isozymes by 50 %). However, it was found that COX-2 selectivity is a continuous variable since some tNSAIDs, such as diclofenac, show comparable COX-1/COX-2 $IC_{50}$ ratios to celecoxib (diclofenac: 24; celecoxib: 30) (García-Rodríguez et al. 2008). Since all these drugs are not specific for COX-2, the degree of COX-2 selectivity obtained in vivo (known as achieved COX-2 selectivity) depends on the dose administered (Capone et al. 2007). In addition to different pharmacodynamic features, NSAIDs are characterized by different pharmacokinetics (PK) parameters, such as half-life, which, by driving the extent and duration of patient drug exposure, are important determinants of their therapeutic and toxic effects in vivo.

## 3 Efficacy of Coxibs in CRC Chemoprevention Trials

tNSAIDs and coxibs have shown to be effective in CRC chemoprevention (Cha and Dubois 2007; Wang and Dubois 2010b). A most plausible mechanism involves their shared capacity to inhibit COX-2-dependent $PGE_2$ (reviewed in detail in Chap. 2).

$PGE_2$ has a predominant role in promoting colorectal tumor growth (Wang and Dubois 2010a and b). It is the most abundant PG detected in human CRC (Bennett and Del Tacca 1975; Jaffe 1974; Rigas et al. 1993). $PGE_2$ modulates a number of signal transduction pathways that may affect proliferation, programmed cell death (apoptosis), angiogenesis, immune response, cellular adhesion, differentiation, and tumor invasion (Ferrandez et al. 2003; Wang and Dubois 2010a).

Increased expression of COX-2 probably occurs during all stages of the multistep progression of CRC, from the first genetically altered cell, all throughout the different steps from hyperplasia, dysplasia, to carcinoma, and even metastasis (DuBois et al. 1996; Hao et al. 1999; Shiff and Rigas 1999). Overexpression of COX-2 also increases cell migration and proliferation in intestinal epithelial cells (Koehne and Dubois 2004; Wang and Dubois 2010b). COX-2 has been linked with several premalignant and malignant lesions of epithelial origin in lung, breast, colon, and stomach (Dannenberg et al. 2001). Eberhart and colleagues showed that COX-2 genes are highly elevated in most human CRCs compared with the normal mucosa (Eberhart et al. 1994). Additionally, it has been observed an increased expression of COX-2 in CRC, while COX-1 expression seems to be unaltered

(Kargman et al. 1995). This finding was confirmed by other studies that observed an increased COX-2 expression (Rao and Reddy 2004; Sinicrope 2006).

The advanced knowledge towards the association between COX-2 and CRC led many scientists and clinicians to investigate whether the inhibition of this pathway could provide some reduction in CRC risk. Data from several studies have directly and indirectly shown that the anticarcinogenic properties of NSAIDs occur through inhibition of COX-2 but other indirect mechanisms could be also involved (Ferrandez et al. 2003; Baek et al. 2001; Goel et al. 2003; Pan et al. 2008; Jana 2008; Chan 2002; Husain et al. 2002). In fact, it was shown that cells that do not express COX-2 also undergo apoptosis in response to exposure to NSAIDs (Arber 2008). However, these studies were performed in vitro by using higher concentrations than those obtained in vivo. Thus, it seems to be unlikely that these COX-independent mechanisms may be involved in the antitumorigenic effect of NSAIDs detected at therapeutic doses.

The first clinical trial in cancer prevention using the selective COX-2 inhibitor celecoxib was carried out in the setting of familial adenomatous polyposis (FAP) patients with intact colon in 2000 year (Steinbach et al. 2000). Patients with FAP have a nearly 100 % risk of developing CRC. The aim of this trial was to evaluate the chemopreventive effects of celecoxib. This trial was a randomized, double blind, placebo controlled. Patients were randomly selected to put on two different plural, dosages of celecoxib (400 or 100 mg/BID) or placebo for six months. Patients underwent endoscopy at the beginning and end of the trial and the main endpoint was the average polyposis reduction from baseline. Upon completion of the study, a significant reduction in polyp burden (by 30 %) was observed in patients who received 400 mg of celecoxib twice daily whilst around 12–15 % reduction was observed in the group receiving celecoxib with 100 mg/BID and placebo, respectively. Based on these results, the FDA approved the use of celecoxib at 800 mg daily as an oral adjunct therapy for the treatment of patients with FAP in 1999. However, more recently, Pfizer has voluntarily withdrawn the indication for reduction of colorectal polyps in patients with FAP for celecoxib, because it was unable to provide confirmatory data regarding clinical benefit due to slow enrolment in an ongoing clinical trial.

Another trial performed with rofecoxib and a mean follow up of 16 months, focused on assessing the maintenance of colon free of polyps in FAP. The trial encompassed only eight patients who were put on rofecoxib (25 mg/day) for 30 months and sigmoidoscopy/colonoscopy was done at entry and every six months. The number, size, and histologic grade of all polyps were assessed, and the polyps were removed during each endoscopic procedure. The efficacy of the combined approach of endoscopy and chemoprevention was shown with a highly significant reduction in the rate of polyp formation (by 70–100 %) at the end of the study. The investigators concluded that long-term use of rofecoxib was well tolerated and effective in inhibiting polyp formation in polyposis patients (Hallak et al. 2003).

In addition, three studies were carried out to examine the efficacy and safety of coxibs in preventing the recurrence of sporadic colorectal polyps. The design of these trials was multi-center, prospective, randomized, and placebo-controlled trial studies and all required continuous treatment for approximately three years, with a 2-year extension to evaluate drug safety. Each study recruited between 1,500 and 2,600 patients who had undergone a recent adenoma removal. The Adenomatous Polyp Prevention On Vioxx (APPROVe) trial was a randomized, double blind, placebo-controlled trial of the efficacy of oral rofecoxib, 25 mg/day, to prevent colorectal adenomas (Baron et al. 2006; Bresalier et al. 2005). For regulatory purposes, the main aim of the study was a three years trial with rofecoxib among subjects at high risk of developing adenomas, meeting the following criteria: having an adenoma 1 cm or greater in diameter, an adenoma with villous or tubulovillous histology, two or more adenomas, younger than 55 years at first adenoma diagnosis and/or history of colon cancer among first degree relatives. The study recruited a total of 2,586 patients. Participants were assigned to receive rofecoxib 25 mg daily (1,257 patients) or placebo (1,299 patients). The authors found that rofecoxib significantly reduce the risk of recurrent adenomas among patients with a recent adenoma history. However, the study was terminated a few months before the planned end of the trial following the advice of the External Safety and Monitoring Board because of a higher rate of CV events in the rofecoxib group.

The Adenoma Prevention with Celecoxib (APC) trial was a randomized, placebo-controlled trial that investigated whether celecoxib reduces the occurrence of endoscopically detected colorectal adenomas (Bertagnolli et al. 2006). This trial included 2,035 randomized patients with a recently removed adenomatous polyp. They were at high risk of recurrent adenomas (e.g., based on a history of either multiple adenomas or removal of a single adenoma more than 5 mm in diameter), and were randomized to either placebo or celecoxib (200 or 400 mg/BID). These patients were followed up for a mean of 33 months while on treatment. The cumulative incidence of detection of one or more adenomas by year 3 was 60.7 % in patients receiving placebo versus 43.2 % for those receiving celecoxib 200 mg/BID (risk ratio, 0.67; 95 % CI, 0.59–0.77; $P < 0.001$) and 37.5 % for those receiving 400 mg of celecoxib twice a day (risk ratio, 0.55; 95 % CI, 0.48–0.64; $P < 0.001$). These authors concluded that celecoxib was an effective agent for the prevention of colorectal adenomas but, because of potential CV events, could not be routinely recommended for this indication.

The Prevention of Sporadic Adenomatous Polyps (PreSAP) trial was also a randomized, placebo controlled, double-blind study of the COX-2 inhibitor celecoxib given daily in a single 400 mg dose conducted in parallel to the APC trial for the same indication: 1,561 patients from 107 medical centers in 32 countries from six continents were randomized (3:2) to receive either celecoxib (400 mg) or placebo. Celecoxib was associated with a relative risk (RR) of 0.64 for adenomas detected during a 3-year period. A reduced risk was already apparent at the first year follow-up colonoscopy. The adenoma recurrence rate was 33 % in the celecoxib group versus 49.3 % in the placebo group ($P < 0.0001$) (Arber et al. 2006).

All the results from these cancer prevention trials with coxibs generated major expectations. However, many concerns on their CV safety arose at the same time (Solomon et al. 2005). In 2004, rofecoxib was withdrawn unilaterally by Merck from the market due to increased CV toxicity observed in APPROVe (Baron et al. 2006; Bresalier et al. 2005). Also, a few months later the FDA issued a "black box" warning for valdecoxib (Bextra, Pfizer) due to increased CV risk in patients undergoing coronary artery bypass (Nussmeier et al. 2005).

With regards to observational epidemiological data, few studies have investigated the link between exposure to coxibs on colorectal occurrence and recurrence. A nested case-control analysis carried out by Rhame et al. showed that exposure to at least three months of rofecoxib or nonselective NSAIDs (all doses) had a significant protective effect, also these authors found a trend towards a greater reduced risk with high-dose than low doses (Rhame et al. 2002).

## 4 CV Toxicity of Coxibs

### 4.1 Risk Estimates: Data from Trials and Observational Studies

Some of the first coxib trials were focused in quantifying the expected improved safety profile (mainly on GI safety) among long-term users of these drugs compared to selected tNSAIDs with an average follow-up duration of one year. The control group consisted of naproxen, ibuprofen or diclofenac and/or placebo if possible, but for some instances like RA patients, the use of placebo was not an option. The first study showing an increased risk of myocardial infarction (MI) associated with a coxib was the VIGOR trial. This trial was initially designed to compare the GI safety of rofecoxib (50 mg/day) and naproxen (500 mg/BID) in patients with RA. Although rofecoxib demonstrated a lower risk of GI events, the finding of a 4 to 5-fold increased risk of MI among users of rofecoxib marked an inflection bent in the assessment of the safety profile of these drugs (Bombardier et al. 2000). However, this effect was mainly described as not related to an increased risk of rofecoxib itself, but to an intrinsic and previously unnoticed major cardio-preventive effect of naproxen (Bombardier et al. 2000). This hypothesis carried on for quite some time despite the following two facts. Firstly, though naproxen at high doses certainly confers a profound and persistent inhibition of platelet COX-1 (Capone et al. 2004), due to its long half-life (i.e 17 h) (Burke et al. 2006), this blockade, unlike the one produced by low-dose ASA, which affects irreversibly COX-1, is time dependent and reversible. Secondly, even in the unlikely event that naproxen would share the same beneficial effect than ASA (which is estimated to reduce the risk in secondary prevention between 20 and 30 %) (Patrono et al. 2008), it could never explain a five-fold increased risk observed among rofecoxib users compared to naproxen users (Bombardier et al. 2000). An increasing number of observational studies and several RCTs analyzing the CV risk profile of coxibs and some tNSAIDs made their appearance over the next decade after the VIGOR results were first published. Eventually, some years along the road all NSAIDs, including tNSAIDs and not just coxibs, were shown to increase, to different degrees, the risk of ischemic CV events and, in particular, of AMI.

The overall results of CLASS, a parallel study performed to compare GI safety of celecoxib (400 mg/BID), diclofenac (75 mg/BID), and ibuprofen (800 mg/TID) failed to detect a significant difference in GI or CV events between various treatment arms (Silverstein et al. 2000). This study was subject to many methodological criticisms that could explain in part these results. The TARGET trial (that was actually comprised by two sub-studies) recruited around 18,000 osteoarthritis patients randomized to lumiracoxib (400 mg), naproxen (500 mg/BID), or ibuprofen (800 mg/TID) during one year (Farkouh et al. 2004). Overall, this study was unable to find significant differences in MI risk neither between lumiracoxib and ibuprofen (RR, 95 % CI: 0.66, 0.21–2.09) nor between lumiracoxib and naproxen (RR, 95 % CI: 1.77, 0.82–3.84). It should be noted that these results were based on a limited number of events (a total of 33 cases) (Farkouh et al. 2004). Some other clinical trials were designed with the main objective to study a reduction in the risk of CRC. However, these trials reported an increased CV risk associated to coxibs and some had an early termination.

APPROVe was a study with three years of planned follow up, assessing as primary endpoint the recurrence of adenomatous polyps in patients with antecedents of colorectal adenomas in patients receiving rofecoxib (25 mg/day) or placebo (Baron et al. 2006). The study was terminated prematurely due to elevated incidence of CV events in the rofecoxib arm (RR: 1.92, 1.19–3.11) (Bresalier et al. 2005). Two similar studies were conducted for celecoxib, the APC, and the Pre-SAP comparing varying doses of celecoxib (APC: 200 mg/BID and 400 mg/BID; Pre-SAP: 400 mg/daily) with placebo (Solomon et al. 2005; Solomon et al. 2006a). Some preliminary results of APC, suggesting a dose-related two-fold increased CV mortality of celecoxib compared to placebo and this motivated the termination of APC when the study was close to be completed. Additionally, a meta-analysis including these and other RCTs not considered here with either shorter follow up, smaller sample sizes, or both, estimated that coxibs were associated with a 42 % increased risk of serious vascular events compared to placebo (RR, 95 % CI:1.42, 1.13–1.78) (Kearney et al. 2006).

Among observational studies assessing NSAIDs and CV risk, most of them were conducted in large cohorts using automated databases as the primary source of information and only a small number were hospital-based case-control studies.

These studies had several strengths like the ability to identify population-based controls from the underlying study cohort, large sample sizes, and the absence of recall bias since exposure was ascertained prospectively (i.e. before the event actually occurred). However, it should be noted that most of these studies had the limitation of not being able to capture over-the-counter (OTC) drug use. However, there is no reason to believe that OTC use was more common in cases than controls. The study performed by Ilkanoff et al. studied this issue and estimated that excluding users of OTC NSAIDs from the unexposed group would result in around 10 % change away from the null (Ilkhanoff et al. 2005).

Among the few observational studies that did not use automated databases, two studies were conducted in a network of 36 hospitals in the Philadelphia area (Kimmel et al. 2004, 2005) and a reanalysis of data from a clinical trial, the physician health study (PHS) (1989), carried out in the 1980s to evaluate the overall efficacy of ASA in reducing the incidence of primary MI. Most studies analyzed first MI or first MI hospitalization as the main endpoint, but there were some studies that either did not exclude cases with antecedents of MI prior to the study period (Kimmel et al. 2005; Ray et al. 2002) or specifically followed patients from a first MI to a second CV event or death (Gislason et al. 2006; Curtis et al. 2003; MacDonald and Wei 2003).

Three different meta analyses have been published to date summarizing the results from observational studies (Kimmel et al. 2004, 2005; Mamdani et al. 2003; García Rodríguez et al. 2004; Solomon et al. 2004; Graham et al. 2005; McGettigan et al. 2006; Singh et al. 2005, 2006; Sturkenboom et al. 2005; Gislason et al. 2006; Curtis et al. 2003; MacDonald and Wei 2003; Hernandez-Diaz et al. 2006; Singh et al. 2006; McGettigan and Henry 2006; Kurth et al. 2003; Ray et al. 2002; Solomon et al. 2002; Watson et al. 2002; Schlienger et al. 2002; Lévesque et al. 2005; Johnsen et al. 2005; Hippisley-Cox and Coupland 2005; Fischer et al. 2004; Bak et al. 2003). Among them, the RR (95 % CI) associated to tNSAIDs ranges from 1.08 (0.95–1.22) to 1.19 (1.08–1.31). Some observational studies were not included in these meta analyses (García-Rodríguez et al. 2008; Andersohn et al. 2006; Varas-Lorenzo et al. 2009; Velentgas et al. 2006; Suissa et al. 2006; Ray et al. 2009; Solomon et al. 2006b; Helin-Salmivaara et al. 2006; Bueno et al. 2010). One of them had a very large sample size. This is a nation-wide Finnish study of discharge summaries and included a total of 33,309 incident cases of MI (Helin-Salmivaara et al. 2006). Overall the results of this study are congruent with previously detailed summarized data. The risk of MI associated with individual NSAIDs went from a 1.06 (0.83–1.34) for celecoxib to 2.21 (1.18–4.14) for etoricoxib.

In APPROVe trial, time to event associated with coxib use compared to placebo suggested that the deleterious effect appeared only after 18 months of initiating treatment (Bresalier et al. 2005). This finding generated a great deal of controversy, because previous studies with shorter follow up were also successfully able to detect an increased risk (Bombardier et al. 2000). New data from an extended follow-up of the APPROVe study was lately published (Baron et al. 2008), and the authors reported that the increased CV risk observed among individuals exposed to rofecoxib persisted for some time after discontinuation: the RR was 1.95 (0.97–3.93) in the first year after discontinuation. To confirm this finding, we used data from a nested case-control study performed by our group, and identified individuals who discontinued NSAID use between 7 and 365 days before the study index date (García-Rodríguez et al. 2008). Overall we found that among those discontinuing NSAID recently, long-term NSAID users for one year or more, RR was 1.58 (1.27–1.96). We also found a similar RR of AMI among patients currently exposed to NSAIDs with duration of more than one year (1.45, 1.27–1.65). These results suggest that tNSAIDs could also carry a persisting risk for a limited period of time after treatment discontinuation. Yet, the exact nature between NSAID duration and the CV hazard remains uncertain.

## 4.2 Mechanisms of CV Toxicity of Coxibs

The most plausible hypothesis of the CV hazard associated with the administration of coxibs is that they affect COX-2-dependent $PGI_2$ generation, while not affecting platelet function (García-Rodríguez et al. 2008; Grosser et al. 2006). In fact, a cardioprotective phenotype can be obtained by the administration of low-dose ASA through its capacity to almost completely ($\geq$95 %) (Reilly and FitzGerald 1987) and persistently suppress platelet $TXA_2$ generation and function throughout dosing interval (Patrono et al. 2008), while leaving almost unaffected vascular $PGI_2$ generation. ASA is an irreversible inhibitor of COX-1 and COX-2, through selective acetylation of a specific serine residue of Ser529 and Ser516, respectively (Patrono et al. 2008). However, ASA has a short half-life (approximately 20 min), thus when administered at low doses (75–100 mg) once daily, it preferentially inhibits platelet COX-1 in the presystemic circulation. Since platelets are anucleated cells with limited capacity to synthesize proteins de novo, the irreversible inhibition of COX-1 persists for all platelet lifespan (i.e. 7–10 days). This ability to permanently inhibit $TXA_2$ production in platelets places ASA in a unique position to be used in coronary heart disease prevention (Patrono et al. 2008; see also Chap. 3).

Other nonselective NSAIDs, which are reversible inhibitors of COXs, cause a profound inhibition of COX-2-dependent $PGI_2$ (García-Rodríguez et al. 2008; Patrignani et al. 2008b). Despite they can also inhibit COX-1 and therefore $TXA_2$ production in platelets, this effect is incomplete and short-lasting (since most of them have a short half-lives) (Burke et al. 2006). The only tNSAID which shows an antiplatelet effect is naproxen at high doses, because it has a long half-life (Burke et al. 2006) and the capacity to inhibit almost completely platelet COX-1 in the interval between doses (Capone et al. 2004).

A study recently published by our group provides some useful insight to this issue (García-Rodríguez et al. 2008). The study included 8,852 cases of nonfatal MI and 20,000 population controls and was performed using the computerized British primary care database THIN (García-Rodríguez et al. 2008). We found that the degree of inhibition of COX-2 was the most important predictor of AMI risk by tNSAIDs and coxibs. In fact, we did not find any correlation of RR of AMI with COX-2 selectivity or the degree of COX-1 inhibition. These results confirm the hypothesis that CV hazard is common to almost all NSAIDs. In fact, tNSAIDs and coxibs profoundly inhibit COX-2 while not affecting platelet function.

In summary, we found that CV hazard is shared by coxibs and tNSAIDs. However, it is likely that the magnitude of the risk may vary between different individual NSAIDs as a result of the extent of inhibition of COX-2 (which is an index of drug potency/exposure) at common doses administered in the general population, in the absence of a complete suppression of TX-dependent platelet function. Results from RCTs and observational studies are remarkably consistent and show a gradient in risk that is partly a function of the degree of reduction of COX-2-dependent $PGI_2$. Following this line of reasoning, we can conclude that

CV risk is maximum for NSAIDs which, at therapeutic doses, suppress almost completely COX-2 not accompanied by almost complete suppression of platelet COX-1, such as diclofenac which is usually administered at high doses to overcome its short half-life. The risk seems to be moderate for other NSAIDs such as ibuprofen, which is for the most part used at low dose, and is lower for NSAIDs that exert an antiplatelet effect, such as high-dose naproxen.

The accumulated knowledge of the peculiarities of CV and GI adverse effects enables the customized selection of a specific NSAID among the vast number of members of this therapeutic class. The same NSAID may not be suitable for everyone depending on the different baseline personal characteristics and the regimen of use. This is probably true for most commonly used drugs and should not be seen as a problem but as a opportunity of rational drug use that is made possible in this area due to the vast experience of use and research with this class of drugs.

It is worth remembering that another possible mechanism by which tNSAIDs (but not coxibs) might cause a CV hazard, is for their possible capacity to interfere with the irreversible antiplatelet effects of ASA. The existence of this pharmacodynamic interaction was initially suggested more than 25 years ago (Livio et al. 1982). Later Catella-Lawson et al. confirmed this hypothesis (Catella-Lawson et al. 2001). They conducted a crossover experiment in which a low-dose ASA was administered followed by a single dose of ibuprofen 400 mg 2 h later, or in reverse order, during six consecutive days. They found that the interference of ibuprofen on ASA antiplatelet effect could be bypassed by giving subjects ASA 2 h before ibuprofen. However, in a second study, they simulated a more clinically relevant ibuprofen dosing regimen. Ibuprofen was administered three times per day, and an enteric-coated preparation of low-dose ASA was administered once daily, as it is commonly used for cardioprotection in patients taking NSAIDs. Under these circumstances, the administration of ASA before the morning dose of ibuprofen failed to circumvent the interaction.

The possible pharmacodynamic interaction between low-dose ASA and naproxen was investigated in two studies, in healthy subjects, using the prescribed dose of 500 mg/BID (Capone et al. 2005) or (OTC) dose of 220 mg BID (Anzellotti et al. 2011). In both studies, it was found that chronic dosing with ASA given 2 h before naproxen was not associated with a significant change in the complete inhibition of platelet $TXB_2$ generation and inhibition of $TXA_2$-dependent platelet aggregation up to 24 h after dosing. However, when Anzellotti et al. (2011) studied the time course of recovery of platelet $TXA_2$ biosynthesis after drug discontinuation (up to 72 h) of ASA alone versus sequential administration of ASA and naproxen, they clearly showed that the administration of naproxen given 2 h before or after ASA reduced the capacity of ASA to cause an almost complete and irreversible inactivation of COX-1. The interference was reduced when naproxen was given 2 h after ASA than in reverse order. However, results of the clinical impact of the interaction between ASA and tNSAIDs were inconsistent among observational studies (MacDonald and Wei 2003; Curtis et al. 2003; Kurth et al. 2003; Kimmel et al. 2004; García Rodríguez et al. 2004; Hippisley-Cox and Coupland 2005; Patel and Goldberg 2004; Hudson et al. 2005).

**Table 1** Ongoing clinical trials with celecoxib in CRC and FAP

| Condition | Main characteristics of patients | Intervention | Phase | Primary end-point | Estimated primary completion date |
|---|---|---|---|---|---|
| *Official title: a phase* III *trial of* 6 *versus* 12 *treatments of adjuvant FOLFOX plus celecoxib or placebo for patients with resected stage* III *colon cancer* (NCT01150045) | | | | | |
| CRC | Patients with stage III disease ($\geq$18 years old) | FOLFOX chemotherapy (Fluorouracil, leucovorin calcium, oxaliplatin) plus celecoxib or placebo | III | Disease-free survival | February 2013 |
| *Official title*: *a phase* III *placebo-controlled trial of celecoxib in genotype positive subjects with FAP* (NCT00585312) | | | | | |
| Adenomatous *Polyposis Coli* | Pediatric patients (10–17 years old) | Celecoxib versus placebo | III | Time from randomization to treatment failure over a 5-year period | January 2019 |
| *Official title*: *a phase* II *trial using a combination of oxaliplatin, capecitabine, and celecoxib with concurrent radiation for patients with newly diagnosed resectable rectal cancer* (NCT00250835) | | | | | |
| Rectal Cancer | Patients with biopsy proven T3-4N0-2M0 rectal cancer ($\geq$18 years old) | Oxaliplatin, capecitabine and Celecoxib with Radiation | II | Pathologic complete response rate | April 2012 |

## 4.3 Ongoing Randomized Clinical Trials with Coxibs/NSAIDs

Despite COX-2 continues to be an important anticancer target (see Chap. 2), the CV toxicity associated with coxib administration (Grosser et al. 2006) limits their use as chemopreventive agent. As reported in the table, only a few RCTs with celecoxib are currently ongoing with the aim to assess its effectiveness to improve conventional chemotherapy or radiotherapy in patients with advanced stages of CRCs. In addition, a placebo-controlled RCT is currently in progress to test whether celecoxib (16 mg/kg/day, for five years) can be used to prevent colon polyp recurrence in children (age 10–17 years) with FAP (Table 1).

It is ongoing a large RCT to compare the relative CV safety profile of chronic treatment with celecoxib, ibuprofen, or naproxen, in patients with high CV risk [prospective randomized evaluation of celecoxib integrated safety versus ibuprofen or naproxen (PRECISION) trial; Clinical Trials.gov Identifier: NCT00346216]. This is a multicenter, multinational study that uses a randomized, double blind, triple dummy, 3-arm (celecoxib, ibuprofen, or naproxen) parallel group design. Patients receiving low-dose ASA ($\leq$325 mg daily) at the time of randomization were permitted to continue this therapy regardless of their CV risk (Becker et al. 2009). However, it is noteworthy that results from clinical pharmacology studies have shown that ibuprofen and naproxen, but not COX-2 selective inhibitors, may interfere with the inhibition of platelet COX-1 by ASA (Catella-Lawson et al. 2001; Capone et al. 2005; Anzellotti et al. 2011). This pharmacodynamic interaction of ibuprofen and naproxen with low-dose ASA might mitigate its cardioprotective effect; on the contrary, this interference with low-dose ASA does not occur with celecoxib (Renda et al. 2006). Thus, the administration of low-dose aspirin and the different interference of aspirin capacity to completely suppress platelet COX-1 by tNSAIDs and celecoxib may represent an important limitation to the interpretation of the clinical outcomes of the PRECISION study.

## 5 Conclusions and Perspectives

The promising use of coxibs in chemoprevention was halted abruptly due to lack of meeting one of the required criteria of an ideal chemopreventive agent: an acceptable safety profile. In this context, low-dose ASA, may have a place for chemoprevention of CRCs. Coxibs or tNSAID, however, might still be reserved for younger patients with FAP who have a very small background CV risk. However, in recent studies, enhanced $TXA_2$ biosynthesis was detected in colon tumorigenesis, in humans (Sciulli et al. 2005). Thus, it remains to be addressed whether the coincident depression of vascular $PGI_2$, in a context of enhanced $TXA_2$ biosynthesis, may curb the chemopreventive efficacy of COX-2 inhibitors, such as celecoxib.

The possible use of coxibs to prevent CRC will depend mainly on research progresses in biomarkers able to identify patients uniquely susceptible of developing thrombotic events by inhibition of COX-2. Recent data suggest that there is an association between polymorphisms of human prostacyclin receptor (hIP) and the development of thrombosis and atherogenesis (Arehart et al. 2008). Moreover, combined analysis of the results of our clinical pharmacology studies performed with COX inhibitors shows that there is a linear relationship between whole blood COX-2 inhibition ex vivo and prostacyclin inhibition in vivo (García-Rodríguez et al. 2008). Thus, further studies should be performed to verify whether the assessment of whole blood COX-2 ex vivo –alone or in combination with the measurement of urinary levels of 2,3-dinor-6-keto-$PGF_{1\alpha}$ (a biomarker of prostacyclin biosynthesis in vivo)—in association with genetic biomarkers (such as polymorphisms in the hIP receptor) may be surrogate end points to CV hazard by pharmacological inhibition of COX-2.

Recently, Chan et al. (2011) found that, in the APC trial cohort, the CV hazard can be stratified using high-sensitivity C-reactive protein (hsCRP) (a circulating inflammatory biomarker of chronic conditions including CV disease). They found that among individuals with elevated level ($\geq$3.0 mg/l) of hsCRP use of high-dose celecoxib (400 mg/BID) was associated with an increased RR of CV events. On the contrary, the average RR of CV events was low [1.11 (95 % CI: 0.61–2.02)] in patients on high-dose celecoxib and with an hsCRP level less than 3.0 mg/l.

Experimental data support prothrombotic activity of CRP in animal models (Danenberg et al. 2003) and humans (Bisoendial et al. 2007). CRP may induce thrombosis through the disruption of thromboregulation. In fact, CRP supress as it is used with may $PGI_2$ synthase and reduce the homeostatic increase in $PGI_2$ biosynthesis following vascular injury while potentially augmenting $TXA_2$ activity through an increase in the expression of TX receptors (TP) (Grad et al. 2009). Thus, elevated CRP levels may predispose to CV risk, by a similar mechanism to that by which COX-2 inhibitors confer CV risk. In experimental animals, ASA administration counteracted CRP-induced thrombosis (Grad et al. 2009); thus, it should be tested in clinical studies whether low-dose ASA may reduce CV risk in patients with elevated CRP levels. Altogether, these results suggest that enhanced hsCRP may be a useful biomarker for selecting patients for cancer prevention trials and for determining the risk of COX inhibitors in clinical practice (Oates 2011). However, it is necessary to perform appropriate clinical studies to validate this possibility.

Further research is needed to develop new drugs and discover new pathways in CRC. Our aim should be also to design large-scale chemoprevention trials and observational studies, assessing anticancer efficacy and CV toxicity in association with the evaluation of different biomarkers in the general population, and evaluate the optimal dosage and duration of NSAIDs with special interest in low-dose ASA.

**Acknowledgments** This work was supported by research founding from the European Community Sixth Framework Programme (Eicosanox grant LSMH-CT-2004-005033). We apologize to our colleagues for not being able to reference all primary work due to space limitations.

## References

Andersohn F, Suissa S, Garbe E (2006) Use of first- and second-generation cyclooxygenase-2-selective nonsteroidal antiinflammatory drugs and risk of acute myocardial infarction. Circulation 113:1950–1957

Antman EM, Bennett JS, Daugherty A et al (2007) Use of nonsteroidal antiinflammatory drugs: an update for clinicians: a scientific statement from the American heart association. Circulation 115:1634–1642

Anzellotti P, Capone ML, Jeyam A et al (2011) Low-dose naproxen interferes with the antiplatelet effects of aspirin in healthy subjects: recommendations to minimize the functional consequences. Arthritis Rheum 63:850–859

Arber N (2008) Cyclooxygenase-2 inhibitors in colorectal cancer prevention: point. Cancer Epidemiol Biomarkers Prev 17:1852–1857

Arber N, Eagle CJ, Spicak J et al (2006) Celecoxib for the prevention of colorectal adenomatous polyps. N Engl J Med 355:885–895

Arehart E, Stitham E, Asselbergs FW et al (2008) Acceleration of cardiovascular disease by a dysfunctional prost acyclin receptor mutation: potential implications for cyclooxygenase-2 inhibition. Circ Res 102:986–993

Baek SJ, Kim KS, Nixon JB et al (2001) Cyclooxygenase inhibitors regulate the expression of a TGF-beta superfamily member that has proapoptotic and antitumorigenic activities. Mol Pharmacol 59:901–908

Baigent C, Blackwell L, Collins R et al (2009) Aspirin in the primary and secondary prevention of vascular disease: collaborative meta-analysis of individual participant data from randomised trials. Lancet 373:1849–1860

Bhatt DL, Scheiman J, Abraham NS et al (2008) ACCF/ACG/AHA 2008 expert consensus document on reducing the gastrointestinal risks of antiplatelet therapy and NSAID use. In: A report of the American college of cardiology foundation task force on clinical expert consensus documents, vol 52, pp 1502–1517

Bak S, Andersen M, Tsiropoulos I et al (2003) Risk of stroke associated with nonsteroidal anti-inflammatory drugs: a nested case-control study. Stroke 34:379–386

Baron JA, Sandler RS, Bresalier RS et al (2006) A randomized trial of rofecoxib for the chemoprevention of colorectal adenomas. Gastroenterology 131:1674–1682

Baron JA, Sandler RS, Bresalier RS et al (2008) Cardiovascular events associated with rofecoxib: final analysis of the Approve trial. Lancet 372:1756–1764

Bautista D, Obrador A, Moreno V et al (1997) Ki-ras mutation modifies the protective effect of dietary monounsaturated fat and calcium on sporadic colorectal cancer. Cancer Epidemiol Biomarkers Prev 6:57–61

Becker MC, Wang TH, Wisniewski L et al (2009) Rationale, design, and governance of prospective randomized evaluation of celecoxib integrated safety versus ibuprofen or naproxen (PRECISION), a cardiovascular end point trial of nonsteroidal antiinflammatory agents in patients with arthritis. Am Heart J 157:606–612

Bennett A, Del Tacca M (1975) Proceedings: prostaglandins in human colonic carcinoma. Gut 16:409

Bertagnolli MM, Eagle CJ, Zauber AG et al (2006) Celecoxib for the prevention of sporadic colorectal adenomas. N Engl J Med 355:873–884

Bisoendial RJ, Kastelein JJP, Peters SLM et al (2007) Effects of CRP infusion on endothelial function and coagulation in normocholesterolemic and hypercholesterolemic subjects. J Lipid Res 48:952–960

Bombardier C, Laine L, Reicin A et al (2000) Comparison of upper gastrointestinal toxicity of rofecoxib and naproxen in patients with rheumatoid arthritis. VIGOR study group. N Engl J Med 343:1520–1528

Boursi B, Arber N (2007) Current and future clinical strategies in colon cancer prevention and the emerging role of chemoprevention. Curr Pharm Des 13:2274–2282

Bresalier RS, Sandler RS, Quan H et al (2005) Cardiovascular events associated with rofecoxib in colorectal adenoma. Chemoprevencion trial. N Engl J Med 352:1092–1102

Brun J, Jones R (2001) Nonsteroidal anti-inflammatory drug-associated dyspepsia: the scale of the problem. Am J Med 110:12S–13S

Buchanan FG, DuBois RN (2006) Connecting COX-2 and wnt in cancer. Cancer Cell 9:6–8

Bueno H, Bardají A, Patrignani P et al (2010) Spanish case-control study to assess NSAID-associated ACS risk investigators. Use of non-steroidal antiinflammatory drugs and type-specific risk of acute coronary syndrome. Am J Cardiol 105:1102–1106

Burke A, Smyth EM, FitzGerald GA (2006) Analgesic-antipyretic agents; pharmacotherapy of gout. In: Brunton LL, Lazo JS, Parker KL (eds) Goodman and Gilman's the pharmacological basis of therapeutics, 11th edn. McGraw-Hill, New York

Campos FG, Logullo Waitzberg AG et al (2005) Diet and colorectal cancer: current evidence for etiology and prevention. Nutr Hosp 20:18–25

Capone ML, Sciulli MG, Tacconelli S et al (2005) Pharmacodynamic interaction of naproxen with low-dose aspirin in healthy subjects. J Am Coll Cardiol 45:1295–1301

Capone ML, Tacconelli S, Di Francesco L et al (2007) Pharmacodynamic of cyclooxygenase inhibitors in humans. Prostaglandins Other Lipid Mediat 82:85–94

Capone ML, Tacconelli S, Sciulli MG et al (2004) Clinical pharmacology of platelet, monocyte, and vascular cyclooxygenase inhibition by naproxen and low-dose aspirin in healthy subjects. Circulation 109:1468–1471

Catella-Lawson F, Reilly MP, Kapoor SC et al (2001) Cyclooxygenase inhibitors and the antiplatelet effects of aspirin. N Engl J Med 345:1809–1817

Cha YI, DuBois RN (2007) NSAIDs and cancer prevention: targets downstream of COX-2. Annu Rev Med 58:239–252

Chan AT, Sima SS, Zauber AG (2011) C-reactive protein and risk of colorectal adenoma according to celecoxib treatment. Cancer Prev Res 4:1172–1180
Chang CH, Shau WY, Kuo CW et al (2010) Increased risk of stroke associated with nonsteroidal anti-inflammatory drugs: a nationwide case-crossover study. Stroke 41:1884–1890
Chan FK, Chung SC, Suen BY et al (2001) Preventing recurrent upper gastrointestinal bleeding in patients with *Helicobacter pylori* infection who are taking low-dose aspirin or naproxen. N Engl J Med 344:967–973
Chan TA (2002) Nonsteroidal anti-inflammatory drugs, apoptosis, and colon-cancer chemoprevention. Lancet Oncol 3:166–174
Cheng I, Caberto CP, Lum-Jones A et al (2011) Type two diabetes risk variants and colorectal cancer risk: the multiethnic cohort and PAGE studies. Gut (May 20 [Epub ahead of print])
Choi NK, Park BJ, Jeong SW et al (2008) Nonaspirin nonsteroidal anti-inflammatory drugs and hemorrhagic stroke risk: the acute brain bleeding analysis study. Stroke 39:845–849
Choti MA, Sitzmann JV, Tiburi MF et al (2002) Trends in long-term survival following liver resection for hepatic colorectal metastases. Ann Surg 235:759–766
Curtis JP, Wang Y, Portnay EL et al (2003) Aspirin, ibuprofen, and mortality after myocardial infarction: retrospective cohort study. BMJ 327:1322–1323
Dannenberg AJ, Altorki NK, Boyle JO et al (2001) Cyclo-oxygenase 2: a pharmacological target for the prevention of cancer. Lancet Oncol 2:544–551
Danenberg H, Szalai A, Swaminathan R et al (2003) Increased thrombosis following injury in human C-reactive protein transgenic mice. Circulation 108:512–515
Di Francesco L, Totani L, Dovizio M et al (2009) Induction of prostacyclin by steady laminar shear stress suppresses tumor necrosis factor-alpha biosynthesis via heme oxygenase-1 in human endothelial cells. Circ Res 104:506–513
DuBois RN, Radhika A, Reddy BS et al (1996) Increased cyclooxygenase-2 levels in carcinogen-induced rat colonic tumors. Gastroenterology 110:1259–1262
Eberhart CE, Coffey RJ, Radhika A et al (1994) Up-regulation of cyclooxygenase 2 gene expression in human colorectal adenomas and adenocarcinomas. Gastroenterology 107:1183–1188
Farkouh ME, Kirshner H, Harrington RA et al (2004) Comparison of lumiracoxib with naproxen and ibuprofen in the therapeutic arthritis research and gastrointestinal event trial (TARGET), cardiovascular outcomes: randomised controlled trial. Lancet 364:675–684
Ferrandez A, Prescott S, Burt RW (2003) COX-2 and colorectal cancer. Curr Pharm Des 9:2229–2251
Fischer LM, Schlienger RG, Matter CM et al (2004) Discontinuation of non-steroidal anti-inflammatory drug therapy and the risk of acute myocardial infarction. Arch Intern Med 164:2472–2476
FitzGerald GA, Patrono C (2001) The coxibs, selective inhibitors of cyclooxygenase-2. N Engl J Med 345:433–442
Fuchs CS, Giovannucci EL, Colditz GA et al (1999) Dietary fiber and the risk of colorectal cancer and adenoma in women. N Engl J Med 340:169–176
Garcia Rodriguez LA, Ruigomez A, Wallander MA et al (2000) Detection of colorectal tumor and inflammatory bowel disease during follow-up of patients with initial diagnosis of irritable bowel syndrome. Scand J Gastroenterol 35:306–311
García Rodríguez LA, Varas-Lorenzo C, Maguire A et al (2004) A non-steroidal anti-inflammatory drugs and the risk of myocardial infarction in the general population. Circulation 109:3000–3006
García-Rodríguez LA, Tacconelli S, Patrignani P (2008) Role of dose potency in the prediction of risk of myocardial infarction associated with nonsteroidal anti-inflammatory drugs in the general population. JACC 52:1628–1636
Giouleme O, Diamantidis MD, Marios Katsaros G (2011) Is diabetes a causal agent for colorectal cancer? Pathophysiological and molecular mechanisms. World J Gastroenterol 17:444–448
Giovannucci E (2002) Modifiable risk factors for colon cancer. Gastroenterol Clin North Am 31:925–943
Gislason GH, Jacobsen S, Rasmussen JN et al (2006) Risk of death or reinfarction associated with the use of selective cyclooxygenase-2 inhibitors and nonselective nonsteroidal antiinflammatory drugs after acute myocardial infarction. Circulation 113:2906–2913

Goel A, Chang DK, Ricciardiello L et al (2003) A novel mechanism for aspirin-mediated growth inhibition of human colon cancer cells. Clin Cancer Res 9:383–390
Grad E, Golomb M, Koroukhov N et al (2009) Aspirin reduces the prothrombotic activity of C-reactive protein. J Thromb Haemost 7:1393–1400
Graham DJ, Campen D, Hui R et al (2005) Risk of acute myocardial infarction and sudden cardiac death in patients treated with cyclo-oxygenase two selective and non-selective non-steroidal anti-inflammatory drugs: nested case-control study. Lancet 365:4996–5002
Greenberg ER, Baron JA, Tosteson TD et al (1994) A clinical trial of antioxidant vitamins to prevent colorectal adenoma. Polyp prevention study group. N Engl J Med 331:141–147
Grosser T, Fries S, FitzGerald GA (2006) Biological basis for the cardiovascular consequences of COX-2 inhibition: therapeutic challenges and opportunities. J Clin Invest 116:4–15
Haag MD, Bos MJ, Hofman A et al (2008) Cyclooxygenase selectivity of nonsteroidal anti-inflammatory drugs and risk of stroke. Arch Intern Med 168:1219–1224
Hallak A, Alon-Baron L, Shamir R et al (2003) Rofecoxib reduces polyp recurrence in familial polyposis. Dig Dis Sci 48:1998–2002
Hao X, Bishop AE, Wallace M et al (1999) Early expression of cyclo-oxygenase-2 during sporadic colorectal carcinogenesis. J Pathol 187:295–301
Headrick JR, Miller DL, Nagorney DM et al (2001) Surgical treatment of hepatic and pulmonary metastases from colon cancer. Ann Thorac Surg 71:975–980
Helin-Salmivaara A, Virtanen A, Vesalainen R et al (2006) NSAID use and the risk of hospitalization for first myocardial infarction in the general population: a nationwide case-control study from Finland. Eur Heart J 27:1657–1663
Hennekens CH, Buring JE, Manson JE et al (1996) Lack of effect of long-term supplementation with beta carotene on the incidence of malignant neoplasms and cardiovascular disease. N Engl J Med 334:1145–1159
Hernández-Díaz S, García Rodríguez LA (2000) Association between nonsteroidal anti-inflammatory drugs and upper gastrointestinal tract bleeding/perforation. An overview of epidemiologic studies published in the 1990s. Arch Intern Med 160:2093–2099
Hernandez-Diaz S, Varas-Lorenzo C, Garcia Rodriguez LA (2006) Non-steroidal antiinflammatory drugs and the risk of acute myocardial infarction. Basic Clin Pharmacol Toxicol 98:266–274
Hippisley-Cox J, Coupland C (2005) Risk of myocardial infarction in patients taking cyclo-oxygenase-2 inhibitors or conventional non-steroidal anti-inflammatory drugs: population based nested case-control analysis. BMJ 330:1366–1372
Hong WK, Lippman SM, Itri LM et al (1990) Prevention of second primary tumors with isotretinoin in squamous-cell carcinoma of the head and neck. N Engl J Med 323:795–801
Hudson M, Baron M, Rahme E et al (2005) Ibuprofen may abrogate the benefits of aspirin when used for secondary prevention of myocardial infarction. J Rheumatol 32:1589–1593
Husain SS, Szabo IL, Tamawski AS (2002) NSAID inhibition of GI cancer growth: clinical implications and molecular mechanisms of action. Am J Gastroenterol 97:542–553
Ilkhanoff L, Lewis JD, Hennessy S et al (2005) Potential limitations of electronic database studies of prescription non-aspirin non-steroidal anti-inflammatory drugs (NANSAIDs) and risk of myocardial infarction (MI). Pharmacoepidemiol Drug Saf 14:513–522
Jaffe BM (1974) Prostaglandins and cancer: an update. Prostaglandins 6:453–461
Jana NR (2008) NSAIDs and apoptosis. Cell Mol Life Sci 65:1295–1301
Janne PA, Mayer RJ (2000) Chemoprevention of colorectal cancer. N Engl J Med 342:1960–1968
Jiang Y, Ben Q, Shen H et al (2011) Diabetes mellitus and incidence and mortality of colorectal cancer: a systematic review and meta-analysis of cohort studies. Eur J Epidemiol [Epub ahead of print]
Johnsen SP, Pedersen L, Friis S et al (2003) Nonaspirin nonsteroidal anti-inflammatory drugs and risk of hospitalization for intracerebral hemorrhage: a population-based case-control study. Stroke 34:387–391
Johnsen SP, Larsson H, Tarone RE et al (2005) Risk of hospitalization for myocardial infarction among users of rofecoxib, celecoxib, and other NSAIDs. Arch Intern Med 165:978–984

Kargman SL, O'Neill GP, Vickers PJ et al (1995) Expression of prostaglandin G/H synthase-1 and -2 protein in human colon cancer. Cancer Res 55:2556–2559
Kearney PM, Baigent C, Godwin J et al (2006) Do selective cyclo-oxygenase-2 inhibitors and traditional non-steroidal anti-inflammatory drugs increase the risk of atherothrombosis? Meta-analysis of randomised trials. BMJ 332:1302–1308
Kimmel SE, Berlin JA, Reilly M et al (2004) The effects of nonselective non-aspirin non-steroidal anti-inflammatory medications on the risk of nonfatal myocardial infarction and their interaction with aspirin. J Am Coll Cardiol 43:985–990
Kimmel SE, Berlin JA, Reilly M et al (2005) Patients exposed to rofecoxib and celecoxib have different odds of nonfatal myocardial infarction. Ann Intern Med 142:157–164
King MC, Wieand S, Hale K et al (2001) National surgical adjuvant breast and bowel project tamoxifen and breast cancer incidence among women with inherited mutations in BRCA1 and BRCA2: national surgical adjuvant breast and bowel project (NSABP-P1) breast cancer prevention trial. JAMA 286:2251–2256
Koehne CH, Dubois RN (2004) COX-2 inhibition and colorectal cancer. Semin Oncol 3:12–21
Kurth T, Glynn RJ, Walker AM et al (2003) Inhibition of clinical benefits on first myocardial infarction by nonsteroidal anti-inflammatory drugs. Circulation 108:1191–1195
Lai KC, Lam SK, Chu KM et al (2002) Lansoprazole for the prevention of recurrences of ulcer complications from long-term low-dose aspirin use. N Engl J Med 346:2033–2038
Laine L (2001) Approaches to nonsteroidal anti-inflammatory drug use in the high-risk patient. Gastroenterology 120:594–606
Lanas A, Scheiman J (2007) Low-dose aspirin and upper gastrointestinal damage: epidemiology, prevention and treatment. Curr Med Res Opin 23:163–173
Larsson S, Orsini N, Wolk A (2005) Diabetes mellitus and risk of colorectal cancer: a meta-analysis. J Natl Cancer Inst 97:1679–1687
Lev-Ari S, Maimon Y, Strier L et al (2006) Down-regulation of prostaglandin E2 by curcumin is correlated with inhibition of cell growth and induction of apoptosis in human colon carcinoma cell lines. J Soc Integr Oncol 4:21–26
Lévesque LE, Brophy JM, Zhang B (2005) The risk for myocardial infarction with cyclooxygenase-2 inhibitors: A population study of elderly adults. Ann Internal Med 142:481–489
Lin KJ, Hernandez-Diaz S, Garcia Rodriguez LA (2011) Acid suppressants reduce risk of gastrointestinal bleeding in patients on antithrombotic or anti-inflammatory therapy. Gastroenterology 141:71–79
Lipkin M, Newmark H (1985) Effect of added dietary calcium on colonic epithelial-cell proliferation in subjects at high risk for familial colonic cancer. N Engl J Med 313:1381–1384
Livio M, Del Maschio A, Cerletti C et al (1982) Indomethacin prevents the long-lasting inhibitory effect of aspirin on human platelet cyclo-oxygenase activity. Prostaglandins 23:787–796
MacDonald TM, Wei L (2003) Effect of ibuprofen on cardioprotective effect of aspirin. Lancet 361:573–574
Mamdani M, Rochon P, Juurlink D et al (2003) Effect of selective cyclooxygenase two inhibitors and naproxen on short-term risk of acute myocardial infarction in the elderly. Arch Intern Med 163:481–486
Massó González EL, Patrignani P et al (2010) Variability among nonsteroidal antiinflammatory drugs in risk of upper gastrointestinal bleeding. Arthritis Rheum 62:1592–1601
McGettigan P, Han P, Henry D (2006) Cyclooxygenase-2 inhibitors and coronary occlusion: exploring dose-response relationships. Br J Clin Pharmacol 62:358–365
McGettigan P, Henry D (2006) Cardiovascular risk and inhibition of cyclooxygenase: a systematic review of the observational studies of selective and nonselective inhibitors of cyclooxygenase 2. JAMA 296:1633–1644
Nussmeier NA, Whelton AA, Brown MT et al (2005) Complications of the COX-2 inhibitors parecoxib and valdecoxib after cardiac surgery. N Engl J Med 352:1081–1091
Oates JA (2011) Cardiovascular risk markers and mechanisms in targeting the COX pathway for colorectal cancer prevention. Cancer Prev Res 4:1145–1148

Pan MR, Chang HC, Hung WC (2008) Non-steroidal anti-inflammatory drugs suppress the ERK signaling pathway via block of Ras/c-Raf interaction and activation of MAP kinase phosphatases. Cell Signal 20:1134–1141
Parkin DM, Pisani P, Ferlay J (1999) Global cancer statistics. CA Cancer J Clin 49:33–64
Patel TN, Goldberg KC (2004) Use of aspirin and ibuprofen compared with aspirin alone and the risk of myocardial infarction. Arch Intern Med 164:852–856
Patrignani P, Capone ML, Tacconelli S (2008a) NSAIDs and cardiovascular disease. Heart 94:395–397
Patrignani P, Tacconelli S, Capone ML (2008b) Risk management profile of etoricoxib: an example of personalized medicine. Ther Clin Risk Manage 4:983–997
Patrignani P, Panara MR, Greco A et al (1994) Biochemical and pharmacological characterization of the cyclooxygenase activity of human blood prostaglandin endoperoxide synthases. J Pharmacol Exp Ther 271:1705–1712
Patrignani P, Sciulli MG, Manarini S et al (1999) COX-2 is not involved in thromboxane biosynthesis by activated human platelets. J Physiol Pharmacol 50:661–667
Patrono C, Baigent C, Hirsh J et al (2008) Antiplatelet drugs: American college of chest physicians evidence-based clinical practice guidelines (8th edn). Chest 133(6 Suppl):199S–233S
Patrono C, Ciabattoni G, Pinca E et al (1980) Low dose aspirin and inhibition of thromboxane B2 production in healthy subjects. Thromb Res 17:317–327
Rao CV, Reddy BS (2004) NSAIDs and chemoprevention. Curr Cancer Drug Targets 4:29–42
Ray W, Stein C, Hall K et al (2002) Non-steroidal anti-inflammatory drugs and the risk of serious coronary heart disease: an observational study. Lancet 359:118–123
Ray WA, Varas-Lorenzo C, Chung CP et al (2009) Cardiovascular risks of non-steroidal anti-inflammatory drugs in patients following hospitalization for serious coronary heart disease. Circ Cardiovasc Qual Outcomes 2:155–163
Reilly IA, FitzGerald GA (1987) Inhibition of thromboxane formation in vivo and ex vivo: implications for therapy with platelet inhibitory drugs. Blood 69:180–186
Renda G, Tacconelli S, Capone ML et al (2006) Celecoxib, ibuprofen and the antiplatelet effect of aspirin in patients with osteoarthritis and ischemic heart disease. Clin Pharmacol Ther 80:264–274
Rhame E, Pilote L, LeLorier J (2002) Association between naproxen use and protection against acute myocardial infarction. Arch Intern Med 162:1111–1115
Rigas B, Goldman IS, Levine L (1993) Altered eicosanoid levels in human colon cancer. J Lab Clin Med 122:518–523
Roumie CL, Mitchel EFJ, Kaltenbach L, Arbogast PG, Gideon P, Griffin MR et al (2008) Nonaspirin NSAIDs, cyclooxygenase 2 inhibitors, and the risk for stroke. Stroke 39:2037–2045
Schlienger R, Jick H, Meier C (2002) Use of nonsteroidal anti-inflammatory drugs and the risk of first-time acute myocardial infarction. Br J Clin Pharmacol 54:327–332
Sciulli MG, Filabozzi P, Tacconelli S et al (2005) Platelet activation in patients with colorectal cancer. Prostaglandin Leukot Essent Fatty Acid 72:79–83
Sciulli MG, Seta F, Tacconelli S et al (2003) Effects of acetaminophen on constitutive and inducible prostanoid biosynthesis in human blood cells. Br J Pharmacol 138:634–641
Shiff SJ, Rigas B (1999) The role of cyclooxygenase inhibition in the antineoplastic effects of nonsteroidal antiinflammatory drugs (NSAIDs). J Exp Med 190:445–450
Silverstein FE, Faich G, Goldstein JL et al (2000) Gastrointestinal toxicity with celecoxib vs nonsteroidal anti-inflammatory drugs for osteoarthritis and rheumatoid arthritis: the CLASS study: a randomized controlled trial. JAMA 284:1247–1255
Simmons DL, Botting RM, Hla T (2004) Cyclooxygenase isozymes: the biology of prostaglandin synthesis and inhibition. Pharmacol Rev 56:387–437
Singh G, Mithal A, Triadafilopoulos G (2005) Both selective COX-2 inhibitors and non-selective NSAIDs increase the risk of acute myocardial infarction in patients with arthritis: selectivity is with the patient not the drug class. Ann Rheum Dis 64(suppl III):85–86
Singh G, Wu O, Langhorne P, Madhok R (2006) Risk of acute myocardial infarction with nonselective non-steroidal anti-inflammatory drugs: a meta-analysis. Arthritis Res Ther 8:R153–R161

Sinicrope FA (2006) Targeting cyclooxygenase-2 for prevention and therapy of colorectal cancer. Mol Carcinog 45:447–454
Smyth EM, Grosser T, Wang M, Yu Y et al (2009) Prostanoids in health and disease. J Lipid Res 50(Suppl):S423–S428
Solomon D, Glynn R, Levin R (2002) Nonsteroidal anti-inflammatory drug use and acute myocardial infarction. Arch Intern Med 162:1099–1104
Solomon D, Schneeweiss S, Glynn R et al (2004) Relationship between selective cyclooxygenase-2 inhibitors and acute myocardial infarction in older adults. Circulation 109:2068–2073
Solomon DH, Avorn J, Sturmer T et al (2006a) Cardiovascular outcomes in new users of coxibs and nonsteroidal antiinflammatory drugs: high-risk subgroups and time course of risk. Arthritis Rheum 54:1378–1389
Solomon SD, McMurray JJ, Pfeffer MA et al (2005) Adenoma prevention with celecoxib (APC) study investigators. Cardiovascular risk associated with celecoxib in a clinical trial for colorectal adenoma prevention. N Engl J Med 352:1071–1080
Solomon SD, Pfeffer MA, McMurray JJ et al (2006b) Effect of celecoxib on cardiovascular events and blood pressure in two trials for the prevention of colorectal adenomas. Circulation 114:1028–1035
Steering Committee of the Physicians' Health Study Research Group (1989) Final report on the aspirin component of the ongoing physicians' health study. Steering committee of the physicians' health study research group. N Engl J Med 321:129–135
Steinbach G, Lynch PM, Phillips RK et al (2000) The effect of celecoxib, a cyclooxygenase-2 inhibitor, in familial adenomatous polyposis. N Engl J Med 342:1946–1952
Sturkenboom MCJM, Dieleman J, Verhamme K et al (2005) Cardiovascular events during use of COX-2 selective and non-selective NSAIDs. Pharmacoepidemiol Drug Saf 14:S57
Suissa S, Bernatsky S, Hudson M (2006) Antirheumatic drug use and the risk of acute myocardial infarction. Arthritis Rheum 55:531–536
Thrift AG, McNeil JJ, Forbes A et al (1999) Risk of primary intracerebral haemorrhage associated with aspirin and non-steroidal anti-inflammatory drugs: case-control study. BMJ 318:759–764
Trock B, Lanza E, Greenwald P (1990) Dietary fiber, vegetables, and colon cancer: critical review and meta-analyses of the epidemiologic evidence. J Natl Cancer Inst 82:650–661
Vane R (1971) Inhibition of prostaglandin synthesis as a mechanism of action for aspirin-like drugs. Nat New Biol 31:250–260
Varas-Lorenzo C, Castellsague J, Stang MR et al (2009) The use of selective cyclooxygenase-2 inhibitors and the risk of acute myocardial infarction in Saskatchewan, Canada. Pharmacoepidemiol Drug Saf 18:1016–1025
Velentgas P, West W, Cannuscio CC et al (2006) Cardiovascular risk of selective cyclooxygenase-2 inhibitors and other non-aspirin non-steroidal anti-inflammatory medications. Pharmacoepidemiol Drug Saf 15:641–652
Wactawski-Wende J, Kotchen JM, Anderson GL et al (2006) Calcium plus vitamin D supplementation and the risk of colorectal cancer. N Engl J Med 354:684–696
Wang D, Dubois RN (2010a) Eicosanoids and cancer. Nat Rev Cancer 10:181–193
Wang D, Dubois RN (2010b) The role of COX-2 in intestinal inflammation and colorectal cancer. Oncogene 29:781–788
Watson D, Rhodes T, Holmes R (2002) Lower risk of thromboembolic cardiovascular events with naproxen among patients with rheumatoid arthritis. Arch Intern Med 162:1105–1110
Weir HK, Thun MJ, Hankey BF et al (2003) Annual report to the nation on the status of cancer, 1975–2000, featuring the uses of surveillance data for cancer prevention and control. J Natl Cancer Inst 95:1276–1299
Willett WC, Stampfer MJ, Colditz GA et al (1990) Relation of meat, fat, and fiber intake to the risk of colon cancer in a prospective study among women. N Engl J Med 323:1664–1672
Wu K, Willett WC, Fuchs CS et al (2002) Calcium intake and risk of colon cancer in women and men. J Natl Cancer Inst 94:437–446

# COX-2 Active Agents in the Chemoprevention of Colorectal Cancer

Sarah Kraus, Inna Naumov and Nadir Arber

**Abstract**

Chemopreventive strategies for colorectal cancer (CRC) have been extensively studied to prevent the recurrence of adenomas and/or delay their development in the gastrointestinal tract. The non-steroidal anti-inflammatory drugs (NSAIDs) and selective cyclooxygenase (COX)-2 inhibitors have been proven as promising and the most attractive candidates for CRC clinical chemoprevention. The preventive efficacy of these agents is supported by a large number of animal and epidemiological studies which have clearly demonstrated that NSAID consumption prevents adenoma formation and decreases the incidence of, and mortality from CRC. On the basis of these studies, aspirin chemoprevention may be effective in preventing CRC within the general population, while aspirin and celecoxib may be effective in preventing adenomas in patients after polypectomy. Nevertheless, the consumption of NSAID and COX-2 inhibitors is not toxic free. Well-known serious adverse events to the gastrointestinal, renal and cardiovascular systems have been reported. These reports have led to some promising studies related to the use of lower doses and in combination with other chemopreventive agents and shown efficacy. In the intriguing jigsaw puzzle of cancer prevention, we now have a definite positive answer for the basic question

S. Kraus · I. Naumov · N. Arber (✉)
The Integrated Cancer Prevention Center, Tel Aviv Sourasky Medical Center,
Tel Aviv University, Tel Aviv, Israel
e-mail: narber@post.tau.ac.il

S. Kraus · I. Naumov · N. Arber
The Sackler Faculty of Medicine, Tel Aviv University, Tel Aviv, Israel

N. Arber
TelAviv Sourasky Medical Center, Yechiel and Helen Lieber Professor for Cancer Research
Tel Aviv University, 6 Weizman St, 64239 Tel Aviv, Israel

A. T. Chan and E. Detering (eds.), *Prospects for Chemoprevention of Colorectal Neoplasia*,
Recent Results in Cancer Research 191, DOI: 10.1007/978-3-642-30331-9_5,

"if", but several other parts of the equation-proper patient selection, the ultimate drug, optimal dosage and duration are still missing.

## Contents



Colorectal cancer (CRC) is a major health concern worldwide. In 2011 alone, 1,200,000 new cases of CRC and more than 600,000 deaths from the disease are predicted. Sporadic CRC has a natural history of evolution from normal mucosa to adenoma to overt cancer that spans on average 10–20 years, thereby providing a window of opportunity for effective intervention and prevention. CRC can be prevented by lifestyle modification (i.e. regular physical activity, smoking abstinence, and healthy nutrition) and screening and surveillance strategies. However, although these strategies are standard clinical practice, their impact is limited due to low adherence. The number of deaths due to this disease remains alarmingly high, and makes CRC prevention paramount.

Chemoprevention interferes with the process of carcinogenesis by targeting key molecular pathways that provides a promising approach to reduce the incidence of and mortality from cancer. Chemoprevention of CRC involves the use of a variety of natural or chemical compounds that can delay, prevent, or even reverse the adenoma to carcinoma process in the colon. CRC fits the criteria for chemopreventive intervention as adenomatous polyps are identifiable and treatable therefore, allowing implementation of therapeutic and preventative strategies (Arber 2008).

Based on reports of chemopreventive activity in the literature and/or efficacy data from in vitro models of carcinogenesis, several agents have been studied including, phytochemicals, vitamins, minerals, inhibitors of proliferation, metabolic inducers, non-steroidal anti-inflammatory drugs (NSAIDs), and differentiation agents. Representative examples include, folic acid, calcium, estrogen, vitamin D, olpitraz, curcumin, selenium, green tea, ursodiol, statins, and fiber, which have been encouraging, but shown modest efficacy in humans.

The most promising drugs are aspirin and NSAIDs, and much of their effect has been attributed to their potent inhibition of the cyclooxygenase (COX) enzymes (Fig. 1).

The COX enzyme is probably the most common therapeutic drug target in human history. Aspirin, a COX Inhibitor, has been used for almost 4000 years, and large amounts of these compounds are consumed each year. Research in this area has been dominated by investigations into the COX enzymes, also known as prostaglandin-endoperoxide synthases, which are central and rate-limiting enzymes in the biosynthesis of prostaglandins (Arber 2008; Tuynman 2004). Three COX isoforms have been identified: COX-1, COX-2, and COX-3.

COX-1 and COX-2 are located on different chromosomes and their expression is tightly regulated (Tuynman 2004). COX-1 is mapped to chromosome 9q32-q33.2, is encoded by the *PTGS1* gene, and constitutively expressed in normal

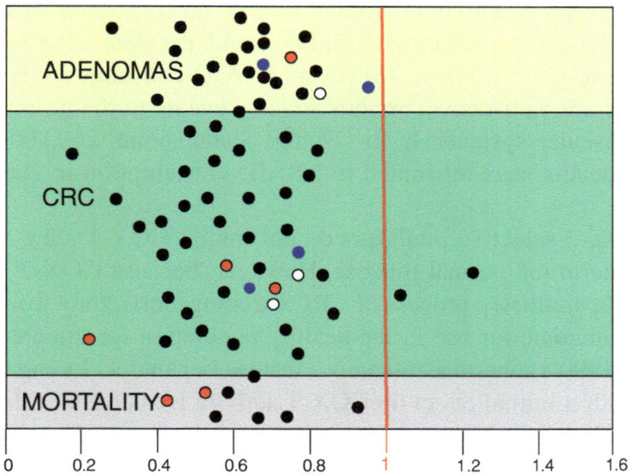


**Fig. 1** Relative risk of colorectal neoplasia in individuals using aspirin, NSAIDs and COX-2 inhibitors

tissues. It serves as a 'housekeeper' of mucosal integrity. COX-1 is the central enzyme in the biosynthetic pathway to prostaglandins from arachidonic acid, it produces prostacyclins, prostaglandins, and thromboxane, which protect gastric mucosa and play a key role in platelet aggregation and renal microvasculature dynamics. COX-2 is mapped to chromosome 1q25.2-q25.3, and is encoded by the *PTGS2* gene, an immediate early response gene that is highly inducible by either neoplastic or inflammatory stimuli. COX-2 is involved in the synthesis of prostaglandins and thromboxanes, which are regulators of processes that are relevant to cancer development. It is generally accepted that alterations in COX-2 expression and the abundance of its enzymatic product prostaglandin $E_2$ ($PGE_2$) have key roles in influencing the development of CRC.

COX-3, a third distinct COX isozyme is a COX-1 variant formed by intron retention, a form of alternative splicing (Chandrasekharan 2002). COX-3 shares all the catalytic features of COX-1 and -2; however, its exact role is yet to be fully understood (Chandrasekharan 2002).

Relative to normal mucosa, COX-2 overexpression occurs in about half of CR adenomas and in 85% of human CRCs, making COX-2 an attractive therapeutic target (Elder et al. 2002; Sheehan et al. 1999). Moreover, the fact that COX-2 expression is up-regulated in both pre-malignant and malignant CR tissue has also potential implications for the prevention of this type of cancer. Already 40 years ago, NSAIDs were hypothesized to inhibit the growth of CRC after a significant decrease in $PGE_2$ was observed in CRC tissue compared to the normal surrounding mucosa (Bennett and Del Tacca 1975; Jaffe 1974). The preventive efficacy of this class of agents is supported by more than 300 animal studies. Most significantly,

70 out of 72 epidemiological studies clearly demonstrated that NSAID/aspirin consumption prevents adenoma formation and decreases the incidence of, and mortality from, CRC (Fig. 1). However, NSAID consumption is not free of toxicities. There are well-known serious adverse events to the gastrointestinal, renal, and cardiovascular systems. In the United States alone, 260,000 hospitalizations and 26,000 deaths were attributed to NSAID consumption in 2002 (Grover et al. 2003).

Since COX-2-selective inhibitors do not inhibit COX-1, they are not generally believed to harm the normal mucosa. However, because COX-2 is overexpressed throughout the multistep process of CRC carcinogenesis, they would seem to be an ideal drug candidate for use in the healthy population for the prevention of CRC. In the early 1990's, pharmaceutical companies began developing COX-2 selective inhibitors with minimal effect on COX-1 activity (Arber 2008). In 1999 and 2000 three international, multicenter, prospective, randomized, placebo-controlled trials in the secondary prevention of CRC were launched (Baron et al. 2006; Bertagnolli et al. 2006, 2009; Bresalier et al. 2005). These clinical trials demonstrated the efficacy of COX-2 inhibitors as a strategy for reducing cancer incidence, although associated side effects and in particular cardiovascular (CVS) side effects prevented their routine use in the general population.

In the Prevention of Colorectal Sporadic Adenomatous Polyps (PreSAP) study, 1,561 patients from 107 sites in 32 countries were recruited. Celecoxib reduced adenoma recurrence by a third after one and three years ($p < 0.001$). Celecoxib was particularly potent in inhibiting the recurrence of advanced adenoma by 51 % (Arber et al. 2006). The Adenoma Prevention with Celecoxib (APC) trial enrolled 2,035 patients that were randomized to receive placebo, celecoxib 200 or 400 mg bid. In patients taking celecoxib, polyp recurrence was reduced by 33 and 45 % for patients taking 400 and 800 mg of the drug, respectively ($p < 0.0001$). The relative risk of advanced adenomas was even more drastically reduced: by 57 and 66 %, respectively ($p < 0.0001$) (Bertagnolli et al. 2006). It was shown that compared to placebo, patients taking celecoxib had fewer and smaller adenomas as well as reduction in overall tumor burden. In a third study the Adenomatous Polyp Prevention on Vioxx (APPROVe), 2,547 participants were randomized to receive rofecoxib at 25 mg qd or placebo. A 25 % reduction in polyp recurrence was seen after one and three years, the effect on advanced adenoma was almost identical (RR-0.76 (95 % CI 0.69–0.83)) (Lagaos 2006).

However, all three studies were terminated earlier than planned due to substantial concern of increased cardiovascular system (CVS) toxicity, as seen by an increase in cardiovascular events (Bertagnolli et al. 2009; Bresalier et al. 2005). The CVS toxicity seen in the APPROVe trial prompted Merck to withdraw rofecoxib from the market; this decision was made even before the efficacy of the drug was evaluated. In the APC trial, the CVS toxicity, as evaluated by an independent cardiovascular adjudicating committee, increased from 1.0 % ($n = 7/679$) for placebo to 2.5 % ($n = 16/685$), and 3.4 % for celecoxib (200 and 400 mg bid, respectively) ($p < 0.01$). As a result, the NCI to suspended the trial. Lastly, the proportion of all patients experiencing CVS toxicity in the PreSAP trial increased from 1.9 % ($n = 12/628$) for placebo to 2.5 % ($n = 23/933$) for celecoxib (400 mg qd) ($p =$ NS).

The CVS toxicity persisted 1 year after rofecoxib was discontinued (APPROVe) (Lagaos 2006) and 2 years after celecoxib was discontinued (PreSAP and APC) (Bertagnolli et al. 2006; Arber et al. 2006) trials. Of note is the disparity in CVS toxicity from celecoxib between the APC and PreSAP trials (Arber 2008). A plausible explanation for this discrepancy is the difference in dosages. The APC trial gave celecoxib twice daily, for a total daily dose of 400 or 800 mg. It stands to reason that a greater dose increases the likelihood of an adverse reaction. Another plausible explanation for the discrepancy is that the 400 mg given once daily in the PreSAP trial was less toxic than the 200 mg given twice daily in the APC trial because of the relatively short half-life of celecoxib.

The actual extent of the CVS risk associated with COX-2 selective inhibitors remains unclear (Arber 2008). The trials were not designed to assess for cardiovascular events and it was difficult to control for confounding variables. Most importantly, the number of events was very low, and the vast majority of patients tolerated celecoxib without the related toxicity throughout the study (Bertagnolli 2007). The polyp recurrence rate reduction was the same after one and three years in all three studies. Cardiovascular toxicity started to increase only after 12–18 months. This suggests the possibility that use of COX-2 inhibitors for 1 year may be sufficient to prevent polyp recurrence, before toxicity appears. The gastrointestinal toxicity of celecoxib in the PreSAP and APC trials has also been recently adjudicated (Arber et al. 2011). There was no significant difference between the drug and placebo for the entire 3 year duration of the study. The discovery of CVS toxicity related to COX-2 specific inhibitors has made the development of new agents in this field difficult. However, to ignore potential benefit from chemoprevention is to accept a higher than necessary death rate from CRC.

The exact mechanism by which COX-2 inhibitors exert their anticancer properties is currently unknown. As mentioned above, the involvement of COX-2 in CR tumorigenesis has been attributed to its role in the production of $PGE_2$ which its levels were found elevated in CR cancers. Thus, deregulation of the COX-2/$PGE_2$ pathway appears to affect CR tumorigenesis via a number of distinct mechanisms involving promotion of tumor maintenance and progression, induction of metastatic spread, and others (Greenhough et al. 2009). There are at least seven mechanisms underlying the pro-tumorigenic effects of COX-2; (Tuynman 2004):

1. Inhibition of apoptosis
2. Increase of proliferation
3. Stimulation of angiogenesis
4. Induction of invasiveness
5. Modulation of inflammation
6. Conversion of carcinogens
7. Suppression of the immune system.

COX-2 inhibitors can also act through COX-2-independent pathways. They can induce apoptosis in cancer cells not expressing the COX-2 enzyme. A variety of non-COX-2 targets for COX-2 inhibitors have been suggested, such as, NF-kB, peroxisome proliferator activating receptor -$\delta$ and -$\gamma$, protein kinase G, and Bcl-XL (Grover et al. 2003; Rao and Reddy 2004; Sinicrope 2006; Arber and Levin 2008).

Personalized medicine has remained an elusive goal and its utilization in chemoprevention is greatly anticipated. If COX-2 inhibition is the principal mechanism through which NSAIDs work, then these agents should be targeted at tumors that overexpress COX-2. Previous studies have shown that aspirin reduces the risk of CRC in COX-2 expressing cancers, but is not effective in COX-2 negative cancers (Chan et al. 2007). The efficacy and toxicity of COX-2 inhibitors may be affected by polymorphisms in COX-2, COX-2 targets, and related metabolizing enzymes (Arber 2008; Ulrich and Bigler 2006). It was suggested that polymorphisms in, COX-2 itself and metabolizing enzymes such as, uridine diphosphatidyl glucotransferase, may increase chemopreventive efficacy by up to 50 % (Macarthur et al. 2005; Lin et al. 2002). Moreover, polymorphisms in COX-2, and particularly -1195A > G may modulate the genetic susceptibility for CRC onset in some cases (Pereira et al. 2010). Another COX-2 polymorphism (rs4648319) was found to modify the effect of aspirin, supporting a role for COX-2 in the etiology of CRC and as a possible target for aspirin chemoprevention (Barry et al. 2009). It appears that polymorphisms in COX-2 targets or metabolizing enzymes may affect COX-2 efficacy and/or toxicity. However, the current literature on these interactions is still very limited (e.g., COX1 P17L or COX2 -765G > C). Reliable detection of gene-COX-2 interactions will require greater sample sizes, consistent definitions of COX-2 use, and evaluation of the outcome of chemoprevention studies. Nevertheless, these studies suggest that this genetically based higher-risk group definition may help to shift the balance between risk and benefits for the use of COX-2 inhibitors in chemoprevention that is currently hampered by adverse side effects (Pereira et al. 2010).

Obviously, the entire picture should be put in place, e.g. overall well-being, morbidity, and mortality. For example, the risk–benefit balance of aspirin for CRC prevention should be carefully weighted in conjunction with its ability to prevent other cancers, its well-established benefits in vascular disease, as well as its potential positive effects in subjects at high risk for Alzheimer disease (Agarwal et al. 1999; Reddy et al. 2006). All of these make aspirin an attractive candidate for personalized medicine.

Modern medicine favors combinatorial therapy. The goal being to increase efficacy, which tends to be modest with single compounds, while minimizing toxicity, by combining low doses of different agents. In rats with carcinogen-induced aberrant crypt foci, a combination of sulindac and statin significantly reduced the number of aberrant crypt foci to a greater degree than each of the drugs alone (Mamdani et al. 2004; Meyskens et al. 2008). The combination of the turmeric extract, curcumin, with low doses of celecoxib (2–5 μM) potentiates the growth inhibitory effect of either drug alone. This synergistic effect is clinically important since it can be achieved in human serum following standard anti–inflammatory or anti-neoplastic dosages of celecoxib (200–400 mg per day) (Zell et al. 2009).

The study by Meyskens and colleagues represents the first clinical validation concept of using more than one drug for effective chemoprevention (Etminan et al.

2003). The authors have clearly shown that unwanted adverse effects can be prevented by using low doses of difluoromethylornithine (DFMO)- 500 mg and sulindac- 150 mg once daily, for 36 months in 375 patients with history of resected ($\geq$3 mm) adenomas. The recurrence of one or more adenomas was 41.1 % in the placebo arm and 12.3 % in the treatment arm (RR, 0.30; 95 % CI, 0.18–0.49; $P < 0.001$). Advanced adenoma was seen in 8.5 or 0.7 % of the patients, respectively (RR, 0.085; 95 % CI, 0.011–0.65; $p < 0.001$. Serious adverse events (grade $\geq$3) occurred in 8.2 % of patients in the placebo group, and 11 % in the active intervention group ($p = 0.35$) (Etminan et al. 2003). In a later study, Meyskens et al. demonstrated that a high cardiovascular risk score at baseline may confer an increased risk of CVS events associated with DFMO treatment combined with sulindac, and a low baseline score may not increase this risk (Bond et al. 2010).

When contemplating the use of COX-2 inhibitors, six issues to consider include:

1. Moderate (personal or family history of colorectal neoplasia) to high-risk for CRC (FAP or HNPCC subjects)
2. Low cardiovascular risk patients
3. Non-high gastrointestinal risk patients
4. COX-2 expressing tumors
5. Polymorphisms in COX-2 targets and metabolizing enzymes
6. In the appropriate sub-group of patients with high cardiovascular risk and low gastrointestinal risk, celecoxib may be combined with low dose aspirin

In some subjects polyp recurrence occurred despite optimal colonoscopic surveillance. In the PreSAP, APC, and APPROVe studies adenomas were detected in patients that underwent up to four colonoscopies during a 5-year period, emphasizing the point that a strategy that relies on surveillance colonoscopies may not be sufficient in high-risk subjects. Further studies are needed to determine the incremental benefit that is provided with the addition of an effective chemopreventive agent. In these trials, patients who developed adenomas despite treatment with a chemopreventive agent had fewer and smaller adenomas than those who consumed placebo (Jaffe 1974; Grover et al. 2003; Baron et al. 2006). There is over all consensuses that removal of adenomas can prevent CRC by 80–90 %. Immense resources are investing therefore, in screening colonoscopy. Recently, this paradigm was challenged. While there is firm evidence that colonoscopy can prevent distal CRC, some concerns were raised regarding it is efficacy in preventing proximal CRC. Screening alone may not be sufficient to prevent the disease, even if it is fully implemented, suggesting that combining screening colonoscopy with chemopreventive agents might be the approach to eradicate CRC. Because small tubular adenomas are unlikely to progress to malignancy; these data suggest that addition of celecoxib to a surveillance regimen can be a very effective strategy.

In the intriguing jigsaw puzzle of cancer prevention, we now have a definite positive answer for the basic question "if", but several other parts of the equation-proper patient selection, the ultimate drug, optimal dosage, and duration are still missing.

It is now clinically possible to minimize adverse effects of chemotherapeutic and chemopreventive drugs by implementing combinatorial treatment strategies that will act synergistically. Nonetheless, the entire field of cancer prevention still suffers from neglect, as most efforts are dedicated to seeking optimal therapy of advanced disease. Combinatorial strategies represent a new approach that will counterbalance between cancer prevention and therapeutic approaches.

Whenever we aim for cancer prevention, and in particular in healthy individuals, one must carefully assess the benefit:risk ratio. The profile of efficacy and safety for any given indication varies significantly among subjects. It depends on the severity of the disease on one hand and the tolerance of the individuals receiving the drug on the other hand.

## References

Agarwal B, Rao CV, Bhendwal S et al (1999) Lovastatin augments sulindac-induced apoptosis in colon cancer cells and potentiates chemopreventive effects of sulindac. Gastroenterology 117(4):838–847

Arber N, Eagle CJ, Spicak J et al (2006) PreSAP Trial Investigators. Celecoxib for the prevention of colorectal adenomatous polyps N Engl J Med 55(9):885–895

Arber N (2008) Cyclooxygenase-2 inhibitors in colorectal cancer prevention: point. Cancer Epidemiol Biomarkers Prev 17(8):1852–1857

Arber N, Levin B (2008) Chemoprevention of colorectal neoplasia; the potential for personalized medicine. Gastroenterology 134(4):1224–1237

Arber N, Spicak J, Rácz I et al (2011) Five-year analysis of the prevention of colorectal sporadic adenomatous polyps trial. Am J Gastroenterol 106(6):1135–1146

Baron JA, Sandler RS, Bresalier RS et al (2006) Approve Trial Investigators. A randomized trial of rofecoxib for the chemoprevention of colorectal adenomas Gastroenterology 131(6):1674–1682

Barry EL, Sansbury LB, Grau MV et al (2009) Cyclooxygenase-2 polymorphisms, aspirin treatment, and risk for colorectal adenoma recurrence–data from a randomized clinical trial. Cancer Epidemiol Biomarkers Prev 18(10):2726–2733

Bennett A, Del Tacca M. In: Proceedings prostaglandins in human colonic carcinoma Gut 1975; 16(5):409

Bertagnolli MM, Eagle CJ, Zauber AG et al (2006) Celecoxib for the prevention of sporadic colorectal adenomas. N Engl J Med 355(9):873–884

Bertagnolli MM (2007) Chemoprevention of colorectal cancer with cyclooxygenase-2 inhibitors: two steps forward, one step back. Lancet Oncol 8:439–443

Bertagnolli MM, Eagle CJ, Zauber AG et al (2009) Five-year efficacy and safety analysis of the Adenoma Prevention with Celecoxib Trial Cancer Prev Res 2(4):310–321

Bond J, Graham N, Padovani A et al (2010) Screening for cognitive impairment. Alzheimer's disease and other dementias: opinions of European caregivers, payors, physicians and the general public J Nutr Health Aging 14:558–562

Bresalier RS, Sandler RS, Quan H et al (2005) Cardiovascular events associated with rofecoxib in a colorectal adenoma chemoprevention trial. N Engl J Med 352(11):1092–1102

Chan AT, Ogino S, Fuchs CS (2007) Aspirin and the risk of colorectal cancer in relation to the expression of COX-2 N Engl J Med 356(21):2131–2142

Chandrasekharan NV (2002) D. H. COX-3, a cyclooxygenase-1 varient inhibited by acetaminophen and other analgesic/antipyretic drugs: cloning, structure, and expression. Proc Natl Acad Sci U S A 99(21):13926–13931

Elder DJ, Baker JA, Banu NA et al (2002) Human colorectal adenomas demonstrate a size-dependent increase in epithelial cyclooxygenase-2 expression. J Pathol 198(4):428–434

Etminan M, Gill S, Samil A (2003) Effect of non-steroidal anti-inflammatory drugs on risk of Alzheimer's disease: systematic review and meta-analysis of observational studies. BMJ 327:128

Greenhough A, Smartt HJ, Moore AE et al (2009) The COX-2/PGE2 pathway: key roles in the hallmarks of cancer and adaptation to the tumour microenvironment. Carcinogenesis 30(3):377–386

Grover JK, Yadav S, Vats V et al (2003) Cyclo-oxygenase 2 inhibitors: emerging roles in the gut. Int J Colorectal Dis 18(4):279–291

Jaffe BM (1974) Prostaglandins and cancer: an update. Prostaglandins 6(6):453–461

Lagaos SW (2006) Time-to-event analyses for long-term treatments—the APPROVe trial. N Engl J Med 355(2):113–117

Lin HJ, Lakkides KM, Keku TO et al (2002) Prostaglandin H synthase 2 variant (Val511Ala) in African Americans may reduce the risk for colorectal neoplasia. Cancer Epidemiol Biomarkers Prev 11(11):1305–1315

Macarthur M, Sharp L, Hold GL et al (2005) The role of cytokine gene polymorphisms in colorectal cancer and their interaction with aspirin use in the northeast of Scotland. Cancer Epidemiol Biomarkers Prev 14(7):1613–1618

Mamdani M, Juurlink DN, Lee DS et al (2004) Cyclo-oxygenase-2 inhibitors versus non-selective non-steroidal anti-inflammatory drugs and congestive heart failure outcomes in elderly patients: a population-based cohort study. Lancet 363(9423):1751–1756

Meyskens FL Jr, McLaren CE, Pelot D, et al (2008) Difluoromethylornithine plus sulindac for the prevention of sporadic colorectal adenomas: a randomized placebo-controlled double-blind trial. Cancer Prev Res (Phila) 1(1):32–38

Pereira C, Pimentel-Nunes P, Brandão C et al (2010) COX-2 polymorphisms and colorectal cancer risk: a strategy for chemoprevention. Eur J Gastroenterol Hepatol 22(5):607–613

Rao CV, Reddy BS (2004) NSAIDs and chemoprevention Curr Cancer Drug Targets 4(1):29–42

Reddy BS, Wang CX, Kong AN et al (2006) Prevention of azoxymethane-induced colon cancer by combination of low doses of atorvastatin, aspirin, and celecoxib in F 344 rats. Cancer Res 66(8):4542–4546

Sheehan KM, Sheahan K, O'Donoghue DP et al (1999) The relationship between cyclooxygenase-2 expression and colorectal cancer. JAMA 282(13):1254–1257

Sinicrope FA (2006) Targeting cyclooxygenase-2 for prevention and therapy of colorectal cancer. Mol Carcinog 45(6):447–454

Tuynman JB (2004) P. M. COX-2 inhibition as a tool to treat and prevent colon cancer. Crit Rev Oncol Hematol 52(2):81–101

Ulrich CM, Bigler J (2006) Potter JD. Non-steroidal anti-inflammatory drugs for cancer prevention: promise, perils and pharmacogenetics Nat Rev Cancer 6(2):130–140

Zell JA, Pelot D, Chen WP, et al (2009) Risk of cardiovascular events in a randomized placebo-controlled, double-blind trial of difluoromethylornithine plus sulindac for the prevention of sporadic colorectal adenomas Cancer Prev Res (Phila) 2(3):209–212

# New NSAID Targets and Derivatives for Colorectal Cancer Chemoprevention

Heather N. Tinsley, William E. Grizzle, Ashraf Abadi, Adam Keeton, Bing Zhu, Yaguang Xi and Gary A. Piazza

**Abstract**

Clinical and preclinical studies provide strong evidence that nonsteroidal anti-inflammatory drugs (NSAIDs) can prevent numerous types of cancers, especially colorectal cancer. Unfortunately, the depletion of physiologically important prostaglandins due to cyclooxygenase (COX) inhibition results in potentially fatal toxicities that preclude the long-term use of NSAIDs for cancer chemoprevention. While studies have shown an involvement of COX-2 in colorectal tumorigenesis, other studies suggest that a COX-independent target may be at least partially responsible for the antineoplastic activity of NSAIDs. For example, certain NSAID derivatives have been identified that do not inhibit COX-2 but have demonstrated efficacy to suppress carcinogenesis with potential for reduced toxicity. A number of alternative targets have also been

H. N. Tinsley
Department of Biology, Chemistry, and Mathematics,
University of Montevallo, Montevallo, AL, USA

W. E. Grizzle
Department of Pathology, The University of Alabama at Birmingham,
Birmingham, AL, USA

A. Abadi
Faculty of Pharmacy and Biotechnology, German University of Cairo,
Cairo, Egypt

A. Keeton · B. Zhu · Y. Xi · G. A. Piazza (✉)
Drug Discovery Research Center Mitchell Cancer Institute,
University of South Alabama, 1660 Springhill Avenue, Suite 3029,
Mobile, AL 36604, USA
e-mail: gpiazza@usouthal.edu

A. T. Chan and E. Detering (eds.), *Prospects for Chemoprevention of Colorectal Neoplasia*, 105
Recent Results in Cancer Research 191, DOI: 10.1007/978-3-642-30331-9_6,

reported to account for the tumor cell growth inhibitory activity of NSAIDs, including the inhibition of cyclic guanosine monophosphate phosphodiesterases (cGMP PDEs), generation of reactive oxygen species (ROS), the suppression of the apoptosis inhibitor protein, survivin, and others. Here, we review several promising mechanisms that are being targeted to develop safer and more efficacious NSAID derivatives for colon cancer chemoprevention.

## Contents



## 1 Introduction

Previous studies have demonstrated strong evidence that nonsteroidal anti-inflammatory drugs (NSAIDs) and cyclooxygenase-2 (COX-2) selective inhibitors have cancer chemopreventive activity against a number of cancer types, particularly colorectal cancer. For example, epidemiologic studies of the general population have shown that long-term use of NSAIDs, most notably aspirin, is associated with a significant reduction of risk from death by colorectal cancer (Chan 2002; Thun et al. 2002). Consistent with these observations, clinical studies have shown the ability of certain prescription strength NSAIDs (e.g. sulindac) to reduce the occurrence and cause the regression of precancerous adenomas in patients with familial adenomatous polyposis (Giardiello et al. 1993; Steinbach et al. 2000). A wealth of observations from preclinical studies supports these observations by showing the ability of aspirin and various non-aspirin NSAIDs to inhibit tumor formation in rodent models of chemically induced carcinogenesis.

The NSAIDs, the most common of which are listed in Table 1, are a chemically diverse family of drugs that are available as either over-the-counter medications or by prescription. Long-term use is common for treating pain associated with chronic inflammatory conditions such as arthritis. The basis for the anti-inflammatory activity of NSAIDs is largely attributed to the inhibition of cyclooxygenases, which catalyze the conversion of arachidonic acid to prostaglandins (Vane and Botting 1998). At least two isoforms of the COX enzyme are expressed in humans. COX-1 is a constitutively active form of the enzyme, whereas COX-2 is an inducible form for which expression is induced during various pathophysiological conditions such as chronic inflammation (Vane et al. 1998). As shown in Fig. 1, NSAIDs generally

**Table 1** Common NSAIDs and COX-2 selective inhibitors listed according to structural classification

| Carboxylic acids | | | | Pyrazoles | Oxicams | COX-2 selective |
|---|---|---|---|---|---|---|
| Salicylates | Acetic acids | Propionic acids | Fenamates | | | |
| Acetylsalicylic acid salsalate diflunisal fendosal | Indomethacin acemetacin cinmetacin sulindac tolmetin zomepirac diclofenac fenclofenac isoxepac furofenac fentiazac clidanac oxepinac fenclorac lonazolac metiazinic acid clopirac amfenac benzofenac clometacine etodolac bumadizone clamidoxic acid | Ibuprofen flurbiprofen naproxen ketoprofen fenoprofen benoxaprofen indoprofen pirprofen carprofen oxaprozin pranoprofen suprofen miroprofen tioxaprofen alminoprofen cicloprofen tiaprofenic acid furaprofen butibufen fenbufen furobufen bucloxic acid protizinic acid | Mefenamic acid flufenamic acid meclofenamate niflumic acid toifenamic acid flunixin clonixin | Phenyibutazone feprazone apazone trimethazone mofebutazone kebuzone suxibuzone | Piroxicam isoxicam tenoxicam | Celecoxib rofecoxib valdecoxibe nimesulide NS 398 |

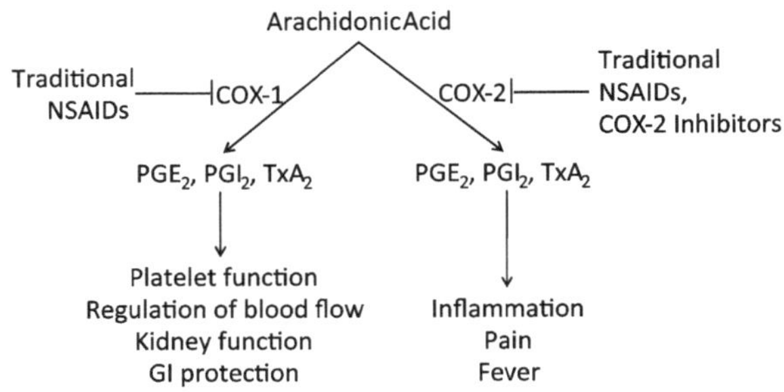


**Fig. 1** Prostaglandins and thromboxanes produced through COX-1 have important physiological functions, whereas the prostaglandins and thromboxanes produced through COX-2 have important pathophysiological functions

inhibit both COX-1 and COX-2 with various degrees of selectivity, while COX-2 selective inhibitors such as celecoxib and rofecoxib have been developed to be highly selective for the inducible COX-2 isoenzyme. Unfortunately, the depletion of physiologically important prostaglandins caused by the suppression of COX-1 or COX-2 is associated with potentially fatal side effects to the gastrointestinal tract, kidneys, and cardiovascular system (Vane and Botting 1998; Vane et al. 1998). While COX-2 selective inhibitors have reduced GI and renal toxicity, their long-term use has been associated with increased risk of heart attack (Chakraborti et al. 2010; Harris 2009; Warner et al. 1999). Consequently, the widespread use of traditional NSAIDs or COX-2 selective inhibitors is precluded, especially in the high dosages administered over extended periods of time that appear to be necessary for effective chemoprevention. While aspirin appears to have unique benefits for colorectal cancer, possibly because of the irreversible nature by which it can bind COX, non-aspirin NSAIDs, especially prescription strength NSAIDs with high potency appear to act by a COX-independent mechanism.

The specific biochemical and cellular mechanism(s) proposed to be responsible for the cancer chemopreventive activity of the NSAIDs is controversial. While there is strong evidence that the mechanism of action involves COX-2 inhibition, there are a number of pharmacological inconsistencies that have led many investigators to conclude that the mechanism is unrelated to COX-2 inhibition (Alberts et al. 1995; Elder et al. 1997; Hanif et al. 1996; Kashfi and Rigas 2005; Piazza et al. 1997a). For example, studies have shown that NSAIDs can inhibit the growth of tumor cells that completely lack the expression COX-2 (Elder et al. 1997; Hanif et al. 1996; Grosch et al. 2001). Other studies have reported that the addition of exogenous prostaglandins cannot rescue cancer cells from the growth inhibitory activity of the NSAIDs, which would be expected if prostaglandin suppression is necessary (Kusuhara et al. 1998; Piazza et al. 1995). Furthermore, as shown in Table 2, the rank order of potency among the NSAIDs to inhibit tumor cell growth does not correlate with their potency to inhibit prostaglandin synthesis (Carter et al. 1989; de Mello et al. 1980; Erickson et al. 1999). For example, sulindac sulfide is appreciably less potent than indomethacin with regard to COX-1 or COX-2 inhibition, but is more potent in terms of its tumor cell growth inhibitory activity (Tinsley et al. 2010). In addition, certain highly specific COX-2 inhibitors such as rofecoxib fail to inhibit tumor cell growth (Soh et al. 2008). Consequently,

**Table 2** Potencies of select NSAIDs and COX-2 selective inhibitors for inhibition of HT-29 colon tumor cell growth, inhibition of purified ovine COX-2, and inhibition of cGMP PDE activity in HT-29 cell lysate

| | IC50 (μM) | | |
|---|---|---|---|
| | Growth inhibition | COX-2 inhibition | cGMP PDE inhibition |
| Tolmetin | 313 | 0.82 | 326 |
| Meclofenamic acid | 85 | 2.9 | 80 |
| Flufenamic acid | 108 | 9.3 | 103 |
| Flurbiprofen | 550 | 5.5 | 504 |
| Celecoxib | 203 | 0.34 | 174 |
| Sulindac | 224 | >300 | 120 |
| Sulindac sulfide | 34 | 6.3 | 20 |
| Sulindac sulfone | 89 | >300 | 96 |

a number of alternative targets have been suggested as potential mediators (Chan 2002; Thun et al. 2002; Shiff and Rigas 1999).

In this review, we consider several important developments in the study of both COX-2-dependent and COX-independent targets that can guide efforts in drug discovery and development strategies for cancer chemoprevention. We also discuss several promising novel NSAID derivatives that have been identified in recent years, which have potential safety and efficacy advantages compared to currently available NSAIDs and COX-2 inhibitors.

## 2 Targeting COX-2

There is strong evidence for the involvement of COX-2 in colon tumorigenesis. For example, COX-2 is overexpressed and prostaglandin levels are elevated in as many as 90 % of sporadic colon carcinomas (Eberhart et al. 1994). Furthermore, the levels of COX-2 expression correlates with colon tumor size and invasiveness (Fujita et al. 1998). The mechanism by which COX-2 may drive tumorigenesis is still unclear but likely involves multiple pathways given that prostaglandins can accelerate cellular growth, inhibit apoptosis, and induce angiogenesis; all key events in carcinogenesis (Shiff and Rigas 1999; Sawaoka et al. 1998; Tsujii et al. 1998). No matter the mechanism, studies have shown that decreasing COX-2 expression in the $Apc^{min}$ mouse model of intestinal carcinogenesis reduces both the size and multiplicity of intestinal polyps (Oshima et al. 1996). Similarly, clinical studies have shown efficacy of celecoxib and rofecoxib, albeit modest, for suppressing the formation of colorectal adenomas in patients with familial adenomatous polyposis as well as the formation of sporadic adenomas (Steinbach et al. 2000; Arber et al. 2006; Baron et al. 2006; Bertagnolli et al. 2006).

While the COX-2 selective inhibitors, rofecoxib and valdecoxib, were removed from the market due to unforeseen cardiovascular toxicity, it is unclear if these side effects are directly linked with COX-2 inhibition, especially since they were less pronounced with celecoxib (Chakraborti et al. 2010). Given that the toxicity may be unrelated to COX-2 but may be compound specific, it is possible that chemical modifications to existing NSAIDs might have potential advantages. Marnett and colleagues, for example, described a series of ester and amide modifications to the carboxylic acid moiety on various NSAIDs, such as indomethacin and meclofenamic acid that increased selectivity for COX-2 (Kalgutkar et al. 2000; 2002). The rational for this approach was based on molecular modeling studies whereby a more restrictive binding domain was noted within the catalytic region of the COX-1 compared with COX-2, which permitted specificity via substitution of the carboxylic acid with bulky neutral residues. A potential concern, however, is that ester and amide linkages may not have sufficient metabolic stability whereby there is the potential to generate the parent NSAID. Studies to demonstrate in vivo antitumor efficacy and reduced toxicity compared with the parent NSAID are therefore needed for future development of this class of compounds.

# 3 COX-Independent Targets

## 3.1 Inhibition of cGMP PDEs

One COX-independent target of NSAIDs that has been used to guide the synthesis of more potent non-COX inhibitory derivatives includes members of the cyclic GMP phosphodiesterase (PDE) superfamily. PDE enzymes are metallophosphohydrolases that hydrolyze the 3′,5′-cyclic phosphate on second messenger cyclic nucleotides, cAMP or cGMP, to 5′-monophosphate. This modification terminates intracellular signaling following activation of cyclic nucleotide coupled receptors (Beavo 1995). The PDE superfamily comprises an estimated 100 distinct protein isoforms divided into 11 protein families, which differ from one another in selectivity for cAMP or cGMP, sensitivity to inhibitors and activators, as well as tissue, cellular, or intracellular distributions (Beavo 1995; Sonnenburg and Beavo 1994). Inhibition of PDE would result in an increase in the magnitude and/or duration of the cAMP and/or cGMP signal depending on the isozyme selectivity of the inhibitor. Increased intracellular cyclic nucleotide levels can activate specific signaling pathways, which, in the case of cGMP, can lead to activation of cGMP-dependent protein kinase (PKG), cyclic nucleotide-gated ion channels, or certain cGMP binding PDEs; all of which play important roles in regulating cellular activity (Beavo 1995; Lincoln and Cornwell 1993).

Studies have suggested that the cGMP pathway may be perturbed during colorectal tumorigenesis. For example, human colon tumors have been shown to express high levels of the cGMP-specific PDE5 isozyme (Tinsley et al. 2010). In addition, Shailubhai and colleagues demonstrated that mRNA levels for the membrane-associated guanylyl cyclase agonist, uroguanylin, are reduced in both colon

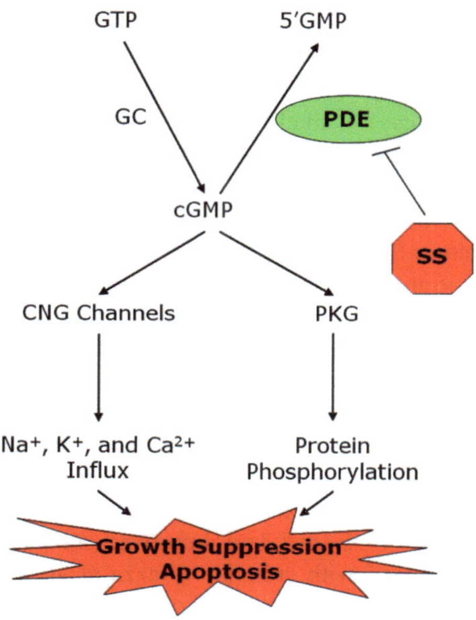


**Fig. 2** Mechanistic model of colon tumor cell growth inhibition mediated by inhibition of cGMP PDE and activation of cGMP signaling

adenomas and adenocarcinomas. Interestingly, oral administration of uroguanylin inhibited tumor formation in the Apc$^{min}$ mouse model of intestinal tumorigenesis, which was associated with increased apoptosis rates within the tumors (Shailubhai et al. 2000). These findings are consistent with the observations that certain cGMP phosphodiesterases may be elevated in colon tumors, leading to reduced cGMP levels, which is necessary to limit tumor cell survival or suppress proliferation. Despite the evidence for a role of cGMP in colon cancer development, the relevant cGMP PDE isozymes that regulate its synthesis and downstream signaling pathways have not been well studied with regard to a role in colon tumorigenesis.

Certain NSAIDs and COX-2 inhibitors can also inhibit cGMP PDE isozymes to increase intracellular cGMP levels and activate cGMP signaling in colon cancer cell lines, as depicted in Fig. 2 (Soh et al. 2000, 2008; Silvola et al. 1982; Thompson et al. 2000; Tinsley et al. 2009). While these effects require high concentrations (Table 2) that cannot be safely achieved in vivo, a strong correlation exists between concentrations of the NSAIDS required to inhibit tumor cell growth in vitro and their ability to inhibit cGMP PDE, especially the cGMP-specific PDE isozyme, PDE5 (Tinsley et al. 2010). In addition, certain known PDE5-specific inhibitors (e.g. MY5445) and non-selective cGMP PDE inhibitors (e.g. MY5445, trequinsin) could also suppress tumor cell growth, as well as knockdown of PDE5 by siRNA or antisense (Tinsley et al. 2011; Zhu et al. 2005). However, other highly selective PDE5 inhibitors (e.g. sildenafil), commonly used for the treatment of erectile dysfunction, required high concentrations compared with those required to inhibit tumor cell growth, which suggest that additional cGMP PDE isozymes may be involved (Tinsley et al. 2011).

Among a number of NSAIDs evaluated for cGMP PDE inhibition, sulindac sulfide was found to be the most active (Tinsley et al. 2010). Since the non-COX inhibitory sulfone form of sulindac can also inhibit cGMP PDE, albeit with less potency, it is likely that the COX inhibitory activity of this class of compounds can be uncoupled from cGMP PDE inhibitory activity (Piazza et al. 1995, 1997b). Initial efforts to synthesize sulindac derivatives that lack COX inhibitory activity, but have improved cGMP PDE inhibitory activity focused on modifications to either the sulfonyl or the carboxylic acid moieties (Thompson et al. 2000). While this approach yielded certain derivatives with high in vitro potency to inhibit colon tumor cell growth and induce apoptosis, poor oral bioavailability and metabolic instability halted further development (Thompson et al. 2000).

In light of information gained from molecular modeling docking sulindac sulfide into the COX active site, our laboratory has focused on chemically modifying the carboxylic acid moiety of sulindac sulfide and substituting with a positive-charged amide to interfere with COX binding (Piazza et al. 2009). This approach yielded an interesting series of compounds that retained ability to inhibit cGMP PDE and had improved anticancer activity both in vitro and in vivo compared with sulindac (Piazza et al. 2009). These derivatives serve to validate cGMP PDE as a target to optimize for anticancer efficacy, while reducing toxicity. Although problems with poor absorption following oral administration necessitated high dosages limited the development of this class of compounds for colorectal cancer chemoprevention, alternative derivatives or formulations with improved oral bioavailability may have advantages.

## 3.2 Generation of Reactive Oxygen Species

Survivin is an apoptosis inhibitor protein that prevents activation of caspases that are important mediators of apoptosis (Altieri 2003a, b; Ambrosini et al. 1997). Not normally found to be expressed in adult tissues, survivin is overexpressed in the vast majority of human cancers and increased levels of this protein strongly correlate with increased tumor stage and a poor prognosis (Altieri 2003a; Ambrosini et al. 1997; Zaffaroni et al. 2005). Furthermore, survivin expression appears to be strongly connected to p53 status and sensitivity to chemotherapy (Hoffman et al. 2002; Li 2005).

Aberrant redox signaling has been documented in cancer, although more work is necessary to determine whether ROS are a driving force in tumorigenesis. For example, abnormally high levels of ROS have been observed in multiple types of cancer (Toyokuni et al. 1995). Furthermore, chronic inflammation, which can promote tumorigenesis, results in elevated levels of ROS. High ROS levels have been reported in tumors and are associated with genomic instability, proliferation, angiogenesis, and aberrant apoptosis, although the effect may be dependent on intracellular levels (Frein et al. 2005; Toyokuni et al. 1995; Halliwell 2007).

Two promising new classes of NSAID derivatives, the nitric oxide NSAIDs (NO-NSAIDs) and the phospho-NSAIDs, demonstrate chemopreventive efficacy through a mechanism that appears to involve the elevation of intracellular ROS levels and activation of proapoptotic redox signaling pathways as described by Rigas and colleagues. The NO-NSAIDs were designed with an NO-releasing moiety attached to a parent compound such as aspirin, sulindac, or naproxen through a chemical linker. The intended design was to increase NO levels in the gut where it could serve a protective function to increase vascular blood supply to reduce the GI toxicity of the parent NSAID (Rigas and Kashfi 2004). Initial studies with the NO-NSAIDs showed enhanced colon cancer chemopreventive activity when compared to the parent compound both in vitro and in vivo (Williams et al. 2004; Yeh et al. 2004). In order to identify the importance of the NO moiety for the enhanced chemopreventive activity, additional modifications were made in which the NO was replaced with a diethylphosphate. Interestingly, these phospho-NSAID derivatives demonstrated similar chemopreventive activity as the NO-NSAIDs, suggesting that release of the NO was not solely responsible for the enhanced activity of these new classes of compounds, but rather a chemical modification to the NSAIDs (Huang et al. 2010; Mackenzie et al. 2010).

Whether the parent NSAID was linked to NO or to the diethylphosphate substituent, the new derivatives caused substantial increases in ROS in tumor cells in vitro and showed advantages in efficacy in animal models of colon cancer (Rigas and Kashfi 2004; Kashfi and Rigas 2007; Rigas and Kozoni 2008; Rigas and Williams 2008; Sun et al. 2011; Xie et al. 2011). While further studies are necessary to develop this class of derivatives, their ability to induce apoptosis of colon tumor cells through activation of redox signaling makes them a promising class of agents for colorectal cancer chemoprevention.

## 3.3 Downregulation of Survivin

Survivin is an apoptosis inhibitor protein that prevents activation of caspases that are important mediators of apoptosis (Altieri 2003a, b; Ambrosini et al. 1997). Not normally found to be expressed in normal adult tissues, survivin is overexpressed in the vast majority of human cancers and increased levels of this protein strongly correlate with increased tumor stage and a poor prognosis (Altieri 2003a; Ambrosini et al. 1997; Zaffaroni et al. 2005). Furthermore, survivin expression appears to be strongly connected to p53 status and sensitivity to chemotherapy (Hoffman et al. 2002; Li 2005).

A number of NSAIDs and COX-2 selective inhibitors have been shown to reduce survivin expression and/or activity in cancer cells, but the best studied of these is celecoxib (Tinsley et al. 2010, 2011; Konduri et al. 2009; Pyrko et al. 2006). Interestingly, the celecoxib derivative 2,5-dimethyl-celecoxib (DMC) lacks COX-2 inhibitory activity but retains the anticancer activity of the parent compound and is actually more potent than celecoxib for suppressing survivin (Pyrko et al. 2006). Even more promising, DMC has shown in vivo chemopreventive efficacy in various models of human cancer (Pyrko et al. 2006; Kardosh et al. 2005).

## 3.4 Other COX-Independent Targets

Additional targets that are known to play a role in colorectal cancer tumorigenesis have also been implicated as targets of NSAIDs. However, the association between these targets and the anticancer activity of the NSAIDs is weaker and has not been established for non-COX-inhibitory derivatives, but nonetheless represent potential targets for future efforts in drug discovery.

One such target is peroxisomal proliferator-activated receptor $\gamma$ (PPAR$\gamma$). PPAR$\gamma$ is overexpressed in colon cancer cells and can inhibit growth and promote differentiation (DuBois et al. 1998; Mueller et al. 1998). Numerous studies have shown that certain NSAIDs can directly bind to and activate PPAR$\gamma$ and that this activity is associated with inhibition of neoplastic growth (Lehmann et al. 1997). However, the activation of PPAR$\gamma$ is not a characteristic shared by all antineoplastic NSAIDs (Lehmann et al. 1997; Lefebvre et al. 1998; Saez et al. 1998).

NF$\kappa$B is another potential COX-independent antineoplastic target of the NSAIDs. NF$\kappa$B is a transcription factor that commonly promotes cellular growth and inhibits apoptosis (Ljungdahl et al. 1997). Increased NF$\kappa$B activity has been observed in multiple types of cancer and can be attributed to a number of alterations including overexpression of NF$\kappa$B or decreased expression of I$\kappa$B, a regulatory protein that sequesters NF$\kappa$B in the cytosol in order to prevent its transcriptional activity (Rayet and Gelinas 1999). Some NSAIDs, particularly the salicylates, have been found to inhibit NF$\kappa$B-mediated transcription, presumably by preventing degradation of I$\kappa$B (Schwenger et al. 1998; Yin et al. 1998). However, these effects are most pronounced among the least active NSAIDs in terms of in vitro colon cancer prevention (Yin et al. 1998).

One of the most novel mechanisms proposed for the anticancer activity of the NSAIDs involves induction of the NSAID-activated gene (NAG-1) as reported by Baek and colleagues. NAG-1 is a member of the transforming growth factor $\beta$ (TGF-$\beta$) superfamily that has both proapoptotic and antiproliferative properties, although the exact mechanism responsible for these effects has not been well defined (Baek et al. 2001a, b). A number of different NSAIDs including indomethacin, aspirin, and ibuprofen have been shown to increase expression of NAG-1 in colon cancer cells and this effect appears to be independent of COX expression (Baek et al. 2001a, 2002). However, there is little association between the anticancer activity of an NSAID and its potency for activating NAG-1 expression, as NAG-1 induction occurs at significantly lower concentrations than those necessary for induction of apoptosis or inhibition of growth (Baek et al. 2002). Furthermore, the effects of the NSAIDs on NAG-1 and the effects of NAG-1 expression have yet to be observed in vivo.

Although not a direct target, microRNA may be another important factor that contributes to the sensitivity of tumor cells to NSAIDs. microRNAs are a set of naturally occurring small RNA molecules that are capable of regulating approximately 30 % of human genes through direct binding with the cognate target genes and are involved in many essential biological processes such as cell growth, differentiation, apoptosis, and tumorigenesis (Carmell et al. 2002; Esquela-Kerscher and Slack 2006), which highlights its clinical applications in tumor diagnosis, prognosis, and therapy (Nakajima et al. 2006; Xi et al. 2006). Our studies, for example, have shown that a panel of microRNAs (miR-10b, -17, -19, -21, and -9) are suppressed in human colon tumor cells treated with sulindac sulfide (Rayet and Gelinas 1999). Interestingly, these microRNAs are known to be elevated during cancer metastasis and invasion (Huang et al. 2009; Ma et al. 2010a, b, 2007; Song et al. 2010; Yu et al. 2010; Zhu et al. 2008) and may mediate the ability of sulindac sulfide to inhibit tumor cell invasion.

Another complicating aspect of determining the mechanisms of the actions of NSAIDs in the prevention of neoplasia is the effects of various types of NSAIDs on inflammation in general. Inflammation in the setting of long standing, continuing damage, inflammation, and repair that occurs in ulcerative colitis and the associated development of colon cancers generates not only increased ROS, but also increased cellular death and proliferation. These associated inflammatory changes may lead to molecular changes in epithelial cells that result in the inhibition of enzymes that repair DNA to molecular changes in signaling pathways associated with the initiation of neoplasia as a result of genetic mutations (Baek et al. 2001b, 2002). Thus, some changes related to the chemopreventive actions of NSAIDs may be related specifically to their anti-inflammatory activity involving COX-inhibition, while others (e.g. tumor cell growth inhibition and apoptosis induction) are more related to their ability to suppress tumorigenesis. Whether the two activities can be fully uncoupled remains to be determined and awaits the development of new derivatives that lack COX inhibitory activity.

## 4 Conclusions

NSAIDs represent a chemically diverse group of drugs that have multiple biological effects, some of which are related to their anticancer activities, while others are responsible for toxicity. Experimental studies over the past 20 years have provided strong evidence that the mechanism responsible for their chemopreventive activity may not require COX inhibition. As such, it should be feasible to develop improved drugs with greater antitumor efficacy and reduced toxicity. Given that the anticancer activity of the NSAIDs is undoubtedly complex, a number of reports have suggested many alternative targets as summarized in Table 3. Traditional NSAIDs and COX-2 selective inhibitors most likely inhibit tumorigenesis through a combination of COX-dependent and COX-independent mechanisms. However, the development of NSAID derivatives that lack COX inhibitory activity have shown promise for improved potency and selectivity to inhibit tumor cell growth. As such, the elucidation of COX-independent mechanisms of the NSAIDs is an important area of research that offers the promise to design a highly specific new class of chemopreventive agents. The greatest challenges will be to identify which molecular target(s) is most important for colon

**Table 3** Summary of drugs and COX-independent targets that have been studied for the chemopreventive activity of the NSAIDs and COX-2 selective inhibitors

| Target | Active NSAIDs | Reference |
|---|---|---|
| cGMP PDE | Sulindac and metabolites | Tinsley et al. (2009, 2010, 2011), Soh et al. (2000, 2008), Silvola et al. (1982), Thompson et al. (2000) |
| | Celecoxib | |
| | Indomethacin | |
| | Meclofenamic acid | |
| | Naproxen | |
| | Tolfenamic acid | |
| | Diclofenac | |
| | NSAID derivatives | |
| ROS | NO-NSAIDs | Huang et al. (2010), Mackenzie et al. (2010), Kashfi and Rigas (2007) |
| | Phospho-NSAIDs | |
| Survivin | Sulindac and metabolites | Tinsley et al. (2009, 2010, 2011), Konduri et al. (2009), Pyrko et al. (2006) |
| | Tolfenamic acid | |
| | Celecoxib and derivatives | |
| PPAR$\gamma$ | Indomethacin | Lehmann et al. (1997) |
| | Fenoprofen | |
| | Ibuprofen | |
| | Flufenamic acid | |
| NF$\kappa$B | Sodium salicylate | Schwenger et al. (1998), Yin et al. (1998) |
| | Aspirin | |
| NAG-1 | Indomethacin and derivatives | Baek et al. (2001b, 2002) |
| | Piroxicam | |
| | Diclofenac | |
| | Aspirin | |
| | Sulindac | |
| microRNA | Sulindac | Rayet and Gelinas (1999) |

tumorigenesis and which chemical scaffold can yield suitable lead compounds for preclinical development with optimal pharmaceutical, efficacy, and toxicity properties.

**Acknowledgments** Funding provided by NIH grants R01 CA131378 and R01 CA148817 and a UAB Breast Cancer SPORE grant.

## References


Alberts DS et al (1995) Do NSAIDs exert their colon cancer chemoprevention activities through the inhibition of mucosal prostaglandin synthetase? J Cell Biochem Suppl 22:18–23

Altieri DC (2003a) Survivin in apoptosis control and cell cycle regulation in cancer. Prog Cell Cycle Res 5:447–452

Altieri DC (2003b) Survivin and apoptosis control. Adv Cancer Res 88:31–52

Ambrosini G, Adida C, Altieri DC (1997) A novel anti-apoptosis gene, survivin, expressed in cancer and lymphoma. Nat Med 3(8):917–921

Arber N et al (2006) Celecoxib for the prevention of colorectal adenomatous polyps. N Engl J Med 355(9):885–895

Baek SJ, Horowitz JM, Eling TE (2001a) Molecular cloning and characterization of human nonsteroidal anti-inflammatory drug-activated gene promoter. Basal transcription is mediated by Sp1 and Sp3. J Biol Chem 276(36):33384–33392

Baek SJ et al (2001b) Cyclooxygenase inhibitors regulate the expression of a TGF-beta superfamily member that has proapoptotic and antitumorigenic activities. Mol Pharmacol 59(4):901–908

Baek SJ et al (2002) Dual function of nonsteroidal anti-inflammatory drugs (NSAIDs): inhibition of cyclooxygenase and induction of NSAID-activated gene. J Pharmacol Exp Ther 301(3):1126–1131

Baron JA et al (2006) A randomized trial of rofecoxib for the chemoprevention of colorectal adenomas. Gastroenterology 131(6):1674–1682

Beavo JA (1995) Cyclic nucleotide phosphodiesterases: functional implications of multiple isoforms. Physiol Rev 75(4):725–748

Bertagnolli MM et al (2006) Celecoxib for the prevention of sporadic colorectal adenomas. N Engl J Med 355(9):873–884

Carmell MA et al (2002) The Argonaute family: tentacles that reach into RNAi, developmental control, stem cell maintenance, and tumorigenesis. Genes Dev 16(21):2733–2742

Carter CA, Ip MM, Ip C (1989) A comparison of the effects of the prostaglandin synthesis inhibitors indomethacin and carprofen on 7,12-dimethylbenz[a]anthracene-induced mammary tumorigenesis in rats fed different amounts of essential fatty acid. Carcinogenesis 10(8):1369–1374

Chakraborti AK et al (2010) Progress in COX-2 inhibitors: a journey so far. Curr Med Chem 17(15):1563–1593

Chan TA (2002) Nonsteroidal anti-inflammatory drugs, apoptosis, and colon-cancer chemoprevention. Lancet Oncol 3(3):166–174

de Mello MC, Bayer BM, Beaven MA (1980) Evidence that prostaglandins do not have a role in the cytostatic action of anti-inflammatory drugs. Biochem Pharmacol 29(3):311–318

DuBois RN et al (1998) The nuclear eicosanoid receptor, PPARgamma, is aberrantly expressed in colonic cancers. Carcinogenesis 19(1):49–53

Eberhart CE et al (1994) Up-regulation of cyclooxygenase 2 gene expression in human colorectal adenomas and adenocarcinomas. Gastroenterology 107(4):1183–1188

Elder DJ et al (1997) Induction of apoptotic cell death in human colorectal carcinoma cell lines by a cyclooxygenase-2 (COX-2)-selective nonsteroidal anti-inflammatory drug: independence from COX-2 protein expression. Clin Cancer Res 3(10):1679–1683

Erickson BA et al (1999) The effect of selective cyclooxygenase inhibitors on intestinal epithelial cell mitogenesis. J Surg Res 81(1):101–107

Esquela-Kerscher A, Slack FJ (2006) Oncomirs–microRNAs with a role in cancer. Nat Rev Cancer 6(4):259–269

Frein D et al (2005) Redox regulation: a new challenge for pharmacology. Biochem Pharmacol 70(6):811–823

Fujita T et al (1998) Size- and invasion-dependent increase in cyclooxygenase 2 levels in human colorectal carcinomas. Cancer Res 58(21):4823–4826

Genestra M (2007) Oxyl radicals, redox-sensitive signalling cascades and antioxidants. Cell Signal 19(9):1807–1819

Giardiello FM et al (1993) Treatment of colonic and rectal adenomas with sulindac in familial adenomatous polyposis. N Engl J Med 328(18):1313–1316

Grosch S et al (2001) COX-2 independent induction of cell cycle arrest and apoptosis in colon cancer cells by the selective COX-2 inhibitor celecoxib. Faseb J 15(14):2742–2744

Halliwell B (2007) Oxidative stress and cancer: have we moved forward? Biochem J 401(1):1–11

Hanif R et al (1996) Effects of nonsteroidal anti-inflammatory drugs on proliferation and on induction of apoptosis in colon cancer cells by a prostaglandin-independent pathway. Biochem Pharmacol 52(2):237–245

Harris RE (2009) Cyclooxygenase-2 (cox-2) blockade in the chemoprevention of cancers of the colon, breast, prostate, and lung. Inflammopharmacology 17(2):55–67

Hoffman WH et al (2002) Transcriptional repression of the anti-apoptotic survivin gene by wild type p53. J Biol Chem 277(5):3247–3257

Huang GL et al (2009) Clinical significance of miR-21 expression in breast cancer: SYBR-Green I-based real-time RT-PCR study of invasive ductal carcinoma. Oncol Rep 21(3):673–679

Huang L et al (2010) Phospho-sulindac (OXT-922) inhibits the growth of human colon cancer cell lines: a redox/polyamine-dependent effect. Carcinogenesis 31(11):1982–1990

Kalgutkar AS et al (2000) Ester and amide derivatives of the nonsteroidal antiinflammatory drug, indomethacin, as selective cyclooxygenase-2 inhibitors. J Med Chem 43(15):2860–2870

Kalgutkar AS et al (2002) Amide derivatives of meclofenamic acid as selective cyclooxygenase-2 inhibitors. Bioorg Med Chem Lett 12(4):521–524

Kardosh A et al (2005) Multitarget inhibition of drug-resistant multiple myeloma cell lines by dimethyl-celecoxib (DMC), a non-COX-2 inhibitory analog of celecoxib. Blood 106(13):4330–4338

Kashfi K, Rigas B (2005) Is COX-2 a 'collateral' target in cancer prevention? Biochem Soc Trans 33(Pt 4):724–727

Kashfi K, Rigas B (2007) The mechanism of action of nitric oxide-donating aspirin. Biochem Biophys Res Commun 358(4):1096–1101

Klaunig JE, Kamendulis LM (2004) The role of oxidative stress in carcinogenesis. Annu Rev Pharmacol Toxicol 44:239–267

Konduri S et al (2009) Tolfenamic acid enhances pancreatic cancer cell and tumor response to radiation therapy by inhibiting survivin protein expression. Mol Cancer Ther 8(3):533–542

Kusuhara H et al (1998) Induction of apoptotic DNA fragmentation by nonsteroidal anti-inflammatory drugs in cultured rat gastric mucosal cells. Eur J Pharmacol 360(2–3):273–280

Lefebvre AM et al (1998) Activation of the peroxisome proliferator-activated receptor gamma promotes the development of colon tumors in C57BL/6 J-APCMin/+ mice. Nat Med 4(9):1053–1057

Lehmann JM et al (1997) Peroxisome proliferator-activated receptors alpha and gamma are activated by indomethacin and other non-steroidal anti-inflammatory drugs. J Biol Chem 272(6):3406–3410

Li F (2005) Role of survivin and its splice variants in tumorigenesis. Br J Cancer 92(2):212–216

Lincoln TM, Cornwell TL (1993) Intracellular cyclic GMP receptor proteins. Faseb J 7(2):328–338

Ljungdahl S, Shoshan MC, Linder S (1997) Inhibition of the growth of 12 V-ras-transformed rat fibroblasts by acetylsalicylic acid correlates with inhibition of NF-kappa B. Anticancer Drugs 8(1):62–66

Ma L, Teruya-Feldstein J, Weinberg RA (2007) Tumour invasion and metastasis initiated by microRNA-10b in breast cancer. Nature 449(7163):682–688

Ma L et al (2010a) Therapeutic silencing of miR-10b inhibits metastasis in a mouse mammary tumor model. Nat Biotechnol 28(4):341–347

Ma L et al (2010b) MiR-9, a MYC/MYCN-activated microRNA, regulates E-cadherin and cancer metastasis. Nat Cell Biol 12(3):247–256

Mackenzie GG et al (2010) Phospho-sulindac (OXT-328), a novel sulindac derivative, is safe and effective in colon cancer prevention in mice. Gastroenterology 139(4):1320–1332
Mueller E et al (1998) Terminal differentiation of human breast cancer through PPAR gamma. Mol Cell 1(3):465–470
Nakajima G et al (2006) Non-coding microRNAs hsa-let-7 g and hsa-miR-181b are associated with chemoresponse to S-1 in colon cancer. Cancer Genomics Proteomics 3(5):317–324
Oshima M et al (1996) Suppression of intestinal polyposis in Apc delta716 knockout mice by inhibition of cyclooxygenase 2 (COX-2). Cell 87(5):803–809
Piazza GA et al (1995) Antineoplastic drugs sulindac sulfide and sulfone inhibit cell growth by inducing apoptosis. Cancer Res 55(14):3110–3116
Piazza GA et al (1997a) Apoptosis primarily accounts for the growth-inhibitory properties of sulindac metabolites and involves a mechanism that is independent of cyclooxygenase inhibition, cell cycle arrest, and p53 induction. Cancer Res 57(12):2452–2459
Piazza GA et al (1997b) Sulindac sulfone inhibits azoxymethane-induced colon carcinogenesis in rats without reducing prostaglandin levels. Cancer Res 57(14):2909–2915
Piazza GA et al (2009) A novel sulindac derivative that does not inhibit cyclooxygenases but potently inhibits colon tumor cell growth and induces apoptosis with antitumor activity. Cancer Prev Res (Phila Pa) 2(6):572–580
Pyrko P et al (2006) Downregulation of survivin expression and concomitant induction of apoptosis by celecoxib and its non-cyclooxygenase-2-inhibitory analog, dimethyl-celecoxib (DMC), in tumor cells in vitro and in vivo. Mol Cancer 5:19
Rayet B, Gelinas C (1999) Aberrant rel/nfkb genes and activity in human cancer. Oncogene 18(49):6938–6947
Rigas B, Kashfi K (2004) Nitric-oxide-donating NSAIDs as agents for cancer prevention. Trends Mol Med 10(7):324–330
Rigas B, Kozoni V (2008) The novel phenylester anticancer compounds: Study of a derivative of aspirin (phoshoaspirin). Int J Oncol 32(1):97–100
Rigas B, Williams JL (2008) NO-donating NSAIDs and cancer: an overview with a note on whether NO is required for their action. Nitric Oxide 19(2):199–204
Saez E et al (1998) Activators of the nuclear receptor PPARgamma enhance colon polyp formation. Nat Med 4(9):1058–1061
Sawaoka H et al (1998) Effects of NSAIDs on proliferation of gastric cancer cells in vitro: possible implication of cyclooxygenase-2 in cancer development. J Clin Gastroenterol 27(Suppl 1):S47–S52
Schwenger P et al (1998) Activation of p38 mitogen-activated protein kinase by sodium salicylate leads to inhibition of tumor necrosis factor-induced IkappaB alpha phosphorylation and degradation. Mol Cell Biol 18(1):78–84
Shailubhai K et al (2000) Uroguanylin treatment suppresses polyp formation in the Apc(Min/+) mouse and induces apoptosis in human colon adenocarcinoma cells via cyclic GMP. Cancer Res 60(18):5151–5157
Shiff SJ, Rigas B (1999) The role of cyclooxygenase inhibition in the antineoplastic effects of nonsteroidal antiinflammatory drugs (NSAIDs). J Exp Med 190(4):445–450
Silvola J et al (1982) Effects of nonsteroidal anti-inflammatory drugs on rat gastric mucosal phosphodiesterase activity. Agents Actions 12(4):516–520
Soh JW et al (2000) Cyclic GMP mediates apoptosis induced by sulindac derivatives via activation of c-Jun NH2-terminal kinase 1. Clin Cancer Res 6(10):4136–4141
Soh JW et al (2008) Celecoxib-induced growth inhibition in SW480 colon cancer cells is associated with activation of protein kinase G. Mol Carcinog 47(7):519–525
Song B et al (2010) MicroRNA-21 regulates breast cancer invasion partly by targeting tissue inhibitor of metalloproteinase 3 expression. J Exp Clin Cancer Res 29:29
Sonnenburg WK, Beavo JA (1994) Cyclic GMP and regulation of cyclic nucleotide hydrolysis. Adv Pharmacol 26:87–114

Steinbach G et al (2000) The effect of celecoxib, a cyclooxygenase-2 inhibitor, in familial adenomatous polyposis. N Engl J Med 342(26):1946–1952
Sun Y et al (2011) Oxidative stress mediates through apoptosis the anticancer effect of phospho-NSAIDs: implications for the role of oxidative stress in the action of anticancer agents. J Pharmacol Exp Ther 338(3):775–783
Thompson WJ et al (2000) Exisulind induction of apoptosis involves guanosine 3',5'-cyclic monophosphate phosphodiesterase inhibition, protein kinase G activation, and attenuated beta-catenin. Cancer Res 60(13):3338–3342
Thun MJ, Henley SJ, Patrono C (2002) Nonsteroidal anti-inflammatory drugs as anticancer agents: mechanistic, pharmacologic, and clinical issues. J Natl Cancer Inst 94(4):252–266
Tinsley HN et al (2009) Sulindac sulfide selectively inhibits growth and induces apoptosis of human breast tumor cells by phosphodiesterase 5 inhibition, elevation of cyclic GMP, and activation of protein kinase G. Mol Cancer Ther 8(12):3331–3340
Tinsley HN et al (2010) Colon tumor cell growth-inhibitory activity of sulindac sulfide and other nonsteroidal anti-inflammatory drugs is associated with phosphodiesterase 5 inhibition. Cancer Prev Res (Phila) 3(10):1303–1313
Tinsley HN et al (2011) Inhibition of PDE5 by Sulindac Sulfide Selectively Induces Apoptosis and Attenuates Oncogenic Wnt/{beta}-Catenin-Mediated Transcription in Human Breast Tumor Cells. Cancer Prev Res (Phila) 4(8):1275–1284
Toyokuni S et al (1995) Persistent oxidative stress in cancer. FEBS Lett 358(1):1–3
Tsujii M et al (1998) Cyclooxygenase regulates angiogenesis induced by colon cancer cells. Cell 93(5):705–716
Vane JR, Botting RM (1998) Mechanism of action of antiinflammatory drugs. Int J Tissue React 20(1):3–15
Vane JR, Bakhle YS, Botting RM (1998) Cyclooxygenases 1 and 2. Annu Rev Pharmacol Toxicol 38:97–120
Warner TD et al (1999) Nonsteroid drug selectivities for cyclo-oxygenase-1 rather than cyclo-oxygenase-2 are associated with human gastrointestinal toxicity: a full in vitro analysis. Proc Natl Acad Sci U S A 96(13):7563–7568
Williams JL et al (2004) NO-donating aspirin inhibits intestinal carcinogenesis in Min (APC(Min/+)) mice. Biochem Biophys Res Commun 313(3):784–788
Xi Y et al (2006) Prognostic values of microRNAs in colorectal cancer. Biomark Insights 2: 113–121
Xie G et al (2011) Phospho-ibuprofen (MDC-917) is a novel agent against colon cancer: efficacy, metabolism, and pharmacokinetics in mouse models. J Pharmacol Exp Ther 337(3):876–886
Yeh RK et al (2004) NO-donating nonsteroidal antiinflammatory drugs (NSAIDs) inhibit colon cancer cell growth more potently than traditional NSAIDs: a general pharmacological property? Biochem Pharmacol 67(12):2197–2205
Yin MJ, Yamamoto Y, Gaynor RB (1998) The anti-inflammatory agents aspirin and salicylate inhibit the activity of I(kappa)B kinase-beta. Nature 396(6706):77–80
Yu Z et al (2010) MicroRNA 17/20 inhibits cellular invasion and tumor metastasis in breast cancer by heterotypic signaling. Proc Natl Acad Sci U S A 107(18):8231–8236
Zaffaroni N, Pennati M, Daidone MG (2005) Survivin as a target for new anticancer interventions. J Cell Mol Med 9(2):360–372
Zhu B et al (2005) Suppression of cyclic GMP-specific phosphodiesterase 5 promotes apoptosis and inhibits growth in HT29 cells. J Cell Biochem 94(2):336–350
Zhu S et al (2008) MicroRNA-21 targets tumor suppressor genes in invasion and metastasis. Cell Res 18(3):350–359

# Aspirin in Prevention of Sporadic Colorectal Cancer: Current Clinical Evidence and Overall Balance of Risks and Benefits

Peter M. Rothwell

**Abstract**

In addition to longstanding evidence from observational studies, evidence from randomised trials of the effectiveness of aspirin for chemoprevention of colorectal cancer has increased substantially in recent years. Trials have shown that daily aspirin reduces the risk of any recurrent colorectal adenoma by 17 % and advanced adenoma by 28 %, and that daily aspirin for about 5 years reduces incidence and mortality due to colorectal cancer by 30–40 % after 20 years of follow-up, and reduces the 20-year risk of all-cause cancer mortality by about 20 %. Recent evidence also shows that the risk of major bleeding on aspirin diminishes with prolonged use, suggesting that the balance of risk and benefit favours the use of daily aspirin in primary prevention of colorectal and other cancers. Updated clinical guidelines are currently awaited.

## Contents



P. M. Rothwell (✉)
Stroke Prevention Research Unit, Nuffield Department of Clinical Neuroscience,
John Radcliffe Hospital, Oxford OX39DU, UK
e-mail: peter.rothwell@clneuro.ox.ac.uk

A. T. Chan and E. Detering (eds.), *Prospects for Chemoprevention of Colorectal Neoplasia*,
Recent Results in Cancer Research 191, DOI: 10.1007/978-3-642-30331-9_7,

# 1 Introduction

Colorectal cancer accounts for about 10 % of all incident cancers about 8 % of all cancer mortality Weitz et al. (2005) and the lifetime risk in developed countries is about 5 %. Sigmoidoscopic and endoscopic screening and polypectomy are partially effective in preventing colorectal cancer, particularly for cancers of the distal colon and rectum (Rex et al. 2009; Atkin et al. 2010), but there is still a substantial clinical need for other supplementary preventive strategies. There is good observational evidence that modifiable lifestyle and dietary factors are important in the aetiology of colorectal cancer, but there remains significant need for pharmacological chemoprevention if a safe and effective agent were available. As detailed by others in this book, aspirin is the most widely studied pharmacological agent for the prevention of colorectal cancer. However, clinical guidelines currently recommended against the routine use of aspirin for colorectal cancer prevention (Cuzick et al. 2009). The aim of this chapter is to first review the evolution of the evidence that aspirin has a clinically useful effect in long-term primary prevention of sporadic colorectal cancer in man and, second, to consider that effect within the context of other indications and effects of aspirin in prevention of vascular disease.

# 2 Aspirin in Prevention of Colorectal Cancer

## 2.1 Observational Studies

Observational studies can reliably identify powerful causal associations (e.g. smoking and lung cancer, cholesterol and coronary heart disease, blood pressure and stroke, radiation exposure and cancer, sleeping position and sudden infant death and male circumcision and incidence of HIV infection), but they have proved less reliable in studying behavioural risk factors that involve an element of choice, such as diet or use of vitamins or, hormone replacement therapy). Nevertheless, much has been learned from observational studies of the association between use of aspirin and risk of colorectal cancer.

In 1988, Kune and colleagues published the first report of an inverse association between use of aspirin and the risk of colorectal cancer in man (Kune et al. 1988). They investigated associations among colorectal cancer and a variety of chronic illnesses, operations and medications in 715 patients with incident, histologically confirmed colorectal cancer and 727 age and sex-matched controls. The authors did not mention any a priori hypotheses about an effect of aspirin, but they found that patients with colorectal cancer were less likely than controls to have used aspirin-containing medications in the past (relative risk 0.53, 95 % confidence interval 0.40–0.71). This association remained significant after adjustment for comorbidities and was consistent for both men and women. A similar association was found for use of other NSAIDS but was confined to colon cancers only. They examined over 30 other potential associations with colorectal cancer and found that hypertension, heart disease, stroke, chronic chest disease, chronic arthritis and use of vitamins supplements were also less common amongst patients with colorectal cancer, whereas haemorrhoids and large bowel polyps were more common amongst cases. However, prior aspirin use remained inversely associated with colorectal cancer in a multivariate model that included all of the statistically significant univariate associations as well as previously identified dietary factors.

The Kune study stimulated considerable interest. A subsequent analysis of 662,424 men and women enrolled in the Cancer Prevention Study II cohort showed that aspirin use at least 16 times per month was associated with a 40 % reduced risk of colon cancer mortality over a 6-year period (Thun et al. 1991). An updated analysis of this cohort observed that daily use of at least 325 mg for at least 5 years was associated with a lower incidence of colorectal cancer compared with non-users (RR, 0.68; 95 % CI, 0.52–0.90) as well as reduced risks of other cancers (Jacobs et al. 2007). Another cohort study of 47,363 men from the Health Professionals Follow-up study showed that regular aspirin users ($\geq$2 times/week) had a 21 % (RR, 0.79; 95 % CI, 0.69–0.90) lower risk of colorectal cancer over 18 years of follow-up (Chan et al. 2008). Similar findings were observed in a cohort of 82,911 women from the Nurses' Health Study; regular aspirin use ($\geq$two 325 mg tablets/week) was associated with a 23 % reduced risk of colorectal cancer (RR, 0.77; 95 % CI, 0.67–0.88) over 20 years of follow-up (Chan et al. 2005a).

By 2007, data on the association between aspirin use and colorectal cancer were available from 11 cohort studies and 19 case-control studies (Flossmann and Rothwell 2007). In a meta-analysis of the case-control studies, there was significantly lower use of aspirin or NSAID in cases than in controls (pooled OR = 0.80, 95 % CI 0.73–0.87, $p < 0.0001$, Fig. 1a), but with substantial heterogeneity between studies ($p < 0.0001$) (Flossmann and Rothwell 2007). Associations tended to be much stronger in smaller studies, with a highly significantly asymmetrical funnel plot (Fig. 1a), which could be misinterpreted as evidence of publication bias and overestimation of any true effect. However, on closer scrutiny the asymmetrical funnel plot appeared to be due to more discriminating definitions of use of aspirin or NSAID in smaller studies, with a strong inverse relation (weighted regression: $r^2 = 0.53$, $p = 0.0005$) between the percentage of the control group defined as users and the relative use of aspirin in cases versus controls (Flossmann and Rothwell 2007).

Fourteen studies stratified analyses by the extent of use of aspirin or NSAID, and when the analysis of all 19 studies was based on the maximum use reported (most regular and/or longest duration) the association with colorectal cancer was much stronger and less heterogeneous (Fig. 1b), and was no longer related to the percentage of controls defined as users ($r^2 = 0.10$, $p = 0.18$). In eight studies where it was possible to look specifically at irregular or occasional use of aspirin or NSAID, there was no association with colorectal cancer (OR = 1.01, 0.93–1.09, $p = 0.87$). Those studies that stratified analyses by both regularity of use and duration of use reported 50–70 % reductions in relative risk of colorectal cancer associated with use of medium to high dose aspirin for over 10 years (Flossmann and Rothwell 2007).

**(a)**

| | Users / Total: Cases | Users / Total: Controls | OR | 95% CI |
|---|---|---|---|---|
| Saskatchewan | 4922 / 5815 | 19980 / 23255 | 0.90 | 0.83-0.98 |
| UK GP Research Database | 1005 / 2002 | 5243 / 10000 | 0.91 | 0.83-1.01 |
| Minnesota, Utah, California | 947 / 2371 | 1488 / 2972 | 0.66 | 0.59-0.74 |
| Case-control Surveillance Study | 866 / 1326 | 3140 / 4906 | 1.06 | 0.93-1.20 |
| Seattle | 911 / 1792 | 862 / 1501 | 0.77 | 0.67-0.88 |
| Massachussets | 395 / 1201 | 457 / 1201 | 0.80 | 0.67-0.94 |
| Cancer Prevention Study II | 333 / 598 | 1923 / 3058 | 0.74 | 0.62-0.89 |
| Roswell Park | 436 / 830 | 769 / 1138 | 0.53 | 0.44-0.64 |
| New York, Ohio | 191 / 511 | 257 / 500 | 0.56 | 0.44-0.73 |
| **Melbourne** | **85 / 713** | **147 / 727** | **0.53** | **0.40-0.71** |
| Insurance Database Canada | 129 / 179 | 2008 / 2568 | 0.72 | 0.51-1.01 |
| North Carolina | 561 / 632 | 971 / 1045 | 0.60 | 0.43-0.85 |
| Italy | 47 / 1357 | 77 / 1891 | 0.85 | 0.58-1.22 |
| Wisconsin | 72 / 184 | 144 / 293 | 0.67 | 0.46-0.97 |
| Liverpool | 36 / 512 | 103 / 512 | 0.30 | 0.20-0.45 |
| Atlanta | 74 / 93 | 163 / 186 | 0.55 | 0.28-1.07 |
| Jinan | 25 / 247 | 18 / 66 | 0.30 | 0.15-0.59 |
| Columbia Presbyterian | 11 / 256 | 33 / 322 | 0.39 | 0.19-0.79 |
| Madrid | 10 / 196 | 40 / 228 | 0.25 | 0.12-0.52 |
| **TOTAL** | **11056 / 20815** | **37823 / 56369** | **0.79** | **0.76-0.81** |

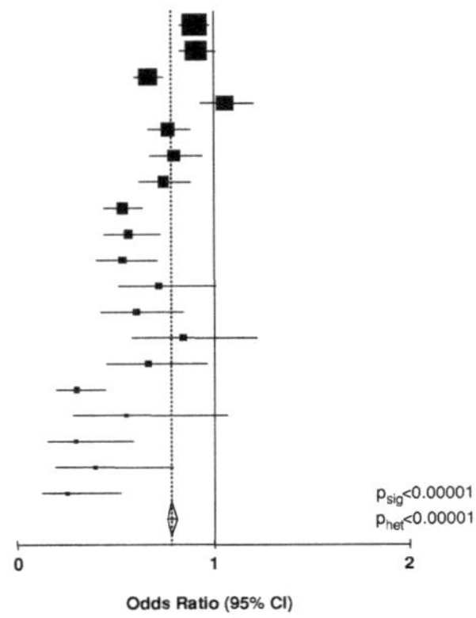


**(b)**

| | Users / Total: Cases | Users / Total: Controls | OR | 95% CI |
|---|---|---|---|---|
| Saskatchewan | 29 / 5815 | 263 / 23255 | 0.44 | 0.30-0.64 |
| UK GP Research Database | 23 / 635 | 155 / 2434 | 0.55 | 0.35-0.86 |
| Minnesota, Utah, California | 196 / 1993 | 346 / 2410 | 0.65 | 0.54-0.78 |
| Case-control Surveillance Study | 6 / 1326 | 51 / 4891 | 0.43 | 0.18-1.01 |
| Seattle | 172 / 1792 | 201 / 1501 | 0.69 | 0.55-0.85 |
| Massachussets | 43 / 1201 | 58 / 1201 | 0.73 | 0.49-1.09 |
| Cancer Prevention Study II | 46 / 598 | 388 / 3058 | 0.57 | 0.42-0.79 |
| Roswell Park | 21 / 830 | 42 / 1138 | 0.68 | 0.40-1.15 |
| New York, Ohio | 23 / 511 | 42 / 500 | 0.51 | 0.30-0.87 |
| **Melbourne** | **85 / 713** | **147 / 727** | **0.53** | **0.40-0.71** |
| Insurance Database Canada | 4 / 179 | 82 / 2568 | 0.69 | 0.25-1.91 |
| North Carolina | 164 / 632 | 330 / 1045 | 0.76 | 0.61-0.95 |
| Italy | 32 / 1357 | 56 / 1891 | 0.79 | 0.51-1.23 |
| Wisconsin | 17 / 184 | 41 / 293 | 0.63 | 0.34-1.14 |
| Liverpool | 36 / 512 | 103 / 512 | 0.30 | 0.20-0.45 |
| Atlanta | 7 / 93 | 29 / 186 | 0.44 | 0.19-1.05 |
| Jinan | 25 / 247 | 18 / 66 | 0.30 | 0.15-0.59 |
| Columbia Presbyterian | 11 / 256 | 33 / 322 | 0.39 | 0.19-0.79 |
| Madrid | 10 / 196 | 40 / 228 | 0.25 | 0.12-0.52 |
| **TOTAL** | **950 / 19070** | **2425 / 48226** | **0.59** | **0.55-0.64** |

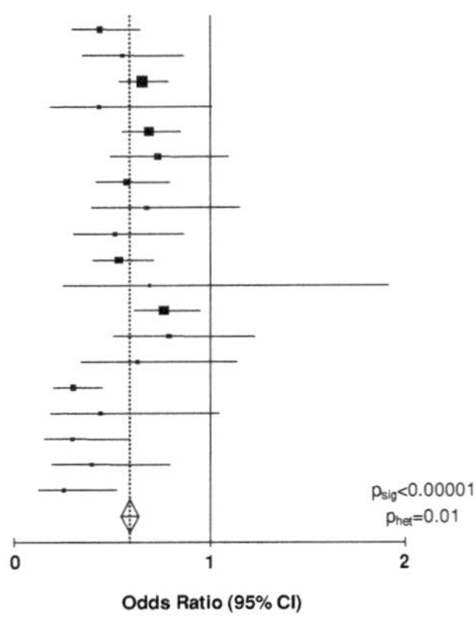


**Fig. 1** **a** Any use of aspirin and/or NSAID in cases of colorectal cancer versus age and sex-matched controls in 19 case-control studies. (Data derived from Flossmann and Rothwell 2007). **b** Maximum use of aspirin and/or NSAID in cases of colorectal cancer versus age and sex-matched controls in 19 case-control studies. (Data derived from Flossmann and Rothwell 2007). The Melbourne Colorectal Cancer Study (Kune et al. 1988), the first such report, is highlighted in bold font

Given the considerable statistical power in these observational studies (the cohort studies included 1,136,110 individuals with over 6,000 colorectal cancers during follow-up and the 19 case-control studies included 20,815 cases of colorectal cancer), they can also be used to address clinically important questions about heterogeneity of effect. For example, the observational data demonstrated no difference in effect of aspirin and other NSAIDs, no difference in relation to age, sex, race or family history, no difference in relation to the site or aggressiveness of the cancer and no fall-off in apparent effect with use for ≥20 years (Flossmann and Rothwell 2007).

## 2.2 Randomised Controlled Trials

There are relatively few data from randomised trials of the effect of aspirin on risk of colorectal cancer compared with the wealth of data from observational studies. The first randomised trial of aspirin was as an adjuvant treatment in patients with established colorectal cancer in the late 1970s and early 1980s. No benefit was seen, but the trial was small and underpowered. Starting in the 1990s, several randomised trials (Baron et al. 2003; Benamouzig et al. 2003; Logan et al. 2008; Sandler et al., 2003) showed that aspirin reduced the recurrence of colorectal adenomas by 20–30 % in patients with previous adenomas or colorectal cancer (Table 1). Meta-analysis of the four trials of aspirin versus placebo, which together included nearly 3,000 patients, showed that aspirin at any dose (81–325 mg/day) reduced the risk of any colorectal adenoma (defined as occurrence after randomisation) by 17 % (RR = 0.83; 95 % CI, 0.72–0.96) over a median post-randomisation follow-up of 33 months (Cole et al. 2009). The risk of advanced colorectal adenomas (defined as 1 cm or larger in size or with high-grade dysplasia or invasive cancer) was reduced by 28 % (RR = 0.72; 95 % CI, 0.57–0.90).

Since adenomas are the precursors of the majority of colorectal cancers (Morson 1984; Levine and Ahnen 2006), these effects of aspirin on risk of recurrent adenoma were encouraging, but with only 2–3 years follow-up the trials were unable to determine any effect on risk of colorectal cancer. A reduction in risk of cancer can not simply be assumed to be an inevitable consequence of the effect of aspirin on recurrence of adenomas. The likelihood of malignant transformation of adenomas that develop despite aspirin versus those that are prevented is uncertain. Although up to 40 % of people in developed countries have one or more colorectal adenomas by age 60 years, less than 10 % of these adenomas progress to cancer. Moreover, it could not be assumed that secondary prevention of adenomas by short-term treatment with aspirin would be maintained on long-term treatment, nor that the same effect would necessarily be seen in patients without a prior history of colorectal neoplasia.

It was still necessary, therefore, to obtain confirmation from randomised trials that aspirin could prevent colorectal cancer in primary prevention. However, a latency of more than 10 years would be expected prior to an effect of aspirin becoming evident, given that the delay between the initiation of development of an adenoma, the point at which aspirin is believed to act and presentation of colorectal cancer is estimated to be 10–15 years (Kozuka et al. 1975; Kelloff et al. 2004). Indeed, two large randomised trials of alternate-day aspirin in primary prevention of vascular disease had shown no effect on risk of colorectal cancer during 10 years of follow-up (Stürmer et al. 1998; Cook et al. 2005), and the

**Table 1** Patient characteristics and effect of aspirin on risk of colorectal adenoma in four randomised trials of daily aspirin versus control (Baron et al. 2003; Benamouzig et al. 2003; Cole et al. 2009; Logan et al. 2008; Sandler et al. 2003)

| | APACC | AFPPS | CALGB | ukCAP |
|---|---|---|---|---|
| Design | Randomised controlled trial | Randomised controlled trial | Randomised controlled trial | Randomised controlled trial |
| | Aspirin (160 or 300 mg/day) or placebo<br>Follow-up: 4 years | Aspirin (81 or 325 mg/day) or placebo<br>Follow-up: 3 years | Aspirin (325 mg/day) or placebo<br>Median follow-up: 12.8 months | Aspirin (300 mg/day) or folate supplement (0.5 mg/day)<br>Follow-up: 3 years |
| Patients (n) | 272 | 1,121 | 635 | 945 |
| Adenoma inclusion criteria | Recent history of colorectal adenomas | Recent history of colorectal adenomas | Previous history of colorectal cancers | Recent history of colorectal adenomas |
| Family history of adenomas (%) | 34.6 | 30.4 | Not reported | 14.1 |
| RR (95 % CI) for any adenoma[a] | 0.95 (0.75–1.21) | 0.88 (0.77–1.02) | 0.61 (0.44–0.86) | 0.79 (0.63–0.99) |
| RR (95 % CI) for advanced adenoma[a] | 0.91 (0.51–1.60) | 0.74 (0.52–1.06) | 0.77 (0.29–2.05) | 0.63 (0.43–0.91) |

[a] Versus placebo or folate (based on colonoscopic follow-up).
AFPPS, Aspirin/Folate Polyp Revention Study; APACC, Association pour la Prévention par l'Aspirine du Cancer Colorectal; CALGB, Colorectal Adenoma prevention study originated in the cooperative trials group cancer and Leukaemia Group B; ukCAP, United Kingdom Colorectal Adenoma Prevention

results of short-term follow-up in cohort studies were similarly unpromising (Flossmann and Rothwell 2007).

Given the likely need for up to 15–20 years follow-up in order to reliably determine the effect of a period of treatment with aspirin on risk of colorectal cancer, new prospective randomised trials were unlikely to be done. It was possible, however, to follow-up patients who had been randomised in previous trials of aspirin in prevention of vascular events in the 1980 and 1990s in order to examine if any delayed effect on incidence or mortality due to colorectal cancer was evident on long-term follow-up after the trials. The first, such, study (Flossmann and Rothwell 2007) reported 20-year follow-up of two UK trials of daily high-dose aspirin versus control, the UK-TIA Aspirin Trial (1,200 vs. 300 mg vs. placebo; Farrel et al. 1991) and the British Doctors Aspirin Trial (500 mg vs. control; Peto et al. 1988). Allocation to aspirin reduced incidence of colorectal cancer (pooled HR = 0.74,

**Table 2** Hazard ratios (95 % CI) for diagnosis of colorectal cancer in a pooled analysis (stratified by trial) of data from the British doctors aspirin trial and the UK-TIA Aspirin trial of long-term follow-up after the scheduled trial treatment period, stratified into 5-year periods (Flossmann and Rothwell 2007)

| Years from randomisation | All patients with scheduled trail treatment of ≥5 years | All complaint[a] patient | Patient with scheduled trial treatment of ≥5 years | All complaint[a] patient |
|---|---|---|---|---|
| 5–9 years[b] | 1.08 (0.55–2.14) p = 0.83 | 0.83 (0.38–1.80) p = 0.63 | 0.93 (0.42–2.09) p = 0.86 | 0.67 (0.25–1.78) p = 0.67 |
| 10–14 years | 0.51 (0.29–0.90) p = 0.02 | 0.43 (0.23–0.79) p = 0.007 | 0.37 (0.20–0.70) p = 0.002 | 0.26 (0.12–0.56) p = 0.0002 |
| 15–19 years | 0.70 (0.43–1.14) p = 0.15 | 0.67 (0.39–1.14) p = 0.14 | 0.69 (0.42–1.15) p = 0.16 | 0.66 (0.37–1.16) p = 0.15 |
| ≥20 years | 0.90 (0.42–1.95) p = 0.79 | 0.85 (0.36–2.03) p = 0.72 | 0.73 (0.33–1.63) p = 0.45 | 0.65 (0.26–1.63) p = 0.35 |

[a] Excluding patients diagnosed with colorectal cancer during the trials
[b] Compliant patients defined as those who were taking allocated trial treatment on at least 50 % of follow-up assessments during the trials
The numbers of colorectal cancers in each time period were: 42 (5–9); 49 (10–14); 68 (15–19); 18 (≥20)

0.56–0.97, $p = 0.02$ overall; 0.63, 0.47–0.85, $p = 0.002$ if allocated aspirin for ≥5 years). However, as predicted, this effect was only seen after a latency of 10 years (0–9 years, HR = 0.92, 0.56–1.49, $p = 0.73$; 10–19 years, HR = 0.60, 0.42–0.87, $p = 0.007$) and was greatest 10–14 years after randomisation in patients who had scheduled trial treatment of ≥5 years (HR = 0.37, 0.20–0.70, $p = 0.002$, Table 2). The authors concluded that use of aspirin ≥300 mg daily for about 5 years was effective in primary prevention of colorectal cancer, with a latency of about 10 years.

These data on the long-term effects of high-dose aspirin were useful proof of principle, but did not change clinical practice because of concern that the adverse effects of long-term use of high-dose aspirin would limit its potential for long-term prevention. Lower doses (75–300 mg daily) reduced the short-term risk of recurrent colorectal adenomas, but effectiveness in long-term primary prevention of colorectal cancer was unknown. Post-trial follow-up was, therefore, done (Rothwell et al. 2010) in three randomised trials of low-dose aspirin versus control, one in primary prevention of vascular events (Medical Research Council's General Practice Research Framework 1998) and two in secondary prevention after TIA or stroke (SALT Collaborative Group 1991; Dutch TIA Trial Study Group 1991).

The effect of allocation to aspirin on the long-term risk of death due to colorectal cancer in the three trials of low-dose aspirin was very similar to that in the trials of high-dose aspirin (Fig. 2) (Rothwell et al. 2010). There was also a significant reduction in long-term incidence of colorectal cancer in patients allocated low-dose aspirin (Fig. 3). A pooled analysis of the four trials of high-dose or low-dose aspirin

| | Deaths due to cancer | | Odds Ratio | 95% CI |
|---|---|---|---|---|
| | Aspirin | Control | | |
| **500-1200mg daily** | | | | |
| British Doctors Study (500mg) | 59 / 3429 | 40 / 1710 | 0.73 | 0.49-1.10 |
| UK-TIA (1200mg) | 11 / 821 | 16 / 817 | 0.68 | 0.31-1.47 |
| **SUBTOTAL** | **70 / 4250** | **56 / 2527** | **0.72** | **0.50-1.03** |
| **75 - 300mg daily** | | | | |
| UK-TIA (300mg) | 8 / 811 | 16 / 817 | 0.50 | 0.21-1.17 |
| TPT (75mg) | 34 / 2545 | 55 / 2540 | 0.61 | 0.40-0.94 |
| SALT (75mg) | 7 / 676 | 10 / 684 | 0.71 | 0.27-1.86 |
| **SUBTOTAL** | **49 / 4032** | **81 / 4041** | **0.60** | **0.42-0.86** |
| **TOTAL** | **119 / 8282** | **137 / 6568** | **0.66** | **0.51-0.84** |

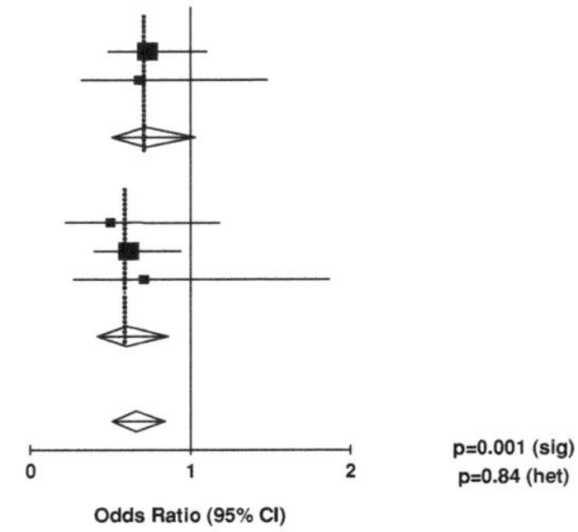


**Fig. 2** Meta-analysis of effect of aspirin on long-term risk of death due to colorectal cancer in randomised trials of aspirin versus control (Data derived form Rothwell et al. 2010). Note to subeditor: the TOTAL line should read as follows in order to avoid double counting of the UK-TIA placebo group: 119/8,282 vs. 121/5,751 OR = 0.66, 95 % CI 0.51 – 0.85, $p = 0.002$ (sig); $p = 0.84$ (het)

versus control (mean duration of scheduled treatment = 6.0 years) was, therefore, performed (Rothwell et al. 2010). Among 14,033 patients, 391 developed colorectal cancer during median follow-up of 18.3 years, with allocation to aspirin reducing the risk of colon cancer (incidence–HR = 0.76, 0.60–0.96, $p = 0.02$; mortality–0.65, 0.48–0.88, $p = 0.005$), but not rectal cancer (0.90, 0.63–1.30, $p = 0.58$; 0.80, 0.50–1.28, $p = 0.35$). Where anatomic subsite data were available, aspirin reduced risk of cancer of the proximal colon (incidence–0.45, 0.28–0.74, $p = 0.001$; mortality–0.34, 0.18–0.66, $p = 0.001$), but not the distal colon (1.10, 0.73–1.64, $p = 0.66$; 1.21, 0.66–2.24, $p = 0.54$): difference–$p = 0.04$ for incidence, $p = 0.01$ for mortality (Fig. 4). Benefit increased with scheduled duration of trial treatment (Rothwell et al. 2010). After scheduled treatment for $\geq$5 years (Fig. 4), aspirin reduced risk of proximal colon cancer by about 70 % (incidence–0.35, 0.20–0.63; mortality–0.24, 0.11–0.52, both $p < 0.0001$) and also reduced risk of rectal cancer (incidence–0.58, 0.36–0.92, $p = 0.02$; mortality–0.47, 0.26–0.87, $p = 0.01$). Results were consistent across trials, with no increase in benefit at doses of aspirin above 75 mg daily, and an absolute reduction in 20-year risk of any fatal colorectal cancer after 5 year's scheduled treatment with 75–300 mg daily of 1.76 % (0.61–2.91, $p = 0.001$). However, there was a trend towards a higher risk of fatal colorectal cancer on 30 versus 283 mg daily on long-term follow-up of the Dutch TIA trial (OR = 2.02, 0.70–6.05, $p = 0.15$) (Rothwell et al. 2010).

The finding of greater effects of aspirin on cancers of the proximal colon versus distal colon and rectum was unexpected and may simply be due to chance. Most observational studies have found no consistent differences in associations among aspirin use and risks of colon cancer versus rectal cancer, and reports of differences in effect by site of colon cancer have been inconsistent (Flossmann and Rothwell 2007). However, the only randomised trial of aspirin in prevention of recurrent adenomas to report results by site did report a 40–50 % reduction in

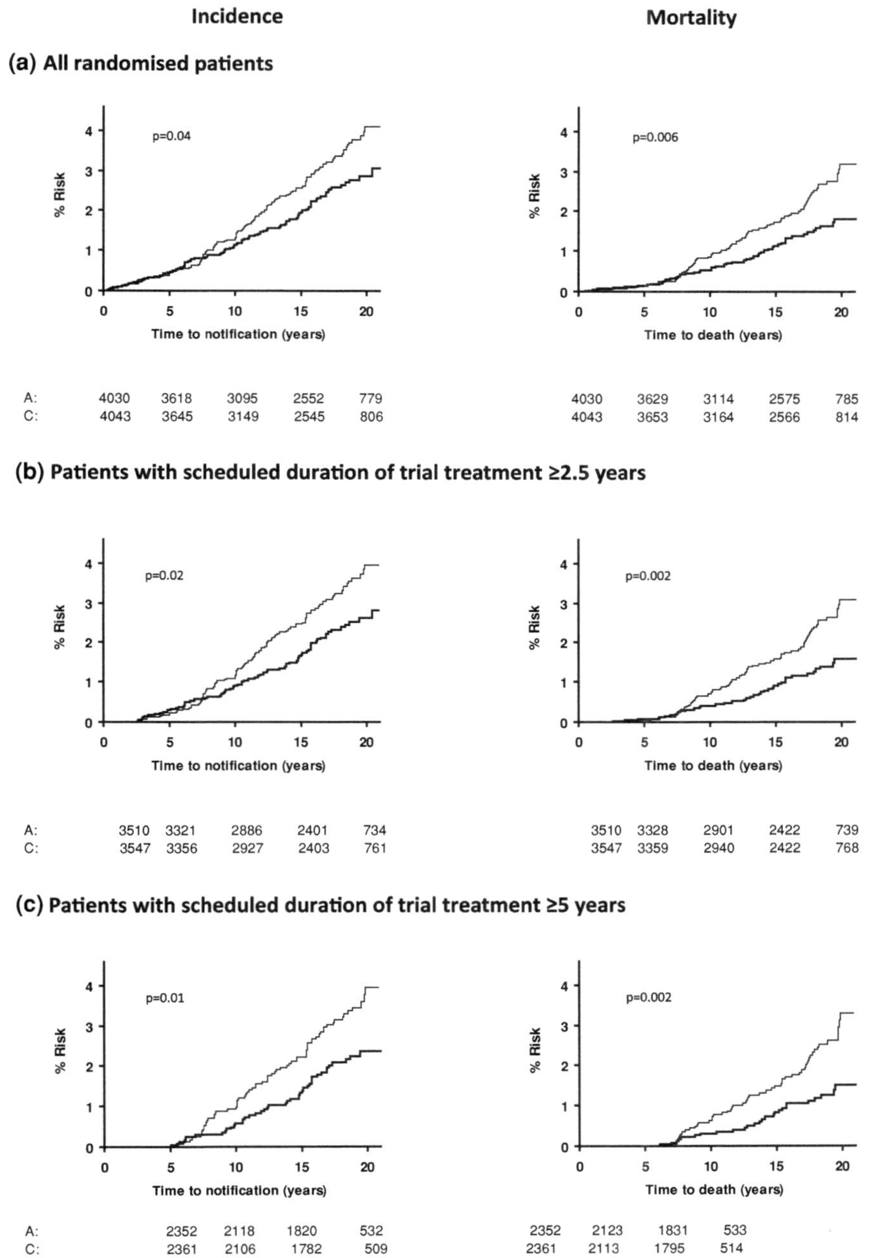


**Fig. 3** Pooled analysis of the effect of aspirin (*thick line*) versus control (*thin line*) on subsequent incidence and mortality due to colorectal cancer in all randomised patients (**a**) in three trials of low-dose (75–300 mg daily) aspirin versus placebo, in those with scheduled duration of trial treatment $\geq$2.5 years (**b**), and in those with scheduled duration of trial treatment $\geq$5 years (**c**) (Rothwell et al. 2010). **a** All randomised patients. **b** Patients with scheduled duration of trial treatment $\geq$2.5 years

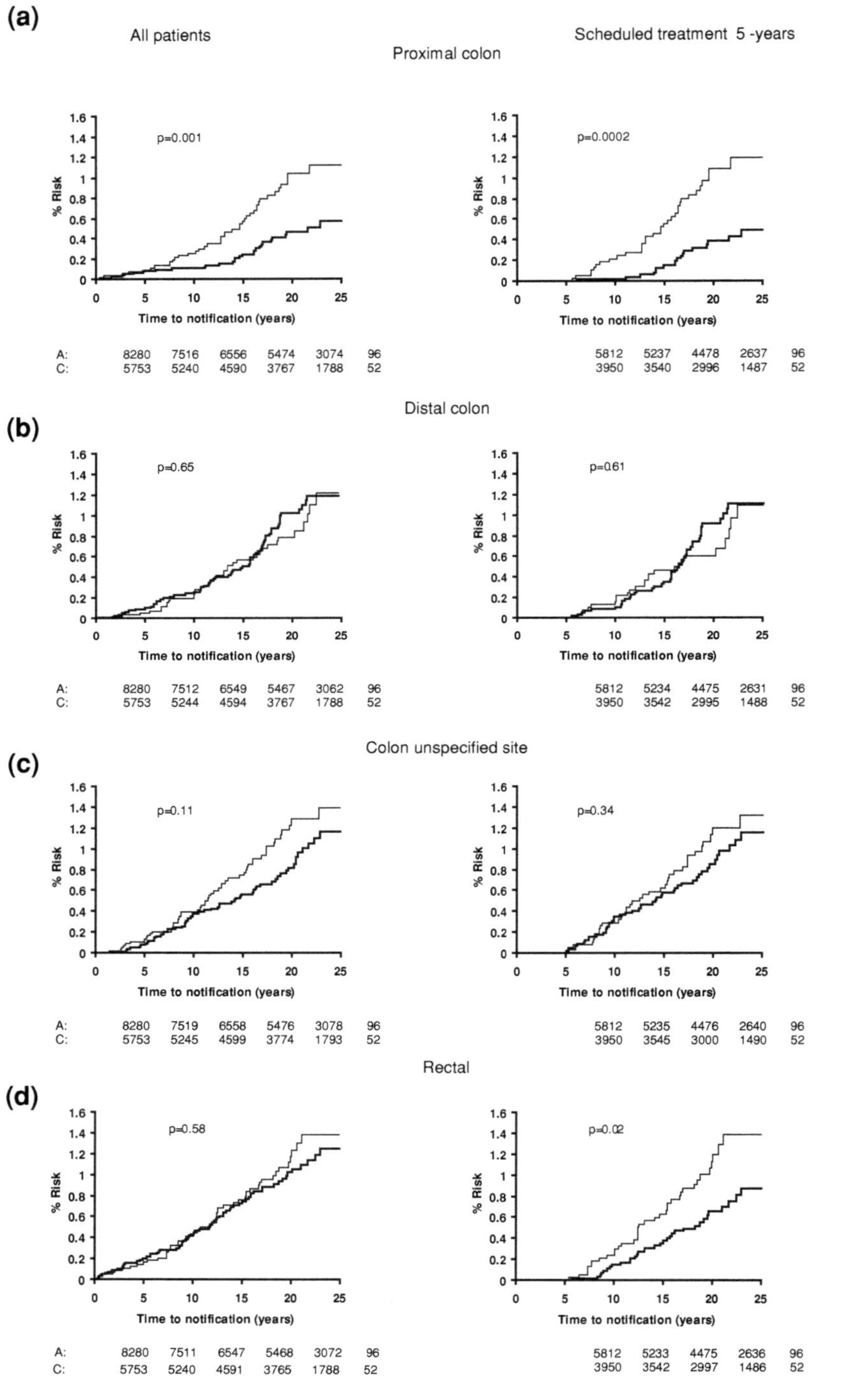


**Fig. 4** Pooled analysis of the effect of aspirin (75–1,200 mg; *thick line*) versus control (*thin line*) on incidence of colorectal cancer by site during and after four randomised patients (Rothwell et al. 2010). **a** Proximal colon. **b** Distal colon. **c** Colon unspecified site. **d** Rectal

proximal colonic adenomas with aspirin and no reduction in distal adenomas (Wallace et al. 2009), and in the analysis of randomised trials of aspirin by Rothwell et al. (2010), the difference in effect of aspirin between proximal and distal colon cancers was statistically significant for both incidence and mortality, was present at all doses of aspirin and consistent in all four trials of aspirin versus control. Moreover, differences in effects of other treatments on proximal versus distal colon tumours are widely accepted (Elsaleh et al. 2000), and there are many differences in normal physiology between the proximal and distal colon (Bufill 1990; Iacopetta 2002), due partly to their different embryological origins and in risk factors for cancers in the two sites, in mechanisms of carcinogenesis, and in the molecular and genetic characteristics of the cancers (Bufill 1990; Iacopetta 2002; Birkenkamp-Demtroder et al. 2005; Yamauchi et al. 2012; Leopoldo et al. 2008), Of potential relevance, expression of COX-2 tends to be greater in tumours of the distal colon and rectum than in tumours of the proximal colon (Birkenkamp-Demtroder et al. 2005; Chapple et al. 2000; Nasir et al. 2004), aspirin, therefore, perhaps achieves less complete inhibition of COX-2 in distal tumours. Follow-up of other aspirin trial cohorts should provide more evidence of the relative effects on proximal versus distal cancers. Irrespective of this, the proven prevention of proximal colonic cancers by aspirin, which would not be identified by sigmoidoscopy and which are often missed on colonoscopy (Singh et al. 2010; Brenner et al. 2010), is clearly important, and suggests that these two approaches to prevention of colorectal cancer may be synergistic.

## 3 Effects on Other Cancers

Thus, the evidence that daily aspirin is effective in the long-term primary prevention of sporadic colorectal cancer is now strong, and is supported by the randomised evidence of a similar effect of aspirin in the high-risk patient group with Lynch syndrome, a hereditary form of colorectal cancer. (see Chap. 9). However, the effect of aspirin on risk of colorectal cancer cannot be interpreted in isolation. Several lines of evidence suggest that aspirin might also reduce risk of other cancers, particularly other cancers of the gastrointestinal (GI) tract (Bosetti et al. 2009; Cuzick et al. 2009; Elwood et al. 2009). A recent study, therefore, analysed individual patient data from all randomised trials of daily aspirin versus control in prevention of vascular events with mean duration of scheduled trial treatment of $\geq 4$ years to determine the effect of allocation to aspirin on the overall risk of cancer death during the trials (Rothwell et al. 2011). In eight eligible trials (25,570 patients; 674 cancer deaths), allocation to aspirin reduced death due to any cancer (pooled OR = 0.79, 0.68–0.92, $p = 0.003$). On analysis of individual patient data (Rothwell et al. 2011), available from seven trials (657 cancer deaths in 23,535 patients), death due to cancer was unaffected during the first 5 year's follow-up, but was reduced during the subsequent 2–3 years of trial follow-up (all cancers −0.66, 0.50–0.87; GI cancers–0.46, 0.27–0.77; both $p = 0.003$). The numbers of cancers were too small to allow reliable conclusions to be drawn about effects on individual primary cancers, but reductions in mortality appeared to be similar for most GI cancers.

In the same study (Rothwell et al. 2011), the effect of aspirin on mortality due to all cancers was also determined in the three large UK trials in which the long-term effects of aspirin on colorectal cancer had been studied previously (Farrell et al. 1991; Medical Research Council's General Practice Research Framework 1998; Peto et al. 1988). In a pooled analysis of individual patient data from the three trials, the 20-year risk of cancer death (1,634 deaths in 12,673 patients in three trials) was reduced in the aspirin groups (all solid cancers—0.80, 0.72–0.88, $p < 0.0001$; GI cancers—0.65, 0.54–0.78, $p < 0.0001$), with benefit increasing (interaction—$p = 0.01$) with scheduled duration of trial treatment ($\geq$7.5 years: all solid cancers—0.69, 0.54–0.88, $p = 0.003$; GI cancers—0.41, 0.26–0.66, $p = 0.0001$). The latent period prior to an effect on deaths was about 5 years for oesophageal cancer and lung cancer, but was more delayed for stomach, colorectal and prostate cancer (Fig. 5; Rothwell et al. 2011). For lung and oesophageal cancer benefit was confined to adenocarcinomas, and the overall effect on 20-year risk of cancer death was greatest for adenocarcinomas (0.66, 0.56–0.77, $p < 0.0001$). Benefit was unrelated to aspirin dose (75 mg upwards), sex or smoking, but increased with age, the absolute reduction in 20-year risk of cancer death reaching 7.08 % (2.42–11.74) at age $\geq$65 years (Rothwell et al. 2011).

Thus, daily aspirin reduced deaths due to several common cancers during and after these trials of aspirin versus control in prevention of vascular events. Benefit increased with duration of treatment and was consistent across the different study populations. However, several questions remained. First, to maximise the potential to detect an effect, the recent analysis of effects of aspirin on all cancer deaths was limited to trials with a mean duration of scheduled treatment $\geq$4 years (Rothwell et al. 2011), limiting statistical power to detect earlier effects on in-trial deaths. Second, the effect of aspirin on cancer incidence was not determined. Third, the two largest trials studied included only men and no data were reported on the effects of aspirin on the risk of cancer in women (Rothwell et al. 2011). Fourth, the key clinical question, the overall balance of risk and benefit of daily low-dose aspirin in primary prevention, was not addressed. Finally, given the need to inform decisions about long-term use of aspirin in prevention of cancer, the evolution of risks and benefits with prolonged use must be determined.

A further report of data from all randomised controlled trials (RCT) of aspirin versus control, irrespective of duration, therefore addressed these areas of uncertainty (Rothwell et al. 2012). To increase reliability of estimates of early effects on cancer death, all known trials of daily aspirin versus control were included. To reduce biases due to selective availability of data or misclassification of cause of death, data on all non-vascular deaths were also analysed. To determine the effect of aspirin on cancer incidence, individual patient data from all trials of daily low-dose aspirin in primary prevention were studied, also looking separately at effects in women. To estimate the likely balance of risk and benefit with prolonged use of aspirin, the time course of effects on cancer incidence, major vascular events and major extracranial bleeds was determined.

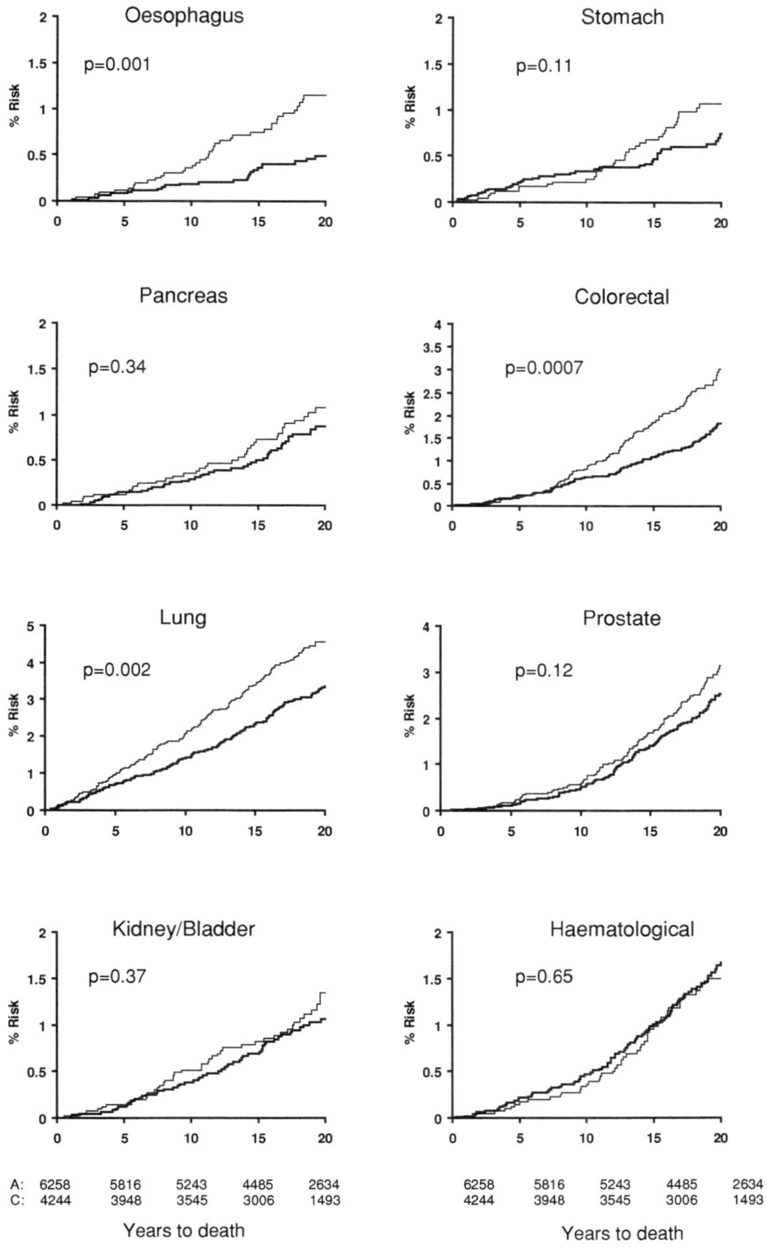


**Fig. 5** Effect of allocation to aspirin (*thick line*) versus control (*thin line*) on the 20-year risk of death due to the most common fatal cancers in the three trials with long-term follow-up (Rothwell et al. 2011). The eight most common cancers are shown and analysis is limited to patients with scheduled duration of trial treatment $\geq 5$ years

**Table 3** Meta-analysis of the effect of aspirin on cancer deaths in 51 trials (77,549 participants) of aspirin versus control in prevention of vascular events stratified by period of follow-up (Rothwell et al. 2012)

| | Number of deaths | | | |
|---|---|---|---|---|
| Years to death | Aspirin | Control | Odds ratio (95% CI) | P |
| *Cancer death only*[a] | | | | |
| 0–2.99 | 292 | 325 | 0.90 (0.76–1.06) | 0.18 |
| 3–4.99 | 161 | 173 | 0.93 (0.75–1.16) | 0.51 |
| ≥5 | 92 | 145 | 0.63 (0.49–0.82) | 0.0005 |
| Unknown | 17 | 21 | | |
| Total | 562 | 664 | 0.85 (0.76–0.96) | 0.008 |
| *Cancer death or non-vascular deaths if cancer data were unavailable*[b] | | | | |
| 0–2.99 | 322 | 364 | 0.88 (0.76–1.03) | 0.10 |
| 3–4.99 | 161 | 173 | 0.93 (0.75–1.16) | 0.51 |
| ≥5 | 92 | 145 | 0.63 (0.49–0.82) | 0.0005 |
| Unknown | 39 | 46 | | |
| Total | 614 | 728 | 0.85 (0.76–0.95) | 0.005 |

[a] Cancer deaths available from 34 trials of aspirin versus control (69,224 participants)
[b] Cancer deaths were unavailable from 17 small trials (8,325 patients). All non-vascular deaths from these trials were, therefore, added to the data on cancer deaths from the other trials

Allocation to daily aspirin reduced deaths due to cancer during the 34 trials (69,224 participants) in which data were available (562 vs. 664, OR = 0.85, 95 % CI 0.76–0.96, $p = 0.008$, Table 3), particularly from 5 years onwards (92 vs. 145; 0.63, 0.49–0.82, $p = 0.0005$), resulting in fewer non-vascular deaths overall (1,021 vs. 1,173; OR = 0.88, 0.78–0.96, $p = 0.003$) in all 51 eligible trials (77,549 participants) (Rothwell et al. 2012). Numbers of deaths due to individual primary cancers were small, but allocation to aspirin did reduce deaths due to colorectal cancer (38 vs. 65, 0.58, 0.38–0.89, $p = 0.008$) and lymphoma (14 vs. 27, 0.52, 0.26–1.00, $p = 0.04$) and tended to reduce deaths due to female reproductive cancers (24 vs. 39; 0.61, 0.36–1.05, $p = 0.058$). In the six trials of daily low-dose aspirin in primary prevention (35,535 participants), aspirin reduced cancer incidence from 3 years onwards (324 vs. 421; 0.76, 0.66–0.88, $p = 0.0003$) in women (132 vs. 176; 0.75, 0.59–0.94, $p = 0.01$) and in men (192 vs. 245; 0.77, 0.63–0.93, $p = 0.008$) (Rothwell et al. 2012).

It is important to note that the aspirin trials included in the analyses reviewed above did not generally include cancer as a primary outcome (Rothwell et al. 2012). However, cancer deaths were recorded in the majority of trials and attribution of cause of death was blinded to treatment allocation. Attribution was usually based on death certification, supported by clinical records, which has been shown to agree well with expert committee review (Ederer et al. 1999; Robinson et al. 2000). In the trials of daily low-dose aspirin in primary prevention, data on non-fatal cancers were derived mainly from patient-reported diagnosis at face-to-face follow-up, usually supported by review of medical records. Post-trial follow-up of the UK trials was based on cancer registration and death certification, which results in very high rates of ascertainment and accuracy for cancer in general (Brewster et al. 2002; Hawkins et al. 1992) and for colorectal cancer specifically (Brewster et al. 1995; Pollock and Vickers 1995).

## 4 Overall Balance of Risk and Benefit

It is, of course, important to consider the effects of aspirin on short and long-term risks of cancer in the context of other effects of treatment, most importantly the reduction in risk of ischaemic vascular events and the increase in risk of bleeding. The most frequently reported serious adverse event associated with regular aspirin use is GI bleeding, with an approximate doubling in risk major GI bleeding associated with use of low-dose aspirin (Weil et al. 1995; Garcia Rodriguez et al. 2001; Antithrombotic Trialists' (ATT) Collaboration 2009). Among individuals without risk factors for GI bleeding (e.g. history of prior ulcer, advanced age), this translates into 1–2 additional GI bleeds per 1,000 patient-years (Antithrombotic Trialists' (ATT) Collaboration 2009). The equivalent excess risk of intracranial bleeds is about 1 per 10,000 patient-years (He et al. 1998; Gorelick and Weisman 2005) and is offset even in primary prevention by the reduction in risk of ischaemic stroke (Patrono et al. 2005; Antithrombotic Trialists' (ATT) Collaboration 2009). The risk of GI bleeding can be reduced by co-prescription of a proton-pump inhibitor (Lai et al. 2002; Chan et al. 2005a, b) and treatment to eradicate H. pylori infection (Lanas et al. 2002), although no large trials of aspirin in prevention of vascular events have tested the impact of such interventions.

Despite the risk of bleeding on aspirin, the overall balance of risk and benefit clearly favours treatment in patients with prior vascular events (secondary prevention), but is less clear-cut in primary prevention (Patrono et al. 2005; Antithrombotic Trialists' (ATT) Collaboration 2009). However, meta analyses carried out without regard to duration study and period of follow-up will be of limited value in informing estimates of the long-term balance of risks and benefits. Given the need to inform decisions about long-term use of aspirin in primary prevention, it is crucial to understand how the effects of aspirin on each of the key outcomes evolves with duration of treatment. In the above study of individual patient data from the six trials of daily aspirin in primary prevention of vascular events (Rothwell et al. 2012), the effects of aspirin on risk of major vascular events, incident cancer and major extracranial bleeds did indeed alter with increasing duration of treatment (Fig. 6). In contrast to cancer incidence, for which the effect of aspirin increased with duration of trial follow-up, effects on major vascular events and major extracranial bleeding diminished over time. The reduced risk of

| | Events / Subjects: Aspirin | Events / Subjects: Control | Odds Ratio | 95% CI | ARR / 1000 / yr | Interaction |
|---|---|---|---|---|---|---|
| **Cancers** | | | | | | |
| 0-2.9 years | 445 / 17745 | 442 / 17790 | 1.01 | 0.88-1.15 | -0.06 | |
| 3-4.9 years | 193 / 16463 | 237 / 16484 | 0.81 | 0.67-0.98 | 2.19 | p=0.04 |
| >5 years | 131 / 4444 | 184 / 4460 | 0.70 | 0.56-0.88 | 4.8 | |
| **Major Vascular Events** | | | | | | |
| 0-2.9 years | 481 / 17745 | 586 / 17790 | 0.82 | 0.72-0.92 | 2.04 | |
| 3-4.9 years | 241 / 16477 | 239 / 16402 | 1.00 | 0.84-1.20 | -0.1 | p=0.07 |
| >5 years | 153 / 4404 | 164 / 4393 | 0.93 | 0.74-1.16 | 0.99 | |
| **Major Extracranial Bleeds** | | | | | | |
| 0-2.9 years | 142 / 17745 | 73 / 17790 | 1.95 | 1.47-2.59 | -1.33 | |
| 3-4.9 years | 45 / 16655 | 33 / 16733 | 1.37 | 0.87-2.14 | -0.59 | |
| >5 years | 16 / 4595 | 26 / 4648 | 0.63 | 0.34-1.16 | 0.96 | p=0.003 |

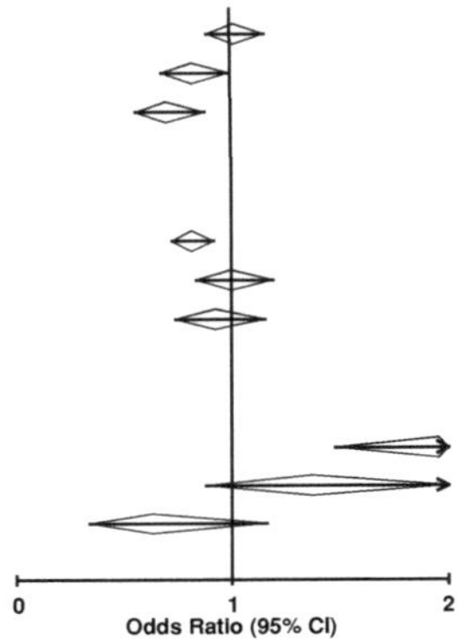


**Fig. 6** Summary meta analyses of the effect of aspirin on risks of incident cancer, major vascular events and major extracranial bleeds during six randomised trials of daily low-dose aspirin versus control in primary prevention of vascular events stratified by period of trial follow-up (0–2.9; 3–4.9; ≥5 years). Data derived from Rothwell et al. (2012). The number of subjects at the start of each period is based on the number of individuals surviving free of the relevant outcome event at the start of the period, such that only first events of each type are included ARR is absolute reduction in risk per 1,000 participants per year. The statistical significance of the interaction between the treatment effect and the period of follow-up is derived from a Cox model in which the time is included as a continuous variable

major vascular events on aspirin was initially offset by an increased risk of major bleeding, but effects of aspirin on both of these outcomes diminished with increasing follow-up (Rothwell et al. 2012), leaving only the reduced risk of cancer (absolute reduction = 3.13, 1.44–4.82, per 1,000 patients/year) from 3 years onwards (Fig. 6). The interaction between time from randomisation and the effect of allocation to aspirin was statistically significant for incident cancer ($p = 0.04$) and for major extracranial bleeds ($p = 0.003$), but not for major vascular events ($p = 0.07$). When analysis was restricted to individuals who remained on allocated trial treatment up until the event the time course of effect of aspirin was similar for risk of major extracranial bleeds ($p = 0.04$) and stronger for major vascular events ($p = 0.03$) (Rothwell et al. 2012).

Also of note from the analysis of the six primary prevention trials (Rothwell et al. 2012) is that the proportion of major extracranial bleeds that were fatal was lower in patients allocated to aspirin versus placebo (8/203 vs. 15/132; OR = 0.32, 0.12–0.83, $p = 0.009$) and this difference remained when analysis was restricted to individuals who were still on allocated trial treatment at the time of the bleed (8/178 vs. 12/97; 0.33, 0.12–0.92, $p = 0.016$). Thus, aspirin undoubtedly increases the risk of non-fatal extracranial bleeds, at least for the first few years of treatment, but does not increase the risk of fatal bleeds.

Analysis of the overall balance of risk and benefit during the six trials showed that aspirin reduced the risk of the composite outcome of major vascular events, cancer or fatal extracranial bleeds (HR $= 0.88$, 0.82–0.94, $p = 0.0002$) and benefit remained when non-fatal extracranial bleeds were added (0.92, 0.86–0.98, $p = 0.01$) (Rothwell et al. 2012). However, such analyses of composite outcomes are simplistic. Many people would consider a non-fatal GI bleed to be less serious, for example, than a stroke or a cancer. Analyses based on disability and death would be preferable, but disability data were not collected in the previous trials (although the ongoing ASPREE trial is collecting disability data). Moreover, analyses should also include the delayed long-term benefit of aspirin in prevention of post-trial colorectal cancer and other cancers (Rothwell et al. 2010, 2011).

## 5 Summary and Outstanding Issues

The reports of the trials of aspirin reviewed above have shown that aspirin (75–325 mg/day for 3 years) reduces the risk of any recurrent colorectal adenoma by 17 % and advanced adenoma by 28 % (Cole et al. 2009) and that use of aspirin for about 5 years reduces incidence and mortality due to colorectal cancer by 30–40 % after 20 years of follow-up (Rothwell et al. 2010), and reduces all-cause cancer mortality by about 20 % (Rothwell et al. 2011). The decline in risk of major bleeds with prolonged use of aspirin in primary prevention (Rothwell et al. 2012) suggests that the balance of risk and benefit will increasingly favour the use of daily aspirin in prevention of cancer with increasing duration of treatment.

It is important to note, however, that these findings only apply to use of daily aspirin. The Women's Health Study, a trial of aspirin 100 mg alternate-days versus control, did not show a reduction in cancer incidence (Cook et al. 2005) and the other large trial of alternate-day aspirin (aspirin 325 mg/every other day; Physicians Health Study–PHS) did not report reductions in cancer death or non-vascular death during the trials and found no reduction in incidence of colorectal cancer at 10 years follow-up (Gann et al. 1993): relative risk of colorectal cancer was 1.03 (95 % CI, 0.83–1.28) in the PHS and 0.97 (95 % CI, 0.77–1.24) in the WHS. Both trials were large (39,876 healthy women in WHS and 22,071 healthy male physicians in PHS) and were, therefore, reasonably well powered to detect effects of aspirin on cancer risk. It is possible that alternate-day dosing may be less effective than daily dosing in inhibiting carcinogenesis, or that the 10-year duration of follow-up reported so far in both the PHS and WHS studies may have been insufficient to detect a difference in colorectal cancer incidence. Analyses of longer-term follow-up of WHS will be published in 2012.

Because the adverse effects of aspirin are to some extent dose-related as noted above, the lowest effective dose required for colorectal cancer prevention remains an important question. In prevention of cardiovascular events, 75–81 mg aspirin daily appears as effective as higher doses. The trials reviewed above showed that 75 mg daily also appears to be as effective in prevention of cancer as high doses, but further data are required on the possible effects of alternate-day aspirin. The trials of aspirin in prevention of recurrent adenoma also showed that there appeared to be little difference in effect within the range of doses studied (81–325 mg daily). Data on dose–response from observational studies are limited and most analyses that have been published have not been stratified by duration of use (Flossmann and Rothwell 2007), which is also crucial given the latent period before an effect of aspirin can be expected.

Insights into the mechanism of action of aspirin in prevention of cancer can also be gained from looking at effects in relation to the formulation of the tablets as well as the dose. For example, the slow-release formulation of aspirin 75 mg daily used in the Thrombosis Prevention Trial (Medical Research Council's General Practice Research Framework 1998) was designed to inhibit platelet function only in the portal venous system and had very little systemic bioavailability due to almost complete de-acetylation on first pass through the liver (Charman et al. 1993). Yet, the long-term reductions in risk of colorectal cancer and other cancers were similar in TPT to those in trials of higher doses of aspirin with more rapid release (Rothwell et al. 2010, 2011). This observation raises the possibility that the effect of aspirin on cancer incidence is mediated via an effect on platelets rather than via a direct effect of aspirin in tumour tissue (see Chap. 2). It follows that other antiplatelet drugs may have similar effects on cancer incidence and that combinations of antiplatelet drugs might be of greater benefit. However, there are no published data on the effects of other antiplatelet drugs on the risk of colorectal cancer and follow-up in trials of combination antiplatelet treatment in prevention of vascular events has been too short to allow any such effects to be studied.

It is important to note that even the combination of the early and late effects of aspirin on cancer death reviewed above will still have only a relatively small impact on all-cause mortality, at least when taken for only about 5 years, as in previous trials (Rothwell et al. 2010, 2011). In a population in which cancer causes 30 % of all deaths; for example, a 20 % relative reduction in 20-year risk of death due to cancer would delay death (people will, of course, die of other causes) in only about 6 % of the population. However, the relative reduction in 20-year risk of cancer death increased with longer duration of trial treatment (Rothwell et al. 2011), reaching a 30 % reduction in patients with scheduled trial treatment of 7.5–10 years. Moreover, these results may well underestimate the benefit that would result from long-term treatment (e.g. from age 50–75 years). Indeed, a late rebound in cancer deaths in the aspirin groups was observed at 10–20 years follow-up of the aspirin trials is clearly present for some cancers (Rothwell et al. 2011).

Overall, the data reviewed above suggest that the benefits of such long-term use of low-dose aspirin may exceed the risks of adverse effects of aspirin. It is possible that the benefits of aspirin use may also exceed those of other established preventive initiatives such as screening for breast or prostate cancer. The balance of risk and benefit may also be increased by efforts to reduce bleeding complications, such as co-prescription of a proton-pump inhibitor (Lai et al. 2002; Chan et al. 2005b) and treatment to eradicate H. pylori infection (Lanas et al. 2002), and by further development of potentially more effective derivatives of aspirin (McIlhatton et al. 2007), or by combination with other drugs. Current recommendations do not support the routine use of aspirin for prevention of colorectal cancer (Cuzick et al. 2009), but the new data from RCTs that have been reported over the last couple of years necessitate an update of clinical guidelines.

## References

Antithrombotic Trialists' (ATT) Collaboration, Baigent C, Blackwell L, Collins R, Emberson J, Godwin J et al (2009) Aspirin in the primary and secondary prevention of vascular disease: collaborative meta-analysis of individual participant data from randomised trials. Lancet 373:1849–1860

Atkin WS, Edwards R, Ines K-H, Wooldrage K, Hart AR et al (2010) Once-only flexible sigmoidoscopy in prevention of colorectal cancer: a multicentre randomised controlled trial. Lancet 375:1624–1633

Baron JA, Cole BF, Sandler RS, Haile RW, Ahnen D, Bresalier R, McKeown-Eyssen G, Summers RW, Rothstein R, Burke CA, Snover DC, Church TR, Allen JI, Beach M, Beck GJ, Bond JH, Byers T, Greenberg ER, Mandel JS, Marcon N, Mott LA, Pearson L, Saibil F, van Stolk RU (2003) A randomized trial of aspirin to prevent colorectal adenomas. N Engl J Med 348:891–899

Benamouzig R, Deyra J, Martin A, Girard B, Jullian E, Piednoir B, Couturier D, Coste T, Little J, Chaussade S (2003) Daily soluble aspirin and prevention of colorectal adenoma recurrence: one-year results of the APACC trial. Gastroenterology 125:328–336

Birkenkamp-Demtroder K, Olsen SH, Sorensen FB, Laurberg S et al (2005) Differential gene expression in colon cancer of the caecum versus the sigmoid and rectosigmoid. Gut 54:374–384

Bosetti C, Gallus S, La Vecchia C (2009) Aspirin and cancer risk: a summary review to 2007. Recent Results Cancer Res 181:231–251

Brenner H, Hoffmeister M, Arndt V, Stegmaier C, Altenhofen L, Haug U (2010) Protection from right- and left-sided colorectal neoplasms after colonoscopy: population-based study. J Natl Cancer Inst 102(2):89–95

Brewster D, Muir C, Crichton J (1995) Registration of colorectal cancer in Scotland: an assessment of data accuracy based on review of medical records. Public Health 109:285–292

Brewster DH, Stockton D, Harvey J, Mackay M (2002) Reliability of cancer registration data in Scotland, 1997. Eur J Cancer 38:414–417

Bufill JA (1990) Colorectal cancer: evidence for distinct genetic categories based on proximal or distal tumour location. Ann Intern Med 113:779–788

Chan AT, Giovannucci EL, Meyerhardt JA, Schernhammer ES, Curhan GC, Fuchs CS (2005a) Long-term use of aspirin and nonsteroidal anti-inflammatory drugs and risk of colorectal cancer. JAMA 2(94):914–923

Chan FK, Ching JY, Hung LC, Wong VW, Leung VK, Kung NN, Hui AJ et al (2005b) Clopidogrel versus aspirin and esomeprazole to prevent recurrent ulcer bleeding. N Engl J Med 352:238–244

Chan AT, Giovannucci EL, Meyerhardt JA, Schernhammer ES, Wu K, Fuchs CS (2008) Aspirin dose and duration of use and risk of colorectal cancer in men. Gastroenterology 134:21–28

Chapple KS, Cartwright EJ, Hawcroft G, Tisbury A, Bonifer C et al (2000) Localisation of cyclooxygenase-2 in human sporadic colorectal adenomas. Am J Pathol 156:545–553

Charman WN, Charman SA, Monkhouse DC, Frisbee SE, Lockhart EA, Weisman S, Fitzgerald GA (1993) Biopharmaceutical characterisation of a low-dose (75 mg) controlled-release aspirin formulation. Br J ClinPharmacol 36:470–473

Cole BF, Logan RF, Halabi S, Benamouzig R, Sandler RS et al (2009) Aspirin for chemoprevention of colorectal adenomas: meta-analysis of the randomised trials. J Natl Cancer Inst 101:256–266

Cook NR, Lee IM, Gaziano JM, Gordon D, Ridker PM, Manson JE, Hennekens CH, Buring JE (2005) Low-dose aspirin in the primary prevention of cancer: the women's health study: a randomized controlled trial. JAMA 294:47–55

Cuzick J, Otto F, Baron JA, Brown PH, Burn J, Greenwald P et al (2009) Aspirin and non-inflammatory drugs for cancer prevention: an international consensus statement. Lancet Oncol 10(5):501–507

Dutch TIA Trial Study Group (1991) A comparison of two doses of aspirin (30 vs. 283 mg a day) in patients after a transient ischemic attack or minor ischemic stroke. N Engl J Med 325:1261–1266

Ederer F, Geisser M, Mongin S, Church T, Mandel J (1999) Colorectal cancer deaths as determined by expert committee and from death certificate. Minnesota Stud J ClinEpidemiol 52:447–452

Elwood PC, Gallagher AM, Duthie GG, Mur LA, Morgan G (2009) Aspirin, salicylates, and cancer. Lancet 373:1301–1309

Elsaleh H, Joseph D, Grieu F, Zeps N, Spry N, Iacopetta B (2000) Association of tumour site and sex with survival benefit from adjuvant chemotherapy in colorectal cancer. Lancet 355:1745–1750

Farrell B, Godwin J, Richards S, Warlow C (1991) The United Kingdom transient ischaemic attack (UK-TIA) aspirin trial: final results. J NeurolNeurosurg Psychiatry 54:1044–1054

Flossmann E (2007) For the British doctors aspirin trial and the UK-TIA aspirin trial. Effect of aspirin on long-term risk of colorectal cancer: consistent evidence from randomised and observational studies. Lancet 369:1603–1613

Gann PH, Manson JE, Glynn RJ, Buring JE, Hennekens CH (1993) Low-dose aspirin and incidence of colorectal tumors in a randomized trial. J Natl Cancer Inst 85:1220–1224

Garcia Rodriguez LA, Hernandez-Diaz S, de Abajo FJ (2001) Association between aspirin and upper gastrointestinal complications: systematic review of epidemiological studies. Br J Pharmacol 52:563–71

Gorelick PB, Weisman SM (2005) Risk of hemorrhagic stroke with aspirin use: an update. Stroke 36:1801–1807

Hawkins MM, Swerdlow AJ (1992) Completeness of cancer and death follow-up obtained through the National health service central register for England and wales. Br J Cancer 66:408–413

He J, Whelton PK, Vu B, Klag MJ (1998) Aspirin and risk of haemorrhagic stroke: a meta-analysis of randomised controlled trials. JAMA 280:1930–1935

Iacopetta B (2002) Are there two sides to colorectal cancer? Int J Cancer 101:403–408

Jacobs EJ, Thun MJ, Bain EB, Rodriguez C, Henley SJ, Calle EE (2007) A large cohort study of long-term daily use of adult-strength aspirin and cancer incidence. J Natl Cancer Inst 99(8):608–615

Kelloff GJ, Schilsky RL, Alberts DS, Day RW, Guyton KZ, Pearce HL, Peck JC, Phillips R, Sigman CC (2004) Colorectal adenomas: a prototype for the use of surrogate end points in the development of cancer prevention drugs. Clin Cancer Res 1(10):3908–3918

Kozuka S, Nogaki M, Ozeki T, Masumori S (1975) Premalignancy of the mucosal polyp in the large intestine: II estimation of the periods required for malignant transformation of mucosal polyps. Dis Colon Rectum 18:494–500

Kune GA, Kune S, Watson LF (1988) Colorectal cancer risk, chronic illnesses, operations, and medications: case control results from the Melbourne colorectal cancer study. Cancer Res 48:4399–4404

Lai KC, Lam SK, Chu KM, Wong BC, Hui WM, Hu WH, Lau GK et al (2002) Lansoprazole for prevention of recurrences of ulcer complications from long-term low-dose aspirin use. NEJM 346:2033–2038

Lanas A, Fuentes J, Benito R, Serrano P, Bajador E, Sainz R (2002) Helicobacter pylori increases the risk of upper gastrointestinal bleeding in patients taking low-dose aspirin. Aliment Pharmacol Ther 16:779–786

Leopoldo S, Lorena B, Cinzia A, Gabriella DC, Angela Luciana B et al (2008) Two types of mucinous adenocarcinoma of the colorectum: clinicopathological and genetic features. Ann Surg Oncol 15:1429–39

Levine JS, Ahnen DJ (2006) Adenomatous polyps of the colon. N Engl J Med 355:2551–2557

Logan RFA, Grainge MJ, Shepherd VC, Armitage NC, Muir KR (2008) Aspirin and folic acid for the prevention of recurrent colorectal adenomas. Gastroenterology 134:29–38

McIlhatton MA, Tyler J, Burkholder S, Ruschoff J, Rigas B, Kopelovich L, Fishel R (2007) Nitric oxide-donating aspirin derivatives suppress microsatellite instability in mismatch repair-deficient and hereditary nonpolyposis colorectal cancer cells. Cancer Res 67:10966–10975

Medical Research Council's General Practice Research Framework (1998) Thrombosis prevention trial: randomised trial of low-intensity oral anticoagulation with warfarin and low-dose aspirin in the primary prevention of ischaemic heart disease in men at increased risk. Lancet 351:233–241

Morson BC (1984) The evolution of colorectal carcinoma. ClinRadiol 35:425–431

Nasir A, Kaiser HE, Boulware D, Hakam A, Zhao H et al (2004) Cyclooxygenase-2 expression in right- and left-sided colon cancer: a rationale for optimisation of cyclooxygenase-2 inhibitor therapy. Clin Colorectal Cancer 3:243–247

Patrono C, García Rodríguez, Landolfi R, Baigent C (2005) Low-dose aspirin for the prevention of atherothrombosis. N Engl J Med 353:2373–2383

Peto R, Gray R, Collins R, Wheatley K, Hennekens C, Jamrozik K, Warlow C, Hafner B, Thompson E, Norton S (1988) Randomised trial of prophylactic daily aspirin in British male doctors. BMJ 296:313–316

Pollock AM, Vickers N (1995) Reliability of data of the thames cancer registry on 673 cases of colorectal cancer: effect of the registration process. Qual Health Care 4:184–189

Rex DK, Johnson DA, Anderson JC, Schoenfeld PS, Burke CA, Inadomi JM (2009) American college of gastroenterology guidelines for colorectal cancer screening 2009 [corrected]. Am J Gastroneterol 104:739–750

Robinson MH, Rodrigues VC, Hardcastle JD, Chamberlain JO, Mangham CM, Moss SM (2000) Faecal occult blood screening for colorectal cancer at Nottingham: details of the verification process. J Med Screen 7:97–98

Rothwell PM, Wilson M, Elwin CE, Norrving B, Algra A, Warlow CP, Meade TW (2010) Long-term effect of aspirin on colorectal cancer incidence and mortality: 20 year follow-up of five randomised trials. Lancet 376: 1741–1750

Rothwell PM, Fowkes GR, Belch JJ, Ogawa H, Warlow CP, Meade TW (2011) Long-term effect of aspirin on deaths due to cancer: pooled analysis of data from randomised controlled trials. Lancet 377:31–41

Rothwell PM, Price JF, Fowkes FG, Zanchetti A, Roncaglioni MC, Tognoni G, Lee R, Belch JF, Wilson M, Mehta Z, Meade TW (2012) Short-term effects of daily aspirin on cancer incidence, mortality and non-vascular death: analysis of the time-course of risks and benefits in 51 randomised controlled trials. Lancet 379:1602–1612

SALT Collaborative Group (1991) Swedish aspirin low-dose trial (SALT) of 75 mg aspirin as secondary prophylaxis after cerebrovascular ischaemic events. Lancet 338:1345–1349

Sandler RS, Halabi S, Baron JA, Budinger S, Paskett E, Keresztes R, Petrelli N, Pipas JM, Karp DD, Loprinzi CL, Steinbach G, Schilsky R (2003) A randomized trial of aspirin to prevent colorectal adenomas in patients with previous colorectal cancer. N Engl J Med 348:883–890

Singh H, Nugent Z, Mahmud SM, Demers AA, Bernstein CN (2010) Predictors of colorectal cancer after negative colonoscopy: a population-based study. Am J Gastroenterol 105(3):663–673

Stürmer T, Glynn RJ, Lee IM, Manson JE, Buring JE, Hennekens CH (1998) Aspirin use and colorectal cancer: post-trial follow-up data from the physicians' health study. Ann Intern Med 128:713–720

Thun MJ, Namboodiri MM, Heath CW (1991) Aspirin use and reduced risk of fatal colon cancer. N Engl J Med 325:1593–1596

Wallace K, Grau MV, Ahnen D, Snover DC, Robertson DJ et al (2009) The association of lifestyle and dietary factors with the risk of serrated polyps of the colorectum. Cancer Epidemiol Biomarkers Prev 18:2310–2317

Weil J, Colin-Jones D, Langman M, Lawson D, Logan R, Murphy M et al (1995) Prophylactic aspirin and risk of peptic ulcer bleeding. BMJ 310:827–830

Weitz J, Koch M, Debus J, Hohler T, Galle PR, Buchler MW (2005) Colorectal cancer. Lancet 365:153–165

Yamauchi M, Morikawa T, Kuchiba A, Imamura Y, Rong Qian Z, Nishihara R, Liao X, Waldron L, Hoshida Y, Huttenhower C, Chan AT, Giovannucci E, Fuchs C, Ogino S (2012) Assessment of colorectal cancer molecular features along bowel subsites challenges the conception of distinct dichotomy of proximal versus distal colorectum Gut. doi: 10.1136/gutjnl-2011-300865

# Nutritional Agents with Anti-Inflammatory Properties in Chemoprevention of Colorectal Neoplasia

Mark A. Hull

**Abstract**

The strong link between inflammation and colorectal carcinogenesis provides the rationale for using anti-inflammatory agents for chemoprevention of colorectal cancer (CRC). Several naturally occurring substances with anti-inflammatory properties, used in a purified 'nutraceutical' form, including omega-3 polyunsaturated fatty acids (PUFAs) such as eicosapentaenoic acid (EPA) and polyphenols such as curcumin and resveratrol, have been demonstrated to have anti-CRC activity in preclinical models. As expected, these agents have an excellent safety and tolerability profile in Phase II clinical trials. Phase III randomized clinical trials of these naturally occurring substances are now beginning to be reported. The omega-3 polyunsaturated fatty acid EPA, in the free fatty acid (FFA) form, has been demonstrated to reduce adenomatous polyp number and size in patients with familial adenomatous polyposis (FAP), a finding which has prompted evaluation of this formulation of EPA for prevention of 'sporadic' colorectal neoplasia. Anti-inflammatory 'nutraceuticals' require further clinical evaluation in polyp prevention trials as they exhibit many of the characteristics of the ideal cancer chemoprevention agent, including safety, tolerability and patient acceptability.

M. A. Hull (✉)
Section of Molecular Gastroenterology, Leeds Institute of Molecular Medicine,
St James's University Hospital, Beckett Street Leeds, West Yorkshire LS9 7TF, UK
e-mail: M.A.Hull@leeds.ac.uk

A. T. Chan and E. Detering (eds.), *Prospects for Chemoprevention of Colorectal Neoplasia*,
Recent Results in Cancer Research 191, DOI: 10.1007/978-3-642-30331-9_8,

## Contents



# 1 Naturally Occurring Substances Used as Pharmaceutical Preparations—'Nutraceuticals'

Man has probably always used naturally occurring substances for medicinal purposes. The analgesic and anti-pyretic properties of willow tree (Salix) bark extract, which were described as far back as the classical ancient civilisations of Rome, Greece, and Egypt, are now believed to be, at least partly, explained by the anti-inflammatory activity of salicin, a $\beta$-glucoside moiety that is metabolised to salicylic acid (the direct metabolite of acetyl-salicylic acid, also known as aspirin) (Vlachojannis et al. 2011).

However, the isolation and purification of specific substances, found in foodstuffs, as pharmaceutical preparations is a relatively new phenomenon, for which the term *nutraceutical* was coined and originally defined as 'a food (or part of a food) that provides medical or health benefits, including the prevention and/or treatment of a disease' (Kalra 2003). More recently, Kalra refined the definition of *nutraceutical* as 'a functional food that aids in the prevention and/or treatment of disease and/or a disorder', in order to distinguish it from the terms dietary supplement or functional food (Kalra 2003). In practice, the use of the above terms remains interchangeable and I will use the term nutraceutical to cover all use of naturally occurring food components for prevention or treatment of CRC, for the purposes of this review. Several nutraceuticals have already been investigated for potential anti-CRC activity in epidemiological, experimental and clinical studies, including folic acid, calcium and micronutrient anti-oxidants such as vitamin E and selenium (WCRF 2007). Other nutraceutical preparations have predominant anti-inflammatory activity and also appear to have efficacy in in vitro and rodent models of CRC, including certain omega ($\omega$)-3 PUFAs, polyphenols and flavonoids. This review will be restricted to discussion of those natural agents that have *combined* anti-inflammatory and anti-CRC activity.

## 2 Anti-inflammatory Agents for Prevention and Treatment of CRC

The link between inflammation and carcinogenesis, particularly in the gastrointestinal tract, is long established (Balkwill and Mantovani 2010). Duration and activity of ulcerative colitis and Crohn's disease are risk factors for development of colorectal epithelial cell dysplasia and CRC (Ullman and Itzkowitz 2011). More recently, the concept that so-called 'sporadic' colorectal carcinogenesis, occurring in the absence of overt colitis, is intimately linked to pro-inflammatory signalling in epithelial and stromal cell compartments of the colorectal adenoma and CRC has become established (Ben-Neriah and Karin 2011). Combined pro-inflammatory and pro-tumorigenic activity is recognised in a large number of cytokines (e.g. interleukin-6, tumour necrosis factor $\alpha$, macrophage migration inhibitory factor; Klampfer 2011), chemokines (CCL2, MCP-1; Popovinova et al. 2009), inflammatory mediators (prostaglandins, NO; Wang and DuBois 2010), as well as transcription factors including nuclear factor $\kappa B$ (Ben-Neriah and Karin 2011) and signal transducer and activator of transcription (STAT) factors (Klampfer 2011).

The evidence that non-steroidal anti-inflammatory drugs (NSAIDs), including aspirin, have anti-CRC activity is overwhelming and is the subject of in-depth review elsewhere in this volume. However, uncertainty regarding the benefit-risk ratio for individuals at different risk of future CRC has limited their clinical evaluation and use to date. In parallel, these concerns have driven study of naturally occurring anti-inflammatory agents, which may have an enhanced safety and tolerability profile, even when administered in 'pharmacological' amounts, compared with synthetic NSAIDs.

## 3 Anti-inflammatory Nutraceuticals with Evidence of Anti-CRC Activity

### 3.1 Omega-3 PUFAs

Omega ($\omega$)-3 PUFAs are naturally occurring long-chain fatty acids. The two main $\omega$-3 PUFAs, C20:5$\omega$3 EPA and C22:6$\omega$3 docosahexaenoic acid (DHA), are predominantly found in oily fish, such as salmon, mackerel and sardines, but are also widely available (usually together as a fish oil preparation) on prescription or 'over-the-counter'.

Fish oil preparations are believed to have several health benefits (Wall et al. 2010). There is evidence that $\omega$-3 PUFAs have anti-inflammatory efficacy in rheumatological conditions (Bhangle and Kolasinski 2011). Omega-3 PUFA intake may also improve cardiovascular outcomes, although recent randomised trials have questioned cardiovascular benefits in certain patient subgroups (De Caterina 2011).

### 3.1.1 Anti-CRC Activity of ω-3 PUFAs

There is now emerging evidence that ω-3 PUFAs have anti-CRC activity. This subject has been reviewed in detail recently (Cockbain et al. 2011). In general, epidemiological data do not support a convincing link between dietary ω-3 PUFA exposure and reduced CRC incidence. In contrast, anti-neoplastic activity of ω-3 PUFA supplementation has been observed consistently in animal models of colorectal carcinogenesis.

#### Observational Evidence that ω-3 PUFAs Prevent CRC

The available observational evidence on the effect of ω-3 PUFA exposure on CRC risk has been summarised and interpreted in detail in the second expert report (SER) of the World Cancer Research Fund and American Institute for Cancer Research (World Cancer Research Fund/American Institute for Cancer Research 2007), which has recently been updated as part of the continuous update project (CUP) of these organisations (WCRF 2011). The 2011 CUP states that there is only limited, suggestive evidence for the beneficial effects of fish intake on future CRC risk (WCRF 2011).

The most recent systematic review of prospective cohort studies of estimated ω-3 PUFA consumption and risk of several cancers identified 38 reports on the association between ω-3 PUFA intake and incidence of 11 types of cancer (MacLean et al. 2006). Nine studies of CRC risk from seven different cohorts were identified but only one demonstrated a statistically significant reduction in CRC risk in the highest ω-3 PUFA intake category compared with the lowest (MacLean et al. 2006).

To date, there has been no epidemiological study of the association between use of prescribed or 'over-the-counter' fish oil supplements and CRC risk.

#### Pre-Clinical Studies of the Anti-CRC Activity of ω-3 PUFAs

Multiple reports using a variety of rodent models of early stage colorectal carcinogenesis, including azoxymethane (AOM)- and dimethylhydrazine-induced colorectal tumorigenesis (using aberrant crypt foci (ACF) or colonic tumours as the primary end-point), as well as the $Apc^{Min/+}$ mouse model of FAP, have demonstrated efficacy of a combination of EPA and DHA (as fish oil substituted for the base fat source in chow; Cockbain et al. 2011), as well as a relatively small number of studies which have described efficacy of either EPA or DHA alone (Cockbain et al. 2011). These studies have consistently demonstrated a 20–50 % decrease in colorectal tumour (or ACF) incidence and a 30–70 % decrease in colorectal tumour number, despite the use of different rodent models and different treatment protocols (Cockbain et al. 2011).

#### The Discrepancy Between Human Observational Data and Pre-Clinical Studies of ω-3 PUFAs

Several explanations have been put forward to explain the discrepancy between human observational data and results from pre-clinical rodent models. Firstly, methodological weaknesses inherent to observational research, including subjective measurement of dietary $\omega$-3 PUFA intake and variable definition of fresh fish intake, may have confounded the epidemiological data. Secondly, 'pharmacological' exposure to $\omega$-3 PUFAs is far higher in rodent models and 'usual' $\omega$-3 PUFA intake via fish may be inadequate to observe anti-CRC activity of $\omega$-3 PUFAs in human populations except in the very highest fish consumers. It is worth noting that the $\omega$-3 PUFA content of 100 g of salmon and sardines is between 1–2 g (Wall et al. 2010). The $\omega$-3 PUFA content of 'lean' fish such as cod and haddock is much lower (approximately 0.25 per 100 g; Wall et al. 2010). Therefore, an extremely high fish intake is required to come close to quantities administered in rodent models (and interventional clinical studies of $\omega$-3 PUFAs; Cockbain et al. 2011). Finally, protocols of some pre-clinical studies of $\omega$-3 PUFAs have failed to control for a concurrent reduction in $\omega$-6 PUFA (such as C22:4$\omega$6 arachidonic acid) administration, which alone could explain reduced tumorigenesis in rodents, rather than anti-neoplastic activity of $\omega$-3 PUFAs (Cockbain et al. 2011).

**Clinical Data Supporting Chemopreventative Activity of $\omega$-3 PUFAs**

Nine independent clinical colorectal mucosal biomarker studies with different designs (but which all tested, with one exception, doses of $\omega$-3 PUFA greater than 2 g daily) have been performed with a reduction in epithelial cell proliferation index observed in all but two studies (Cockbain et al. 2011). Importantly, these biomarker studies demonstrated that oral $\omega$-3 PUFA dosing leads to increased colorectal mucosal $\omega$-3 PUFA levels and confirmed the impression from previous cardiovascular Phase III clinical trials that fish oil supplementation, at doses higher than those expected through dietary means alone, is safe and well tolerated (Cockbain et al. 2011). Uncertainty about the predictive value of changes in colorectal mucosal proliferation index for future CRC risk means that it is currently not possible to draw any firm conclusion about the chemopreventative efficacy of $\omega$-3 PUFAs from these studies.

There have been two clinical studies of $\omega$-3 PUFA supplementation using colorectal adenoma as the surrogate end-point for CRC risk (Akedo et al. 1998; West et al. 2010). A small ($n = 5$) open-label study in Japanese FAP patients demonstrated no change in colorectal polyp number following administration of 2.2 g DHA and 0.6 g EPA daily for more than one year (Akedo et al. 1998). It remains unclear what the planned sample size of this study was and whether the study was terminated prematurely (Akedo et al. 1998). Efficacy of the FFA form of EPA in the $Apc^{Min/+}$ mouse model of FAP (Fini et al. 2010) led to a Phase III randomised placebo-controlled trial of EPA–FFA 2 g daily for 6 months in 55 patients with FAP undergoing sigmoidoscopic surveillance of a rectal stump after total colectomy (West et al. 2010). Patients in the EPA–FFA arm had a significant 22.4 % lower rectal polyp number and a 29.8 % decrease in the sum of polyp diameters in a tattooed area of the rectum in comparison with the changes in polyp number and size over 6 months in the placebo group (West et al. 2010). Importantly, EPA–FFA 2 g daily was safe and well tolerated (West et al. 2010), a finding

**Table 1** Putative mechanisms of the anti-inflammatory and anti-neoplastic activity of $\omega$-3 PUFAs

| |
|---|
| Immunomodulation (reduced T cell activation) |
| Inhibition of cyclooxygenase (COX) activity |
| Production of novel anti-inflammatory lipid mediators, e.g. resolvins |
| Direct fatty acid signaling via GPCRs |
| Alteration of membrane dynamics and cell surface receptor function |
| Alteration of cellular redox state |
| Anti-angiogenesis |

replicated by previous Phase II evaluation of this formulation of EPA in patients with a history of colorectal adenoma (West et al. 2009). The reduction in polyp number and size in the EPA–FFA group compared with the placebo group during the treatment period was similar to that observed in a previous randomised trial in FAP patients of the selective COX-2 inhibitor celecoxib (Steinbach et al. 2000).

Efficacy of EPA in the FFA form in FAP patients has prompted a larger scale randomised trial of EPA–FFA in patients with a history of colorectal adenoma undergoing colonoscopic surveillance within the English bowel cancer screening programme (The seAFOod Polyp Prevention Trial; ISRCTN05926847) which is expected to report in 2016. A fish oil preparation (1 g containing 465 mg EPA and 375 mg DHA daily) is also being tested in the large-scale VITamin D and OmegA-3 Trial (VITAL), which includes cancer as a primary outcome (see Sect. 3.5.1).

### 3.1.2 Mechanisms of the Anti-inflammatory and Anti-Neoplastic Activity of $\omega$-3 PUFAs

There are believed to be several mechanism(s) underlying the anti-inflammatory activity of $\omega$-3 PUFAs, which are likely to contribute to the anti-neoplastic activity of $\omega$-3 PUFAs (Table 1). In general, the in vivo relevance of each of the above putative mechanisms and their relative contributions to the anti-cancer activity of the $\omega$-3 PUFAs remains unclear (Chapkin et al. 2007; Calviello et al. 2007).

Evidence is strongest for a role for inhibition of COX-2-dependent synthesis of prostaglandin (PG) $E_2$ in the anti-CRC activity of $\omega$-3 PUFAs. EPA can act as an alternative substrate for COX-2, instead of the usual substrate, arachidonic acid, leading to a reduction in formation of protumorigenic $PGE_2$ in favour of $PGE_3$ in several cell types including CRC cells (Smith 2005). Recently, a '$PGE_2$ to $PGE_3$ switch' has been demonstrated in colorectal mucosa of rats treated with fish oil (Vanamala et al. 2008). However, reduction of $PGE_2$ synthesis and/or generation of $PGE_3$ following EPA treatment remains to be demonstrated in mouse or human CRC tissue.

It is known that DHA also binds the substrate channel of COX-2 and inhibits COX-2 activity (Vecchio et al. 2010).

In the presence of aspirin, which irreversibly acetylates the COX enzyme, EPA drives COX-2-dependent production of resolvin (Rv) E1 (5*S*,12*R*,18*R*-

trihydroxyeicosapentaenoic acid; Serhan et al. 2008). 18*R*-RvE1 has been detected in plasma of healthy volunteers in ng/ml quantities after aspirin and EPA ingestion [31]. The precursors of E-series resolvins may also be produced independent of COX by direct CYP450 metabolism of EPA (Serhan et al. 2008). Metabolism of DHA can produce D-series resolvins, 17S-docosatrienes termed protectins or 14-lipoxygenase-derived products termed maresins. These newly described families of EPA- and DHA-derived lipid mediators all share anti-inflammatory and inflammation resolution activity in animal models of acute inflammation (Serhan et al. 2008). RvE1 is a ligand for ChemR23 and BLT1 G protein-coupled receptors (GPCRs). It is currently not known whether $\omega$-3 PUFA-derived resolvins exhibit anti-neoplastic activity. However, it is known that ChemR23-dependent RvE1 signalling inhibits NF$\kappa$B activation in leukocytes (Serhan et al. 2008).

EPA and DHA can also act as direct ligands for GPCRs including Gpr120 and Gpr40 (Oh et al. 2010). Gpr120 is not expressed by intestinal epithelial cells, including several human CRC cell lines (Oh et al. 2010). However, Gpr120 activation decreases adipose tissue macrophage M1 polarisation in mice (Oh et al. 2010) suggesting that direct $\omega$-3 PUFA signaling via GPCRs could negatively affect pro-tumourigenic tumour-associated macrophage activity or modulate the systemic host anti-tumour response.

There is some evidence that the incorporation of $\omega$-3 PUFAs into cell phospholipid membranes alters the fluidity, structure and/or function of lipid rafts or calveolae (Schley et al. 2007). The localisation of cell surface receptors, such as epidermal growth factor receptor (EGFR), in lipid rafts is believed to be crucial for downstream receptor signalling controlling proliferation and apoptosis, which in turn could be altered by $\omega$-3 PUFA incorporation (Schley et al. 2007).

PUFAs are highly peroxidisable, generating reactive oxygen species such as the superoxide radical. Therefore, $\omega$-3 PUFAs may have anti-neoplastic activity through alteration in the cellular redox state and increased oxidative stress, leading to cancer cell apoptosis (Sanders et al. 2004).

## 3.2 Curcumin

Curcumin (diferuloylmethane) is a polyphenolic phytochemical, which is extracted from turmeric, a rhizomatous plant of the *Ginger* family used widely in Asian cooking (Aggarwal et al. 2007). Turmeric has been used for medicinal purposes for many centuries. Curcumin powder consists of approximately 75 % curcumin in combination with curcuminoid derivatives that are metabolised to the parent curcumin in vivo. Curcumin is stable in acidic conditions, which are generally observed in the gastrointestinal tract.

### 3.2.1 Anti-inflammatory Activity of Curcumin

Curcumin is believed to have anti-inflammatory activity via several mechanisms (Hanai and Sugimoto 2009; Irving et al. 2011). These include attenuation of NF$\kappa$B signalling, via poorly understood mechanisms including inhibition of I$\kappa$B kinase, and inhibition of synthesis of multiple pro-inflammatory mediators including PGs, nitric oxide (NO) and chemokines (Irving et al. 2011). Curcumin has efficacy in animal models of inflammatory bowel disease (Sugimoto et al. 2002; Billerey-Larmonier et al. 2008). Curcumin also exhibits immunomodulatory properties in vitro and in vivo including modulation of intestinal lymphocyte infiltration in $Apc^{Min/+}$ mice (Churchill et al. 2000).

### 3.2.2 Preclinical Studies of the Anti-CRC Activity of Curcumin

Preclinical evidence for the CRC chemopreventative activity of curcumin has been obtained from chemical carcinogenesis and $Apc^{Min/+}$ rodent models. Dietary curcumin supplementation has been demonstrated to reduce AOM-induced ACF and CRC incidence in mice and rats by 40–60 % (Huang et al. 1994; Rao et al. 1995; Pereira et al. 1996). Rao and colleagues also provided evidence for inhibition of intestinal COX and lipoxygenase (LOX) activity by curcumin (Rao et al. 1995). More recently, similar effects on $Apc^{Min/+}$ mouse adenoma multiplicity have been reported (Perkins et al. 2002).

### 3.2.3 Pharmacokinetics of Curcumin

Curcumin has limited systemic bioavailability following oral dosing. It is poorly absorbed with the majority of the parental molecule and related curcuminoids excreted in faeces (Irving et al. 2011). Curcumin also has a short half-life and is preferentially excreted in bile, with poor renal excretion. Whether the low nanomolar concentrations of curcumin detected in human plasma are sufficient for possible systemic activity of curcumin, or whether local intestinal bioactivity of curcumin restricts anti-neoplastic properties to the gastro-intestinal tract, is not clear (Dhillon et al. 2008). Tissue curcumin levels reach nmol/g concentrations in normal colorectal mucosa and CRC following oral dosing in humans (Garcea et al. 2005). The above pharmacokinetic properties of curcumin have hampered clinical evaluation because of uncertainty regarding appropriate dosing. New pharmacodynamic assays should provide greater understanding of the systemic bioavailability of curcumin and its bioactive metabolites (Ponnurangam et al. 2010).

### 3.2.4 Clinical Data Supporting the CRC Chemopreventative Activity of Curcumin

Phase I and II trials of curcumin in the setting of colorectal adenoma or CRC have used daily dosing from 450 mg to 4 g daily (reviewed in Irving et al. 2011). In all cases, curcumin was well tolerated with few adverse events, mainly minor gastrointestinal disturbances. Higher doses have been administered in clinical studies although adverse events were higher in these studies suggesting a possible limit to tolerable daily dosing. Uncertainty about the relative importance of systemic *versus* topical delivery of curcumin for activity in the intestine means that dosing frequency remains an open question.

A dose of 1440 mg curcumin daily for six months has been tested in 5 patients with FAP, in combination with another polyphenol quercetin (Cruz-Correa et al. 2006). In this open-label study, there was a significant 50–60 % reduction in colorectal adenoma number and size leading to early termination of the trial (Cruz-Correa et al. 2006).

These results have prompted ongoing randomized evaluation of 1–3 g curcumin daily for 12 months in FAP patients. In a separate non-randomised, open-label study, 41 individuals undergoing colonoscopic screening for CRC received either 2 or 4 g curcumin daily for one month prior to measurement of rectal ACF multiplicity. There was a significant 40 % reduction in ACF number in the group taking 4 g daily compared with the 2 g daily group (Carroll et al. 2011).

### 3.2.5 Mechanisms of the Anti-CRC Activity of Curcumin

Several different modes of the anti-neoplastic activity of curcumin have been proposed. However, the contribution of these individual mechanisms to activity in vivo is currently unclear. For example, reduction in intestinal mucosal $PGE_2$ levels previously observed in rodent models (Rao et al. 1995) has not been observed in endoscopically normal rectal mucosa or ACFs following curcumin administration in humans (Carroll et al. 2011).

Curcumin can scavenge or trap oxygen and nitrogen free radicals, which are believed to contribute to DNA mutagenesis during carcinogenesis (Weber et al. 2005). In addition to the anti-inflammatory mechanisms attributed to curcumin noted in Sect. 3.2.1, particularly NF$\kappa$B signalling inhibition and COX/LOX downregulation, several other effects relevant to anti-neoplastic activity have been reported including CRC cell cycle arrest and apoptosis via p53-dependent and -independent mechanisms, anti-angiogenic activity and modulation of the host immune response to tumourigenesis (Irving et al. 2011). It will be important in future clinical trials to measure biomarker end-points relevant to these putative mechanisms of action in order to develop predictive biomarkers of chemoprevention activity in order to personalise treatment (particularly dose) with curcumin.

## 3.3 Resveratrol

Resveratrol (trans-3,4′,5-trihydroxystilbene) is another phytochemical polyphenol with well-recognised anti-oxidant properties (Patel et al. 2010). Predominant dietary sources are grapes, peanuts and cranberries. The anti-inflammatory properties of resveratrol are less well characterized than curcumin (Patel et al. 2010), but dietary supplementation with resveratrol does attenuate dextran sodium sulphate (DSS)-induced colitis in mice (Sanchez-Fidalgo et al. 2010; Cui et al. 2010). Unlike curcumin, it is rapidly and efficiently absorbed along the gastrointestinal tract with predominant metabolism in the liver (Patel et al. 2010).

### 3.3.1 Preclinical Studies of the Anti-CRC Activity of Resveratrol

Resveratrol has been demonstrated to have chemopreventative efficacy in AOM-induced ACF and $Apc^{Min/+}$ mouse models in a similar manner to curcumin (Tessitore et al. 2000; Schneider et al. 2001). Resveratrol also has efficacy against colitis-associated cancer in the DSS–AOM mouse model (Cui et al. 2010). Pharmacokinetic evaluation of an oral resveratrol preparation in CRC patients is ongoing and data from these studies should inform design of Phase II biomarker studies more relevant to CRC chemoprevention.

### 3.3.2 Mechanisms of the Anti-CRC Activity of Resveratrol

The majority of mechanistic studies with resveratrol have provided in vitro data using human CRC cells, which suggest effects on cancer cell cycling and apoptosis (Patel et al. 2010). Alterations in expression levels of cell cycle proteins (D cyclins) and the pro-apoptotic protein Bax have been confirmed in vivo (Tessitore et al. 2000; Schneider et al. 2001).

## 3.4 Other Dietary Polyphenols

Many other dietary polyphenols have been demonstrated to have anti-neoplastic activity but are beyond the scope of this review as they have not been tested in 'nutraceutical' form (Ricciardiello et al. 2011). For example, a complex apple polyphenol extract has recently been demonstrated to have efficacy in the $Apc^{Min/+}$ mouse (Fini et al. 2011). In a recent perspective, Ricciardiello and colleagues have argued that the mixture of naturally occurring anti-inflammatory phytochemical compounds found in high fruit and vegetable diets, particularly polyphenols, may have greater anti-neoplastic efficacy than higher quantities of single agents in nutraceutical form (Ricciardiello et al. 2011).

One promising preparation with anti-inflammatory properties that requires detailed assessment for anti-CRC activity is green tea, which contains a complex mixture of polyphenols termed tea catechins (Chow and Hakim 2011). Administration of green tea extract for 12 months has been demonstrated to reduce incidence of colorectal adenoma (15 vs. 31 % in a non-supplemented control group) in individuals with a past history of colorectal adenoma in a randomised trial of 136 patients (Shimizu et al. 2008). A placebo-controlled colorectal polyp prevention trial testing decaffeinated green tea extract of *Camellia Sinensis*, containing 300 mg (-)epigallocatechin 3-gallate (EGCG) daily in gelatin capsules, is currently underway in patients with previous colorectal neoplasia (NCT01360320).

## 3.5 Other Natural Anti-inflammatory Agents with CRC Chemopreventative Efficacy

### 3.5.1 Vitamin D

A large amount of epidemiological evidence is suggestive that vitamin D intake protects against CRC, although the complex relationship between existing vitamin D status (as measured by serum 25-hydroxy-vitamin D) and the dose required for efficacy is poorly understood (Zhang and Giovannucci 2011; Touvier et al. 2011). More recently, it has become recognised that the active moiety calcitriol (1$\alpha$,25-dihydroxyvitamin $D_3$) has potent anti-inflammatory activity and that this mechanism of action may contribute to anti-cancer activity of vitamin D (Krishnan and Feldman 2011). Calcitriol may decrease COX-2-PG signalling during carcinogenesis via suppression of COX-2 expression, induction of 15-PG dehydrogenase and reduced expression of PG receptors (Krishnan and Feldman 2011). Calcitriol has also been demonstrated to inhibit NF$\kappa$B signalling and have anti-angiogenic activity (Krishnan and Feldman 2011).

Calcitriol or vitamin D analogues have been demonstrated to have activity in the Apc$^{Min/+}$ mouse model (Huerta et al. 2002), as well as inhibit inflammation and carcinogenesis in the AOM–DSS mouse model (Fichera et al. 2007).

The effect of vitamin D supplementation (2000 IU vitamin $D_3$ per day) on cancer incidence at 5 years will be studied in the large-scale 2 $\times$ 2 factorial VITAL study, which includes $\omega$-3 fish oil arms (NCT01169259). The effect of vitamin D (1000 IU per day), with or without 1200 mg elemental calcium (calcium carbonate 3 g daily), on colorectal adenoma incidence at 3–5 year follow-up colonoscopy is currently being tested in the vitamin D/calcium polyp prevention study (NCT00153816).

## 4 Summary

Many natural dietary substances have been demonstrated to have combined anti-inflammatory and anti-neoplastic activity in in vitro studies and preclinical rodent models. These ‘nutraceuticals’ seem to have multiple modes of action, which contribute to their anti-neoplastic activity, and share effects on PG signalling and NF$\kappa$B signalling in particular. A small number of these agents such as EPA, curcumin and EGCG have been, or are now being, evaluated in ‘nutraceutical’ form in Phase II and Phase III clinical trials of CRC chemopreventative activity. The results of these studies are eagerly awaited, not least because these agents display several characteristics of an ideal chemoprevention agent such as excellent safety and tolerability, patient acceptability and cost.

**Acknowledgments** Work in the Hull laboratory is funded by the National Institute for Health Research Efficacy & Mechanism Evaluation Programme, Yorkshire Cancer Research and an unrestricted Scientific Grant from SLA Pharma (UK).

**Conflict of Interest Statement** Mark Hull has received an unrestricted Scientific Grant and a travel grant for conference travel from SLA Pharma (UK), which produces the $\omega$-3 PUFA EPA, in the free fatty acid form.

## References

Aggarwal BB, Sundaram C, Malani N et al (2007) Curcumin: the Indian solid gold. Adv Exp Med Biol 595:1–75

Akedo I, Ishikawa H, Nakamura T et al (1998) Three cases with familial adenomatous polyposis diagnosed as having malignant lesions in the course of a long-term trial using docosahexaenoic acid (DHA)-concentrated fish oil capsules. Jpn J Clin Oncol 28:762–765

Balkwill F, Mantovani A (2010) Cancer and inflammation: implications for pharmacology and therapeutics. Clin Pharmacol Ther 87:401–406

Ben-Neriah Y, Karin M (2011) Inflammation meets cancer, with NF$\kappa$B as the matchmaker. Nature Immunol 12:715–723

Bhangle S, Kolasinski SL (2011) Fish oil in rheumatic diseases. Rheum Dis Clin North Am 37:77–84
Billerey-Larmonier C, Uno JK, Larmonier N et al (2008) Protective effects of dietary curcumin in mouse model of chemically induced colitis are strain dependent. Inflamm Bowel Dis 14:780–793
Calviello G, Serini S, Piccioni E (2007) n-3 polyunsaturated fatty acids and the prevention of colorectal cancer: molecular mechanisms involved. Curr Med Chem 14:3059–3069
Carroll RE, Benya RV, Turgeon DK et al (2011) Phase IIa clinical trial of curcumin for the prevention of colorectal neoplasia. Cancer Prev Res 4:354–364
Chapkin RS, McMurray DN, Lupton JR (2007) Colon cancer, fatty acids and anti-inflammatory compounds. Curr Opin Gastroenterol 23:48–54
Chow HH, Hakim IA (2011) Pharmacokinetic and chemoprevention studies on tea in humans. Pharmacol Res 64:105–112
Churchill M, Chadburn A, Bilinski RT et al (2000) Inhibition of intestinal tumors by curcumin is associated with changes in the intestinal immune cell profile. J Surg Res 89:166–175
Cockbain AJ, Toogood GJ, Hull MA (2011) Omega-3 polyunsaturated fatty acids for the prevention and treatment of colorectal cancer. Gut. doi:10.1136/gut.2010.233718
Cruz-Correa M, Shoskes DA, Sanchez P (2006) Combination treatment with curcumin and quercetin of adenomas in familial adenomatous polyposis. Clin Gastroenterol Hepatol 4:1035–1038
Cui X, Jin Y, Hofseth AB et al (2010) Resveratrol suppresses colitis and colon cancer associated with colitis. Cancer Prev Res 3:549–559
De Caterina R (2011) n-3 fatty acids in cardiovascular disease. N Engl J Med 364:2439–2450
Dhillon N, Aggarwal BB, Newman RA et al (2008) Phase II trial of curcumin in patients with advanced pancreatic cancer. Clin Cancer Res 14:4491–4499
Fichera A, Little N, Dougherty U et al (2007) A vitamin D analogue inhibits colonic carcinogenesis in the AOM/DSS model. J Surg Res 142:239–245
Fini L, Piazzi G, Ceccarelli C et al (2010) Highly purified eicosapentaenoic acid as free fatty acids strongly suppresses polyps in ApcMin/+ mice. Clin Cancer Res 16:5703–5711
Fini L, Piazzi G, Daoud Y et al (2011) Chemoprevention of intestinal polyps in ApcMin/+ mice fed with western or balanced diets by drinking annurca apple polyphenol extract. Cancer Prev Res 4:907–915
Garcea G, Berry DP, Jones DJ et al (2005) Consumption of the putative chemopreventive agent curcumin by cancer patients: assessment of curcumin levels in the colorectum and their pharmacodynamic consequences. Cancer Epidemiol Biomarkers Prev 14:120–125
Hanai H, Sugimoto K (2009) Curcumin has bright prospects for the treatment of inflammatory bowel disease. Curr Pharm Des 15:2087–2094
Huang M-T, Lou Y-R, Ma W et al (1994) Inhibitory effects of dietary curcumin on forestomach, duodenal, and colon carcinogenesis in mice. Cancer Res 54:5841–5847
Huerta S, Irwin RW, Heber D et al (2002) 1α, 25-$(OH)_2$-D3 and its synthetic analogue decrease tumour load in the $Apc^{Min}$ mouse. Cancer Res 62:741–746
Irving GR, Karmokar A, Berry DP et al (2011) Curcumin: the potential for efficacy in gastrointestinal diseases. Best Pract Res Clin Gastroenterol 25:519–534
Kalra EK (2003) Nutraceutical—definition and introduction. AAPS J 5:25
Klampfer L (2011) Cytokines, inflammation and colon cancer. Curr Cancer Drug Targets 11:451–464
Krishnan AV, Feldman D (2011) Mechanisms of the anti-cancer and anti-inflammatory actions of vitamin D. Annu Rev Pharmacol Toxicol 51:311–336
MacLean CH, Newberry SJ, Mojica WA et al (2006) Effects of omega-3 fatty acids on cancer risk. A systematic review. J Am Med Assoc 295:403–415
Oh DY, Talukdar S, Bae EJ et al (2010) GPR120 is an omega-3 fatty acid receptor mediating potent anti-inflammatory and insulin-sensitizing effects. Cell 142:687–698
Patel VB, Misra S, Patel BB et al (2010) Colorectal cancer: chemopreventive role of curcumin and resveratrol. Nutr Cancer 62:958–967

Pereira MA, Grubbs CJ, Barnes LH et al (1996) Effects of the phytochemicals, curcumin and quercetin, upon azoxymethane-induced colon cancer and 7,12-dimethylbenz[*a*]anthracene-induced mammary cancer in rats. Carcinogenesis 17:1305–1311

Perkins S, Verschoyle RD, Hill K et al (2002) Chemopreventive efficacy and pharmacokinetics of curcumin in the Min/+ mouse, a model of familial adenomatous polyposis. Cancer Epidemiol Biomarkers Prev 11:535–540

Ponnurangam S, Mondalek FG, Govind J et al (2010) Urine and serum analysis of consumed curcuminoids using an IkappaB-luciferase surrogate marker assay. In vivo 24:861–864

Popovinova BK, Kostadinova FI, Furuichi K et al (2009) Blockade of a chemokine, CCL2, reduces chronic colitis-associated carcinogenesis. Cancer Res 69:7884–7892

Rao CV, Rivenson A, Simi B, Reddy BS (1995) Chemoprevention of colon carcinogenesis by dietary curcumin, a naturally occurring plant phenolic compound. Cancer Res 55:259–266

Ricciardiello L, Bazzoli F, Fogliano V (2011) Phytochemicals and colorectal cancer prevention-myth or reality? Nature Rev Gastroenterol Hepatol 8:592–596

Sanchez-Fidalgo S, Cardeno A, Villegas I et al (2010) Dietary supplementation of resveratrol attenuates chronic colonic inflammation in mice. Eur J Pharmacol 633:78–84

Sanders LM, Henderson CE, Hong MY et al (2004) An increase in reactive oxygen species by dietary fish oil coupled with the attenuation of antioxidant defenses by dietary pectin enhances rat colonocyte apoptosis. J Nutr 134:3233–3238

Schley PD, Brindley DN, Field CJ (2007) n-3 PUFA alter raft lipid composition and decrease epidermal growth factor receptor levels in lipid rafts of human breast cancer cells. J Nutr 137:548–553

Schneider Y, Duranton B, Gosse F et al (2001) Resveratrol inhibits intestinal tumorigenesis and modulates host-defense-related gene expression in an animal model of human familial adenomatous polyposis. Nutr Cancer 39:102–107

Serhan CN, Chiang N, van Dyke TE (2008) Resolving inflammation: dual anti-inflammatory and pro-resolution lipid mediators. Nat Rev Immunol 8:349–361

Shimizu M, Fukutomi Y, Ninomiya M et al (2008) Green tea extracts for the prevention of metachronous colorectal adenomas: a pilot study. Cancer Epidemiol Biomarkers Prev 17:3020–3025

Smith WL (2005) Cyclooxygenases, peroxide tone and the allure of fish oil. Curr Opin Cell Biol 17:174–182

Steinbach G, Lynch PM, Phillips RKS et al (2000) The effect of celecoxib, a cyclooxygenase-2 inhibitor, in familial adenomatous polyposis. N Engl J Med 342:1946–1952

Sugimoto K, Hanai H, Tozawa K et al (2002) Curcumin prevents and ameliorates trinitrobenzene sulfonic acid-induced colitis in mice. Gastroenterology 123:1912–1922

Tessitore L, Davit A, Sarotto I et al (2000) Resveratrol depresses the growth of colorectal aberrant crypt foci by affecting bax and p21(CIP) expression. Carcinogenesis 21:1619–1622

Touvier M, Chan DS, Lau R et al (2011) Meta-analyses of vitamin D intake, 25-hydroxyvitamin D status, vitamin D receptor poymorphisms and colorectal cancer risk. Cancer Epidemiol Biomarkers Prev 20:1003–1016

Ullman TA, Itzkowitz SH (2011) Intestinal inflammation and cancer. Gastroenterology 140:1807–1816

Vanamala J, Glagolenko A, Yang P et al (2008) Dietary fish oil and pectin enhance colonocyte apoptosis in part through suppression of PPAR$\delta$/$PGE_2$ and elevation of $PGE_3$. Carcinogenesis 29:790–796

Vecchio AJ, Simmons DM, Malkowski MG (2010) Structural basis of fatty acid substrate binding to cyclooxygenase-2. J Biol Chem 285:22152–22163

Vlachojannis J, Magora F, Chrubasik S (2011) Willow species and aspirin: different mechanisms of action. Phytother Res. doi:10.1002/ptr.3386

Wall R, Ross RP, Fitzgerald GF, Stanton C (2010) Fatty acids from fish: the anti-inflammatory potential of long-chain omega-3 fatty acids. Nutr Rev 68:280–289

Wang D, DuBois RN (2010) The role of COX-2 in intestinal inflammation and colorectal cancer. Oncogene 29:781–788

Weber WM, Hunsaker LA, Abcouwer SF et al (2005) Anti-oxidant activities of curcumin and related enones. Bioorg Med Chem 13:3811–3820

West NJ, Belluzzi A, Lund EK et al (2009) Eicosapentaenoic acid (EPA), as the free fatty acid, reduces colonic crypt cell proliferation in patients with sporadic colorectal polyps. Gut 58(Suppl. 2):A68 (abstract)

West NJ, Clark SK, Philips RK et al (2010) Eicosapentaenoic acid reduces rectal polyp number and size in familial adenomatous polyposis. Gut 59:918–925

World Cancer Research Fund/American Institute for Cancer Research (2007) Food, nutrition, physical activity, and the prevention of cancer: a global perspective. AICR, Washington DC

World Cancer Research Fund/American Institute for Cancer Research (2011) Continuous update project interim report summary. Food, nutrition, physical activity, and the prevention of colorectal cancer

Zhang X, Giovannucci E (2011) Calcium, vitamin D and colorectal cancer chemoprevention. Best Pract Res Clin Gastroenterol 25:485–494

# Genetics, Inheritance and Strategies for Prevention in Populations at High Risk of Colorectal Cancer (CRC)

John Burn, John Mathers and D. Tim Bishop

**Abstract**

Hereditary forms of colorectal cancer account for less than 5 % of colorectal cancer but attract disproportionate attention because they offer an opportunity for effective surgical prophylaxis, influence the health of the wider family and give insight into the critical pathways of carcinogenesis. Familial Adenomatous Polyposis (FAP) due to loss of the APC gene and Lynch syndrome or Hereditary Non-Polyposis Colon Cancer (HNPCC) due to breakdown in MisMatch Repair are the principal syndromes of broader interest and both have been the subject of chemoprevention trials. There has been a longstanding interest in non-steroidal anti inflammatories in FAP where trials have shown regression of polyps with the "pro drug"sulindac and the selective COX2 inhibitors though impact on long-term cancer risk is not confirmed. The CAPP1 trial focused on two interventions in a factorial design, aspirin and resistant starch or fermentable fibre. Resistant starch is not absorbed in the small intestine and undergoes colonic fermentation to short-chain fatty acids including butyrate which have anti-cancer effects. Polyposis registry clinicians across Europe recruited adolescents with FAP to receive aspirin (600 mg as 2 tablets/d) and/or 30 g as 2 sachets/d in a 1:1 blend of potato starch and high

J. Burn (✉)
Institute of genetic medicine, Centre for Life Central Parkway,
Newcastle Upon Tyne, NE1 3BZ, UK
e-mail: john.burn@newcastle.ac.uk

J. Mathers
Institute of Ageing and Health, Newcastle University, Newcastle Upon Tyne, NE1 3BZ, UK

D. T. Bishop
Cancer Research UK Genetic Epidemiology Unit, Institute of Molecular Medicine, Leeds University, UK

A. T. Chan and E. Detering (eds.), *Prospects for Chemoprevention of Colorectal Neoplasia*, Recent Results in Cancer Research 191, DOI: 10.1007/978-3-642-30331-9_9, 

amylose maize starch [Hylon VII]) with placebo control for at least a year or until surgery before age 21. Fifty-nine percent (133/227) of recruits had a baseline and at least one other endoscopy. After a median of 17 months , the primary endpoint of a risk of an increased polyp number in the rectum and sigmoid colon was not significantly reduced in either treatment group with relative risks of 0.77 (aspirin; 95 % CI, 0.54–1.10;) and 1.05 (RS; 95 % CI, 0.73–1.49. The diameter of the largest polyp detected tended to be smaller in the aspirin arm. The planned subgroup analyses of patients who elected to continue on study for more than one year found a significant reduction in the size of the largest polyp in the aspirin versus non-aspirin group ($p$ = 0.02), Mean crypt length decreased significantly over time on study in the two combined RS groups, compared with the two combined non-RS groups ($p <$ 0.0001 for interaction), in a model of the interaction between intervention and time. In CAPP2, 1009 Lynch syndrome gene carriers were recruited from 43 international centres. 937 commenced intervention: 600mg enteric coated aspirin and/or 30grams of the resistant starch Novelose in a 2 by 2 factorial placebo controlled design. After a mean of 29 months, intervention, there was no evidence that either agent influenced development of colonic neoplasia. However, the design included double blind follow-up for at least 10 years. After a mean of 55.7 months, and despite regular colonoscopy and polyp removal, 48 recruits developed CRC. Of these, 18 received aspirin and 30 received AP; the HR for CRC for aspirin was 0.63 (CI 0.35–1.13, $p = 0.12$). Five of the 48 people who developed CRC each had two primary colon cancers. Poisson regression analysis to allow for multiple primary events indicated a protective effect: IRR 0.56 (CI 0.32–0.99, $p$ = 0.05). For those who took aspirin (or AP) for a minimum of 2 years (per protocol) the HR was 0.41 (CI 0.19–0.86 $p = 0.02$) and the IRR, 0.37 (CI 0.18–0.78 $p$ = 0.008). Combined analysis of all LS cancers including CRC revealed a similar effect. On intention to treat analysis, the HR was 0.65 (CI 0.42–1.00, $p$ = 0.05 and IRR was 0.59 (CI 0.39–0.90 $p$ = 0.01), while the Per Protocol analysis HR was 0.45 (CI 0.26–0.79 $p = 0.005$,) and IRR was 0.42 (CI 0.25–0.72, $p$ = 0.001). Adverse events in the aspirin and placebo groups were similar with 11 significant gastrointestinal bleeds or ulcers in the aspirin group and 9 in the placebo group. The evidence is now sufficient to recommend aspirin to all Lynch syndrome gene carriers. CAPP3 will recruit 3000 gene carriers into a dose inferiority study to test the relative benefits of 100mg, 300 or 600mg daily doses.

## Contents

## 1 Introduction

All cancer is genetic. It involves a breakdown in the control by a cell's genes of its growth, division, migration and senescence. On rare occasions, predisposition is transmitted as a familial trait, fulfilling the true meaning of the term "genetics". Such families provide an insight into the mechanisms of gene action and have, as a result, attracted research attention which is disproportionate to their frequency. In turn, the recognition that cancer can be a hereditary trait has entered the public consciousness such that people with a family history of cancer are alarmed and their physicians consider genetic investigation. The great majority of such families do not have single gene defect underlying the family history. Twin studies have suggested that up to 35 % of the cause of colorectal cancer can be attributed to genetic makeup (Lichtenstein and Wolfe 2000) but most of this reflects the action of multiple genes of small effect (Tomlinson et al. 2011) Extensive molecular studies have identified several rare but distinct syndromes. These can be divided into conditions characterised by multiple polyps and the much more common "hereditary non-polyposis colon cancer", now renamed Lynch syndrome. The polyposis syndromes are further divided into conditions characterised by hamartomatous polyps like Peutz Jeghers syndrome and Juvenile Polyposis, and those with adenomatous polyps (Clark 2009) (Table 1).

Any of these conditions is amenable to chemoprevention strategies but most are too rare and lack clear relevance to the general population. Two conditions stand out as targets because they are well-defined and can act as a model for common cancers;

1. Familial Adenomatous Polyposis (FAP), formerly known as Adenomatous Polyposis Coli, which results from loss of function of the APC gene on chromosome 5
2. Lynch syndrome or Hereditary Non-Polyposis Colon Cancer (HNPCC) due to breakdown in MisMatch Repair

FAP captured clinical attention in the early twentieth century when it became clear that young people would develop hundreds, sometimes thousands, of adenomatous polyps in the colorectum leading without intervention to inevitable) death from colorectal cancer by early middle age (Burn et al. 1991). Prophylactic

**Table 1** Heritable forms of colorectal polyps and cancer

| Syndrome | Features and inheritance pattern | Gene |
|---|---|---|
| Familial adenomatous polyposis | Over 100 adenomatous polyps in colorectum, onset in teens<br>Gastric polyps<br>Congenital Hypertrophy of the Retinal Pigment Epithelium<br>Jaw cysts<br>Desmoid tumours | APC |
| Attenuated FAP | Later onset more benign course, fewer polyps<br>Autosomal Dominant | Less disruptive mutations |
| Lynch syndrome | Microsatellite unstable tumours in colorectum, endometrium, ovary, stomach, small intestine uroepithelium, brain, skin<br>Autosomal dominant | Mismatch repair genes<br>MLH1<br>MSH2<br>MSH6<br>PMS2 |
| MAP: MutYH-associated polyposis | Multiple Adenomatous colorectal polyps<br>Autosomal Recessive | MutYH1 |
| Juvenile polyposis | Multiple hamartomatous polyps in colorectum<br>Autosomal dominant | SMAD4 |
| Peutz jeghers syndrome | Hamartomatous polyps throughout the GI tract<br>Pigmentation of the mucous membranes, particularly lips | STK11 |
| Cowden syndrome<br>Bannayan-riley-ruvalcaba syndrome | Colonic polyps, breast cancer thyroid cancer | PTEN |
| Hereditary mixed polyposis | Mixed adenomatous and hamartomatous polyps in the colorectum | GREM1 (Jaeger et al. 2012) |

colectomy with ileorectal anastomosis offered hope to these families where the faulty gene is transmitted as a fully penetrant autosomal dominant trait meaning that a child born to an affected parent had a 50 % chance of inheriting the faulty gene and developing the syndrome.

Systematic registries supported early gene mapping efforts and once the gene had been localised to chromosome 5q by a report of a man with FAP and learning difficulties due to a 5q deletion (Herrera et al. 1986) it took only a few months to localise and then identify the APC gene (Bodmer et al. 1987). Molecular genetic studies combined with more sophisticated clinical evaluation based on the detection of extra colonic features, particularly characteristic pigmented lesions of the retina known as congenital hypertrophy of the retinal pigment epithelium (CHRPE) resulted in highly effective family identification and more extensive endoscopic surveillance and prophylactic surgery (Burn et al. 1991).

The status of the disease was raised significantly once it became apparent that the large *APC* gene which harboured the hereditary defects in FAP was also usually mutated in CRC and that mutations were evident in the earliest adenomas. Somatic mutations in the *APC* gene are considered an initiating event in around 85 % of CRCs making FAP patients a powerful model for CRC chemoprevention studies. In essence, the cancer in an FAP gene carrier is identical to the commonest cancers in the general population. The primary difference is that in "sporadic cancer" both alleles of the APC gene must be lost in the same viable cell for neoplasia to get going where as every cell in the FAP gene carrier has one defective copy of the APC gene so only a single mutation is needed and there are millions of opportunities for that second event to occur.

There has been a long-standing interest in non-steroidal anti inflammatories in FAP. Labayle et al. (1991) reported that sulindac causes regression of rectal polyps in a randomized, placebo-controlled, double-blind crossover study in 10 patients with rectal polyps that had been previously treated by colectomy and ileorectal anastomosis. Patients received sulindac, 300 mg/day, or placebo during two 4-month periods separated by a 1-month wash-out phase. One patient was not compliant and was excluded. With sulindac, the authors observed a complete (six patients) or almost complete (three patients) regression of the polyps. With placebo, the authors observed an increase (five patients), no change (two patients), and a relative decrease (two patients) in the number of polyps. The difference between sulindac and placebo was statistically significant ($p < 0.01$). In biopsy specimens of polyps and normal rectal mucosa of six patients, the authors conducted an immunohistochemical study of the cellular proliferation index using the Ki 67 monoclonal antibody (Ki 67 index), at the beginning and at the end of each treatment period. They were not able to show a sulindac-induced modification of the Ki 67 index. The authors conclude that sulindac is effective in inducing the regression of rectal polyps in FAP. Giardiello et al. (1993) conducted a randomized, double-blind, placebo-controlled study of 22 patients with FAP, including 18 who had not undergone colectomy. The patients received sulindac at a dose of 150 mg orally twice a day for nine months or identical-appearing placebo tablets. The number and size of the polyps were evaluated every 3 months for 1 year. A statistically significant decrease in the mean number of polyps and their mean diameter occurred in patients treated with sulindac. When treatment was stopped at 9 months, the number of polyps had decreased to 44 % of baseline values and the diameter of the polyps to 35 % of baseline values ($p = 0.014$ and $p < 0.001$, respectively, for the comparison with the changes in the group given placebo). No patient had complete resolution of polyps. Three months after treatment with sulindac was stopped, both the number and the size of the polyps increased in sulindac-treated patients but remained significantly lower than the values at baseline. No side effects from sulindac were noted.

Nugent et al. (1993) studied sulindac in 24 FAP patients who had previously undergone prophylactic colectomy and had advanced duodenal polyposis; they were entered into a randomized trial to assess the effect of sulindac on duodenal and rectal polyps. Polyp size and number were assessed by videotaped duodenoscopy (and rectoscopy in 14 patients) at entry and after 6 months of treatment; the tapes were compared by two assessors who were unaware of the randomization and the shuffled chronological order of the recordings. Mucosal cell proliferation was measured by in vitro incorporation of 5-bromo-2′-deoxyuridine. Sulindac therapy was associated with a reduction in epithelial cell proliferation in the duodenum (median labelling index (LI) 15.8 versus 14.4 %, $p = 0.003$) and a trend towards duodenal polyp regression ($p = 0.12$). In the rectum, cell proliferation showed a marked reduction (median LI 8.5 versus 7.4 %, $p = 0.018$), and significant ($p = 0.01$) polyp regression was seen. Rectal polyposis was less severe than that in the duodenum and responded more dramatically.

A small study involving 12 FAP patients supported sulindac use (Cruz-Correa et al. 2002). Five women and seven men with men of age 37 years who had undergone ileorectal anastomosis received a mean dose of 158 mg/day for a mean period of $63.4 \pm 31.3$ months (range 14–98) and were followed every 4 months. Half remained polyp-free and there was a significant regression of polyps in all participants ($p = 0.006$). Prevention of recurrence of higher grade adenomas (tubulovillous, villous adenomas) was also observed ($p = 0.004$). At 35 months of follow-up, one patient developed stage III cancer in the rectal stump. The most common side effect was rectal mucosal erosions in six patients. Long-term use of sulindac was deemed to be effective in reducing polyp number and preventing recurrence of higher grade adenomas in the retained rectal segment of most FAP patients focused on the anti-inflammatory sulindac which acts as a pro drug. Metabolism in the gut converts it into the active form. They found a significant impact on polyp formation but there were some concerns about benefits in the long term.

Enthusiasm for the use of sulindac was diminished by reports of cancers emerging in rectal segments despite apparent suppression of polyp formation (Lynch et al. 1995). This may explain the disappointing results from the long-term follow-up analysis by Giardiello et al. (2002); After 4 years of treatment with either 75 or 150 mg sulindac in an RCT, 41 FAP subjects had achieved 76 % compliance. 43 % of the sulindac versus 55 % of the placebo ($p = 0.54$) developed polyps. There was no significant difference in polyp size or mean number.

Cyclo oxygenase exists in two forms, COX1 and COX2; the former is constitutive and its inhibition underlies the gastrointestinal toxicity of aspirin and other non-steroidals. COX2 is upregulated in inflammation prompting a search for agents which were more COX2 selective. The selective COX2 inhibitors proved to be highly effective and well tolerated leading to widespread use in the management of arthritic conditions. Recognition of the upregulation of COX2 in early colorectal cancer prompted studies of the more popular agents as cancer chemopreventives.

Steinbach et al. (2000) investigated the effects of the selective COX2 inhibtor celecoxib in FAP. In a double-blind, placebo-controlled study, they randomly assigned 77 patients to treatment with celecoxib (100 or 400 mg twice daily) or placebo for 6 months. Patients underwent endoscopy at the beginning and at the end of the study. They determined the number and size of polyps from photographs and videotapes; the response to treatment was expressed as the mean percent change from baseline.

At baseline, the mean (±SD) number of polyps in focal areas where polyps were counted was 15.5 ± 13.4 in the 15 patients assigned to placebo, 11.5 ± 8.5 in the 32 patients assigned to 100 mg of celecoxib twice a day and 12.3 ± 8.2 in the 30 patients assigned to 400 mg of celecoxib twice a day. After 6 months, the patients receiving 400 mg of celecoxib twice a day had a 28.0 % reduction in the mean number of colorectal polyps ($p = 0.003$ for the comparison with placebo) and a 30.7 % reduction in the polyp burden (the sum of polyp diameters) ($p = 0.001$), as compared with reductions of 4.5 and 4.9 %, respectively, in the placebo group. The improvement in the extent of colorectal polyposis in the group receiving 400 mg twice a day was confirmed by a panel of endoscopists who reviewed the videotapes. The reductions in the group receiving 100 mg of celecoxib twice a day were 11.9 % ($p = 0.33$ for the comparison with placebo) and 14.6 % ($p = 0.09$), respectively. The incidence of adverse events was similar among the groups. It is noteworthy that the effects were more convincing with the larger 400 mg twice daily dose which exceeds the levels at which the drug is Cox2 selective.

Huang et al. (2011) similar beneficial effects in their study of 54 celecoxib treated FAP carriers with 13 controls. The Kaplan–Meier estimated probability of not having a polypectomy 12 and 60 months post- ileorectal anastomosis in the celecoxib-treated patients ($n = 33$) was 60.6 and 42.2 %, respectively. The estimated probability of not having a polypectomy 6–60 months post-ileal pouch-anal anastomosis the celecoxib-treated patients ($n = 24$) was 100 %. The median total daily dose of celecoxib was 698.9 mg with the majority treated for more than 24 months. There was one case of a rash attributed to the treatment.

## 2 CAPP1

The third major randomised controlled trial in FAP was our own CAPP1 trial commenced in 1993 but was not finally published until 2011 (Burn et al. 2011a). The trial was conceived shortly after the discovery of the genetic basis and our centre had developed an active registry of FAP families, taking responsibility for management of the regular surveillance programme. It was clear that the families were keen to pursue any realistic avenue of polyp and cancer prevention. The high penetrance meant almost all gene carriers would develop disease, enhancing the statistical power of a prevention trial. The acceptance that all gene carriers should be followed by having endoscopy at least annually meant that prevention trials would be much less expensive. Funding was obtained from the European Union Concerted Action programme, giving rise to the initial name Concerted Action Polyposis Prevention. The acronym has persisted but has had a variety of meanings and in future CAPP will stand for Cancer Prevention Programme.

The CAPP1 trial focused on two interventions in a factorial design such that participants were separately randomised to each. The first agent chosen was aspirin based primarily on the early case control and observational studies suggesting its potential efficacy (Kune et al. 1988; Thun et al. 1991) and the nutritional agent, resistant starch or fermentable fibre.

Nine epidemiological studies have investigated the relationship between starch intake and CR neoplasms, with higher starch intakes providing neoplasm reductions in the range of 25–50 % (Young and Leu 2004). The Bingham team (Cassidy et al. 1994) reported a significant negative correlation between population starch intakes and colon-cancer incidence. Resistant starch (RS) is the sum of starch and the products of starch digestion not absorbed in the small intestine of healthy individuals; it undergoes colonic fermentation to short-chain fatty acids including butyrate. RS supplementation can improve a number of potential biomarkers of CRC risk including faecal concentrations of total and secondary bile acids, which it lowers (Hylla et al. 1998; Grubben et al. 2001). Butyrate and non-steroidal anti-inflammatory drugs (NSAIDs) differ radically in the transcriptome and proteome modifications they produce in tumour cells (Williams et al. 2003; van Munster et al. 1994).

CAPP1 aimed to use adenoma development in adolescents with FAP as the primary measure and effects on mucosal crypt dimensions and cell proliferation as secondary biomarkers of CRC chemoprevention. Polyposis registry clinicians across Europe recruited young male and female FAP patients between 10 and 21 years. Restricting eligibility to members of families manifesting classical FAP helped ensure homogeneity. This restriction meant exclusion of people with less damaging mutations which result in Attenuated or Atypical FAP (AFAP for short). Current NSAID therapy, known aspirin sensitivity, major intercurrent illness and pregnancy were grounds for exclusion. The eligibility cut-off at 21-years old was based on concerns that continuation beyond this age might risk delaying preventive surgery.

## 2.1 CAPP1 Trial Design

CAPP1 was a double-blind, randomized trial with four arms: aspirin (600 mg as 2 tablets/d) plus matched placebo, RS (30 g as 2 sachets/d in a 1:1 blend of potato starch and high amylose maize starch [Hylon VII]) plus matched placebo, aspirin plus RS, and placebo plus placebo; this trial employed a 2 × 2 factorial design. The accrual goal was 208 patients, 52 in each of the four intervention arms.

Randomization was in blocks of 16 stratified at the level of European geographical regions. The duration of intervention was from 1 to a potential maximum of 12 years, with a scheduled annual endoscopy. Patients were advised of their option to leave intervention after each annual examination but were invited to remain on intervention up to age 21 years.

The primary trial endpoint was the proportion of patients with an increased polyp count in the rectum and sigmoid colon after intervention. A major secondary endpoint was size of the largest polyp, which was chosen as another quantifiable and objective measure of disease severity. Given the multiple, international centres participating in this trial, it was not feasible to influence the clinical decision on whether the largest polyp was removed or left in situ nor to tattoo any polyps for review at a later examination.

Secondary laboratory endpoints were proliferative-state assessments assayed using three techniques; samples were microdissected to enable direct counts of total numbers (and location) of mitoses in whole crypts. Formalin-fixed biopsies were paraffin-embedded and sectioned routinely prior to immunohistochemical staining by MIB1 to detect Ki67 and by PC10 to detect PCNA (Mills et al. 2001).

## 2.2 CAPP1 Endpoint Ascertainments

Endoscopists counted the actual number of polyps in the rectum and sigmoid colon if there were 10 or fewer and provided an estimate (11–15, 16–20, 21–30, 31–50, 51–100, >100) when more numerous. Data were collected on the total number of polyps (rectum and sigmoid, ascending, transverse, and descending colon), which presented a challenge because of differing endoscopy policies and the challenge of the total number of polyps in an FAP patient, which can run into the thousands. The situation was made more challenging by marked variation across centres in technology used and the extent of examination. We used diagrams with count estimates, the size of the largest polyp seen and withdrawal rectal videos. The video recordings were scored (better, worse or same) by two experienced endoscopists blinded to intervention and the time point of examination.

## 2.3 CAPP1 Laboratory and Statistical Methods

For assessing proliferative-state endpoints six variously fixed biopsies were taken from normal mucosa near the anal verge at the baseline and annual examinations and microdissected to enable direct counts of total numbers (and location) of mitoses in whole crypts, and measurement of crypt width and length.

The study was designed to detect a statistically significant difference in the proportion of patients with an increased polyp number in the rectum and sigmoid colon for aspirin versus non-aspirin groups or in the RS versus non-RS groups. We included the secondary endpoint of the total number of polyps throughout the colon (adjusted for the extent of endoscopy to account for the variable completeness of endoscopy) so as to make more complete use of collected data. Variability in local policy over extent of endoscopy meant that polyps were counted, or estimated when too dense, in differing numbers of colorectal segments.

We estimated that 40 % of the patients in the placebo group would have an increased polyp count at the end of intervention compared to 20 % in the aspirin or RS groups based on published observational studies (Giovannucci et al. 1995). Due to the suggestion in some of these studies that the effect was greater with prolonged use, this study was designed to allow participants to remain on study for as long as possible. The final sample size estimate of 208 patients was based on early data indicating that almost all patients had detectable pathology and was designed to detect the anticipated intervention effect with an 80 % power and alpha level of 0.025.

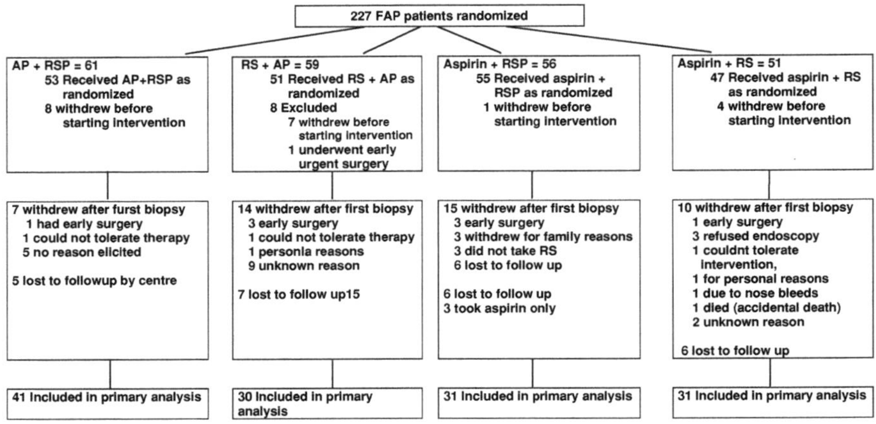


**Fig. 1** CAPP1 consort diagram

A supplementary prespecified secondary analysis was the size of the largest polyp at the end of intervention and assessed in the subset of patients who remained on study for >1 year; these patients were anticipated to be more likely fully compliant and to respond to an active intervention.

## 2.4 CAPP1 Results

Initially, 227 young people aged from 10 to 21 years with intact colons were recruited into the study (1993–2002) and 206 of these started the intervention (Fig. 1). Fifty-nine percent (133/227) had a baseline and at least one other endoscopy and were therefore eligible for data analyses. (Table 2). Some patients remained on intervention for up to 7 years before the study ended.

Withdrawal rates in each intervention group were compatible with random loss. For the 94 patients excluded from analysis, there was a non-significant difference in age at "dropout" between the four intervention groups (ANOVA, $p = 0.06$). Of the patients included in the final analysis, 57 % (76/133) had two colonoscopies, 23 % (30/133) had three colonoscopies, 11 % (15/133) had four and 9 % (12/133) had 5–8 colonoscopies. No polyps were found in 15 % of the colonoscopies; 57 % of the colonoscopies went further than the sigmoid colon.

At baseline, the four intervention groups were well matched; at entry endoscopy, 41 % of patients had one or more polyps removed; these patients tended to be older.

After a median intervention period of 17 months (range 1–73), the primary endpoint of a risk of an increased polyp number in the rectum and sigmoid colon was not significantly reduced in either treatment group with relative risks of 0.77 (aspirin; 95 % CI, 0.54–1.10;) and 1.05 (RS; 95 % CI, 0.73–1.49; Table 3). The diameter of the largest polyp (major secondary endpoint) detected by the endoscopist at the end of intervention tended to be smaller in the aspirin arm ($p = 0.05$

**Table 2** CAPP1 Patient characteristics

| Baseline measures (range of values) | | | Number | Intervention (N)[a] | | | | *P*-value |
|---|---|---|---|---|---|---|---|---|
| | | | | RSP/AP (41) | RS/AP (30) | A/RSP (31) | A/RS (31) | |
| Age | Mean (s.d) | | | 18.2 (7.8) | 17.9 (10.8) | 17.2 (6.9) | 18.8 (7.9) | 0.90 |
| | N | | 133 | 41 | 30 | 31 | 31 | |
| Sex | N (%) | Female | 66 | 19 (46.3) | 21 (70.0) | 12 (41.4) | 14 (45.2) | $X^2(3) = 6.2$, |
| | | Male | 65 | 22 (53.7) | 9 (30.0) | 17 (58.6) | 17 (54.8) | $p = 0.10$ |
| | | Total | 131 | 41 (100) | 30 (100) | 29 (100) | 31 (100) | |
| Number of endoscopies | N | 2 | 76 | 20 | 19 | 21 | 16 | |
| | | 3 | 30 | 12 | 3 | 3 | 12 | |
| | | 4 | 15 | 4 | 5 | 4 | 2 | |
| | | 5 | 8 | 4 | | 3 | 1 | |
| | | 6 | 1 | 1 | | | | |
| | | 7 | 2 | | 2 | | | |
| | | 8 | 1 | | 1 | | | |
| | | Total | 133 | 41 | 30 | 31 | 31 | |
| *Polyp data* | | | | | | | | |
| At least 1 polyp found | N (%) | No | 13 | 1 (2.4) | 5 (17.9) | 3 (10.0) | 4 (13.3) | $X^2(3) = 4.8$, |
| | | Yes | 116 | 40 (97.6) | 23 (82.1) | 27 (90.0) | 26 (86.7) | $p = 0.18$ |
| | | Total | 129 | 41 (100) | 28 (100) | 30 (100) | 30 (100) | |
| Number of polyps in the rectum and sigmoid colon (0, 200) | Mean (s.d) | | | 29.8 (43.0) | 29.7 | 22.7 | 25.6 | 0.53[b] |
| | N | | 129 | 41 | (52.5) 28 | (32.3) 30 | (44.4) 30 | |
| Total number of polyps (0, 425) | Mean (s.d) | | | 56.7 (86.4) | 63.8 | 44.5 | 43.1 | 0.60[b] |
| | N | | 129 | 41 | (115.6) 28 | (90.5) 30 | (76.2) 30 | |
| Size of largest polyp (mm) (0.5, 50) | Mean (s.d) | | | 6.1 (8.2) | 4.2 (2.7) | 4.0 (2.5) | 4.3 (2.4) | 0.63[b] |
| | N | | 110 | 38 | 21 | 27 | 24 | |

(continued)

**Table 2** (continued)

| Baseline measures (range of values) | | Number | Intervention (N)[a] | | | | P-value |
|---|---|---|---|---|---|---|---|
| | | | RSP/AP (41) | RS/AP (30) | A/RSP (31) | A/RS (31) | |
| *Crypts* | | | | | | | |
| Crypt width (74.2, 199.7) | Mean (s.d) | | 121.5 (21.6) | 110.7 (20.3) | 116.8 (24.1) | 111.5 (17.3) | 0.16[b] |
| | N | 113 | 35 | 24 | 25 | 29 | |
| Crypt length (290.4, 765.1) | Mean (s.d) | | 499.4 (84.4) | 467.3 (92.9) | 494.8 (75.6) | 498.6 (69.1) | 0.27[b] |
| | N | 112 | 35 | 24 | 25 | 28 | |
| Mean total CCP (0.2, 37.9) | Mean (s.d) | | 5.3 (4.9) | 6.1 (7.8) | 7.5 (6.1) | 6.1 (4.2) | 0.27[b] |
| | N | 113 | 35 | 24 | 25 | 29 | |

[a] Raw means presented
[b] Log transformed measures used in the tests

and $p = 0.09$ after adjusting for baseline measures; Table 4. The planned subgroup analyses of patients who elected to continue on study for more than 1 year found a significant reduction in the size of the largest polyp in the aspirin versus non-aspirin group ($p = 0.02$, adjusted for baseline; Table 4 and Fig. 2). We found an absence of polyps in the majority of our blinded review of rectal videos (both at baseline and during intervention), even though there were adenomas in the colon making these recordings of little value. The risk of an increased total number of polyps in all examined segments of the colorectum was not reduced in either intervention group, with relative risks of 0.97 (aspirin; 95 % CI, 0.65–1.43;) and 0.96 (RS; 95 % CI, 0.65–1.42;).

Relative risks of effects of intervention on crypt width and length are shown in Table 3 and Fig. 3. Mean crypt length decreased significantly over time on study in the two combined RS groups, compared with the two combined non-RS groups ($P < 0.0001$ for interaction), in a model of the interaction between intervention and time (Fig. 2).

Histological examination of microdissected crypts revealed increases in total CCP of 28 % ($p = 0.12$) in the RS versus non-RS group and 37 % ($p = 0.05$) in the aspirin versus non-aspirin group (Table 3).

## 2.5 CAPP1 Toxicity

No serious adverse effects were recorded. None of the participants reported any problems with symptoms of ulceration or gastrointestinal bleeding. One participant in the aspirin/RS arm withdrew because of persistent nose bleeds. There were no

**Table 3** Relative risks (*RelRs*) and 95 % confidence intervals (*CIs*) from 12 univariate models[a] estimating the effect of intervention by outcome measure

| Outcome measures | No. of obs (no. of patients) | RS versus non-RS | | Aspirin versus non-aspirin | |
|---|---|---|---|---|---|
| | | RelR[b] (95% CI) | *p*-value | RelR (95% CI) | *p*-value |
| Total number of polyps in rectum and sigmoid | 215 (116) | 1.05 (0.73, 1.49) | 0.80 | 0.77 (0.54, 1.10) | 0.16 |
| Crypt width | 95 (58) | 1.03 (0.93, 1.13) | 0.60 | 0.95 (−0.15, 0.04) | 0.28 |
| Crypt length | 95 (58) | 1.01 (0.93, 1.09) | 0.86 | 1.08 (1.00, 1.16) | 0.04 |
| Mean total CCP | 95 (58) | 1.28 (0.94, 1.73) | 0.12 | 1.37 (1.00, 1.86) | 0.05 |
| Mean number of MIB1-positive cells[c] | 116 (78) | 1.02 (0.89, 1.16) | 0.82 | 0.99 (0.87, 1.14) | 0.93 |
| Hemicrypt cells[c,d] | 116 (78) | −0.82 (−5.05, 3.42)[d] | 0.71 | 3.67 (−0.55, 7.90)[d] | 0.09 |

[a] All models adjusted for first result and time on intervention (years)
[b] Estimated as the exponential coefficient of the intervention effect in the random effects model
[c] Adjusted for calendar time to account for possible effect of differences in storage time of these samples before analysis; MIB1 is the antibody used in staining for Ki67
[d] Variable not logged, coefficient not exponentiated

reports of cardiovascular or cerebrovascular events.As expected, some participants randomised to receive RS described bloating; a sense of abdominal distension attributable to the products of fermentation in the bowel. The most common reason cited for withdrawal from study was difficulty in including starch in the habitual diet. There was no statistically significant difference between starch and its matching placebo or aspirin and its matching placebo in rates of withdrawal.

## 2.6 CAPP1 Conclusions

There was a non-significant trend of a reduced number of polyps in the rectum and sigmoid colon (primary endpoint) in the overall aspirin group (aspirin plus placebo and aspirin plus RS) versus the non-aspirin group at the end of intervention. There also was evidence that the size of the largest polyp (secondary endpoint) was reduced in the overall aspirin versus the overall non-aspirin group. Furthermore, among those treated for more than 1 year, the diameter of the largest polyp recorded in the aspirin group (3.0 mm) was only half that recorded in the placebo group (6.0 mm; $p = 0.02$).

**Table 4** Mean size of largest polyp by intervention group at baseline and at the end of intervention with aspirin and/or resistant starch

| | Mean Size of largest polyp[a] (N) | | | | | | | |
|---|---|---|---|---|---|---|---|---|
| | Four intervention group comparison[b] | | | | Aspirin comparison | | Starch comparison | |
| | RSP/ AP[c] | RS/ AP | A/ RSP | A/ RS | Non-aspirin[c] | Aspirin | Non-RS[c] | RS |
| At baseline[d] | 6.9 (31) | 4.3 (20) | 4.0 (25) | 4.6 (19) | 5.8 (51) | 4.3 (44) | 5.6 (56) | 4.4 (39) |
| *p*-value | | 0.12 | 0.07 | 0.41 | | 0.31 | | 0.55 |
| Final largest polyp size for all patients[e] | 6.5 (31) | 4.0 (20) | 3.4 (25) | 4.4 (19) | 5.5 (51) | 3.8 (44) | 5.1 (56) | 4.2 (39) |
| *p*-value | | 0.03 | 0.006 | 0.07 | | 0.05 | | 0.27 |
| *p*-value adjusted for baseline | | 0.10 | 0.03 | 0.11 | | 0.09 | | 0.35 |
| Final largest polyp size for patients treated for more than 1 year | 6.5 (17) | 4.6 (7) | 2.9 (8) | 3.1 (9) | 6.0 (24) | 3.0 (17) | 5.4 (25) | 3.8 (16) |
| *p*-value | | 0.26 | 0.03 | 0.02 | | 0.01 | | 0.17 |
| *p*-value adjusted for baseline | | 0.42 | 0.09 | 0.03 | | 0.02 | | 0.19 |

[a] Raw means presented, log transformed measures used in tests
[b] The *p*-values are from linear regression for the following comparisons: RS/P vs P/P, A/P vs P/P an A/RS vs P/P
[c] Reference group in the linear regression models
[d] 23/133 Patients did not have polyps measured at baseline, and 15/133 patients did not have polyps measured throughout the study. Numbers are based on patients who also have a result post-baseline
[e] Numbers are based on patients who also have a baseline result

## 3 Chemoprevention in Lynch Syndrome: CAPP2

A century has passed since Warthin reported the dominant cancer risk in his seamstress' family, later described by Henry Lynch and colleagues as Family G. (1971) Around the same time a family doctor in the North east of England noticed frequent deaths from colorectal cancer in a family under his care. He eventually traced and reported 45 related cases in what became the "Durham family" (Dunstone and Knaggs 1972). The early 1990s saw a flurry of publications linking such families to a dominant tarit determined by genes on chromosomes 2 and 3 and subsequently making the connection to the mismatch repair system based on the tendency of tumours to manifest microsatellite instability, an inability to correctly replicate repetitive sections of DNA (Boland et al. 1997, 1998; Fishel et al. 1993). It is now recognised that Lynch syndrome, the name preferred to the earlier label of HNPCC or Hereditary Non-Polyposis Colorectal Cancer, is much more common that the collective polyposis syndromes and offers a model system for cases of sporadic

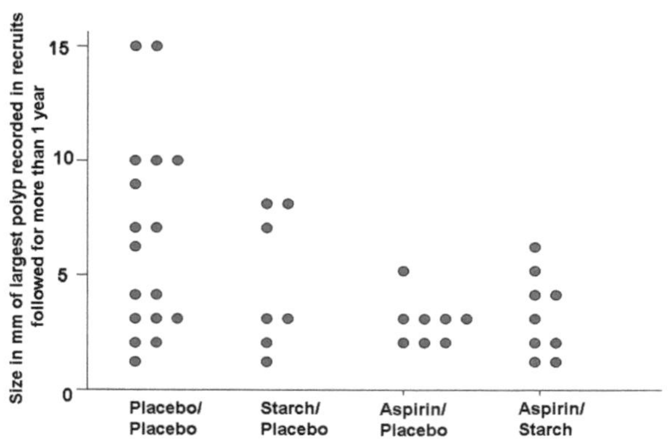


**Fig. 2** Size of largest polyp in patients who stayed in the study for more than 1 year, adjusted for baseline ($p = 0.02$)

colorectal cancer associated with acquired loss breakdown of mismatch repair. The latter group make up about 1 in 6 of all colorectal cancers while Lynch syndrome clinically (de la Chapelle 2004) affects at least 1 in 3,000 adults but may be carried by as many as 1 in 300 people, accounting for at least 1 in 35 of all colorectal cancers. (de la Chapelle 2004; Lynch and Krush 1971; Hampel et al. 2008).

CAPP2 (ISRCTN59521990.) (Burn et al. 2011b) was the first large-scale genetically targeted chemoprevention trial with over 80 % of recruitment-based exclusively on molecular genetic testing for mutations in the mismatch repair genes. CAPP2 was calculated to need 1,000 people with Lynch syndrome (LS) on the presumption that intervention would reduce colorectal neoplasia by 50 %.

Between 1999 and 2005, 1009 eligible gene carriers were recruited from 43 international centres and 937 of these commenced intervention: 600 mg enteric coated aspirin and/or 30grams of the resistant starch Novelose in a 2 × 2 factorial placebo controlled design. After the intervention period lasting a mean of 29 months, there was no evidence that either agent influenced development of colonic neoplasia with most lesions being adenomas (Burn et al. 2008).

Given cohort and case–control evidence of a CRC protective effect of aspirin only after prolonged exposure, the original design of the CAPP2 Study included double blind post-intervention follow-up for at least 10 years.

At the end of the intervention period 128 persons had developed at least one adenoma and 23 had developed CRC. These were pooled for analysis as "neoplasia" since it was considered unlikely that the primary endpoint of CRC would be influenced within 4 years in a population under colonoscopic surveillance. In 2009 when the first recruit reached her 10-year-CAPP2 anniversary, an analysis of cancer incidence was commenced. The baseline population of 861 persons (randomized to aspirin or aspirin placebo in the RCT) was the focus of our recent publication (Burn et al. 2011b).

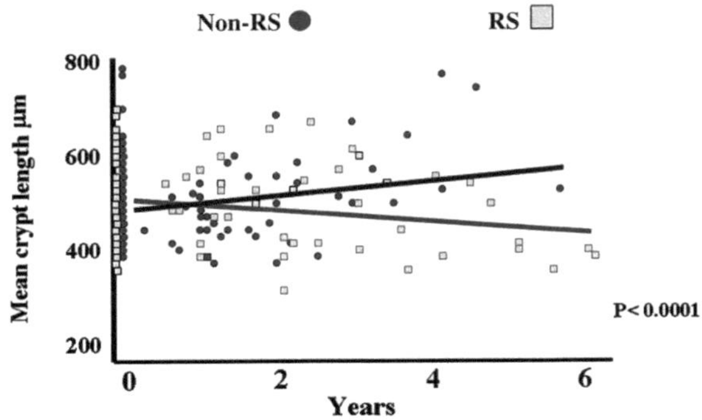


**Fig. 3** Mean length of microdissected crypts over time on study in patients of the resistant starch (*RS*) group (RS plus aspirin placebo, RS plus aspirin) or of the non-RS group (aspirin plus RS placebo, aspirin placebo plus RS placebo). Crypts tended to lengthen with time on study for the non-RS group, whereas they shortened in the RS group (*P*-value for interaction <0.0001)

## 3.1 CAPP2 Trial Design

The study was a 2 × 2 factorial RCT involving intervention for between 1 and 4 years and a preplanned design for 10 years follow-up; at the time of the second analysis, of the 937 persons who commenced treatment, 427 were randomized to aspirin, 434 to aspirin placebo (AP) and the remaining recruits were not randomized for the aspirin intervention having opted not to participate in this study limb ($N = 76$; almost all due to perceived aspirin sensitivity or history of peptic ulceration). All participants in this latter group were randomized to the RS or resistant starch placebo (RSP) intervention only (Fig. 4; Consort diagram).

The 2011 publication focused on the 861 CAPP2 participants randomized to aspirin or AP. Our analysis included (1) the LS syndrome cancers included in the earlier report (Burn et al. 2008) (2) those that occurred subsequent to exit from the intervention phase and (3) all cancers that occurred in persons without an exit colonoscopy which excluded them from the statistical analysis in the 2008 report.

## 3.2 CAPP2 Endpoint Ascertainments

Due to dispersed international recruitment and because routine surveillance was provided by local healthcare teams, records of adenoma occurrence among CAPP2 participants subsequent to the intervention phase were incomplete.

## 3.3 CAPP2 Statistical Methods

Analysis was designed to test the primary hypothesis that aspirin would reduce the development of CRC (as primary outcome) and LS cancers (as secondary outcome) in 861 persons randomized to aspirin. The original protocol invited

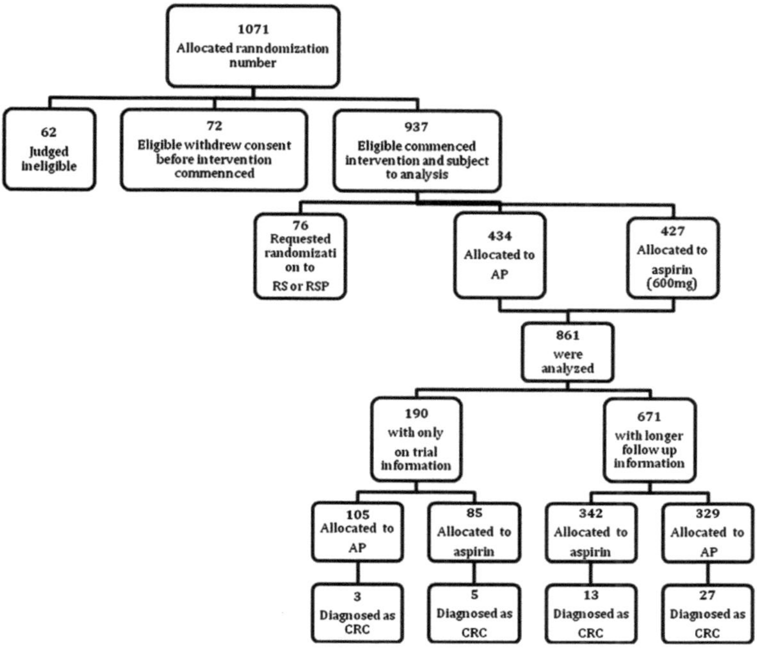


**Fig. 4** CAPP2 consort diagram

participants to continue with the original intervention for a further 2-year cycle following the initial 2 years.

Two approaches were taken: time to first CRC occurrence (the original focus) examined using life-table methods and Cox proportional hazards and second, Poisson regression modelling to investigate primary cancers at multiple anatomical sites, a feature of LS. Poisson regression analysis takes into account the complete cancer history of the participant since randomization in contrast with the more restricted time to first event analysis.

For life-table analysis, end of follow-up was determined as (1) the time of first CRC diagnosis, if affected, or (2) the last recorded date at which the clinical status was known. Analyses included Cox proportional hazards models to estimate gender-adjusted hazard ratios (HR) and 95 % Confidence Intervals and Kaplan–Meier curves to assess non-parametrically the outcome differences between the aspirin and AP interventions. The assumption of proportional hazard was tested to assess compliance.

For the Poisson regression analysis, incidence rate ratios (IRR) for the effect of aspirin adjusted for gender were estimated from log-linear models for the number of primary cancers diagnosed after randomization; exposure time being that from randomization until date of last known clinical status.

**Table 5** Study population: numbers, time on study, time on follow-up and cancer burden according to aspirin use

| | | Aspirin | AP | Total |
|---|---|---|---|---|
| Number of participants | | 427 | 434 | 861 |
| Months on CAPP2 intervention study (mean) (sd, range) | | 25.0 (12.5) (0.8, 60.6) | 25.4 (14.2) (1.1, 74.4) | 25.2 (13.4) (0.8, 74.4) |
| Months since study entry (mean) (sd, range) | | 56.6 (30.9) (0.8, 125.4) | 54.8 (31.8) (1.6, 128) | 55.7 (31.4) (0.8, 128) |
| Number of participants with first CRC | Since randomization | 18 | 30 | 48 |
| | Within 2 years of randomization | 10 | 10 | 20 |
| | More than 2 years from randomization | 8 | 20 | 28 |
| Number of participants with other LS cancers[a] | Since randomization | 16 | 24 | 40 |
| | Within 2 years of randomization | 5 | 9 | 14 |
| | More than 2 years from randomization | 11 | 15 | 26 |
| Number of participants with one or more LS cancers (including CRC) | Since randomization | 34 | 52 | 86 |
| | Within 2 years of randomization | 15 | 19 | 34 |
| | More than 2 years from randomization | 19 | 33 | 52 |
| Number of participants with non-LS cancers | | 19 | 19 | 38 |

[a] Two participants in placebo group had CRC and another LS cancer. These two participants are counted in the rows relating to both CRC and other LS cancers. In the row reporting to all Lynch syndrome cancers, these participants are counted only once

Analyses were conducted on the basis of "Intention to Treat" (i.e. intervention assigned at randomization) and also "Per Protocol" (restricting consideration to those taking aspirin (or AP) for at least 2 years) as defined in the protocol. A secondary planned analysis addressed the category of "LS cancer incidence" including new cancers considered to result from the underlying genetic defect. Designation of LS cancer spectrum was a clinical assessment, blinded to intervention, and based on a review of the LS phenotype (Vasen et al. 2007); endometrial, ovarian, pancreatic, small bowel, gall bladder, ureter, stomach and kidney cancers and cancer of the brain were included. A final analysis examined the total burden of LS-related cancers in those who had been on intervention for at least 2 years (per protocol).

**Table 6** Cox proportional hazards analysis and Poisson regression for CRC cancer (adjusted for gender) based only on those randomized to aspirin or aspirin placebo (AP)

| | Estimate of effect of | CRC HR (95 % CI)[a] | p-value | CRC IRR[c] (95 % CI) | p-value |
|---|---|---|---|---|---|
| Intention to treat | Aspirin vs AP | 0.63 (0.35–1.13) | 0.12 | 0.56 (0.32–0.99) | 0.05 |
| Per protocol analysis | ≥2 years AP[b] | 1.0 | | 1.0 | |
| | <2 years AP[b] | 0.62 (0.25–1.52) | 0.30 | 0.72 (0.32–1.59) | 0.41 |
| | <2 years aspirin[b] | 1.07 (0.47–2.41) | 0.87 | 0.90 (0.42–1.91) | 0.77 |
| | ≥2 years aspirin[b] | 0.41 (0.19–0.86) | 0.02 | 0.37 (0.18–0.78) | 0.008 |
| Cumulative aspirin dose | Units of 100 aspirin[d] | 0.97 (0.94–1.00) | 0.06 | 0.97 (0.94–1.00) | 0.03 |

[a] Cox proportional Hazards analysis based on 48 participants with CRC involving a total of 53 cancer diagnoses: HR = hazard ratio (95 % Confidence Interval)
[b] The threshold for 2 years intervention was consumption of more than 1,400 aspirin tablets; rounded down from a 2-year total of 1,461 tablets to allow for early scheduling of the exit colonoscopy and/or occasional missed dosage
[c] Incidence rate ratio (95 % Confidence Interval) from Poisson regression
[d] Units of 100 aspirin = the total number of aspirin taken divided by 100

## 3.4 CAPP2 Results

The mean observation period was 55.7 months (range 1–128 months) and 1 % of recruits were ≥10 years from randomization by the time of the current analysis (Table 5).

In 190 recruits only “on trial” information was located. Post intervention data were collected on the remaining 671. Demographic data indicate no differences between those traced and not traced in this follow-up in respect of age, gender, randomization category, or geographical location though it is plausible that the development of a cancer made follow-up reporting more complete. There were no significant regional differences in CRC incidence (data not shown, Chi-squared (2) = 5.03, $p = 0.08$).

Overall, 40 people were diagnosed with CRC among those with post intervention information (13/342 allocated to aspirin and 27/329 allocated to AP). Another 8 CRC occurred among 190 (83 male and 107 female) individuals with intervention phase only information, (5/85 and 3/105 for aspirin and AP arm respectively) (Fig. 4).

Evidence emerged of delayed protection by aspirin against cancer. Despite regular colonoscopy and polyp removal, 48 recruits developed CRC after randomization (Table 1). Of these, 18 received aspirin and 30 received AP. For the whole

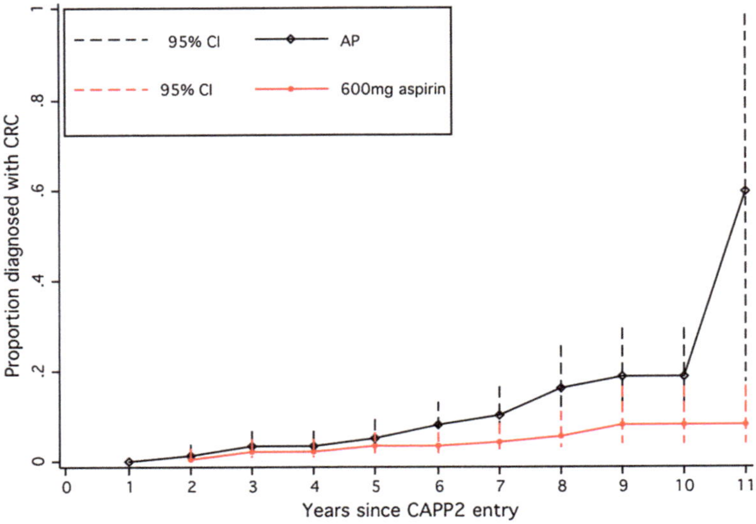


**Fig. 5** Time to first colorectal cancer in those randomized to aspirin compared with those randomized to the aspirin placebo (*AP*). In each case, Kaplan–Meier analysis was restricted to participants who had taken ≥2 years intervention and the analysis was adjusted for gender (HR 0.41 (CI 0.19–0.86), $p = 0.02$). Each point on the plot shows the estimated cumulative incidence by years of follow-up together with the corresponding 95 % confidence interval

post-randomization period, the HR for CRC for aspirin was 0.63 (CI 0.35–1.13, $p = 0.12$) favouring protection in the aspirin group (Table 6). Five of the 48 people who developed CRC each had two primary colon cancers. Of these, one had received aspirin and four AP. Although the Intention to treat time-to-event analysis showed a non-significant protective effect of aspirin, the Poisson regression taking into account the five multiple primary CRC participants (53 CRC) indicated a protective effect: IRR 0.56 (CI 0.32–0.99, $p = 0.05$). Because of this protective effect we re-estimated the protective effect with a Per Protocol analysis and obtained similar results.

Participants who took aspirin (or AP) for a minimum of 2 years [defined as consumption of at least 1,400 (300 mg) tablets]. 258 (30 %) and 250 (29.1 %) participants took aspirin and AP respectively for at least 2 years. The HR for this group was 0.41 (CI 0.19–0.86 $p = 0.02$, Table 6; Fig. 5) and the IRR, 0.37 (CI 0.18–0.78 $p = 0.008$). These results are similar to those for Poisson regression in the ITT analysis.

We explored the effect of compliance on outcome (important because noncompliance may be related to factors that also affect CRC risk) using Per Protocol analysis, and found those who took aspirin for ≥2 years had an incidence rate of 0.06 per 100 person-years compared with 0.13 per 100 person years among those who took aspirin <2 years. A similar analysis within the placebo group found no significant difference in CRC incidence between those who took AP for ≥2 years (0.14 per 100 person years) compared with those took AP for <2 years (0.10 per 100 person years).

**Table 7** Cox proportional hazards analysis and poisson regression for non-CRC Lynch syndrome cancers (adjusted for gender) based only on those randomized to aspirin or aspirin placebo (AP)

| | Estimate of effect of | Non-CRC Lynch cancer | | Non-CRC LS cancer | |
|---|---|---|---|---|---|
| | | HR (95 % CI)[a] | p-value | IRR[c] (95 % CI) | p-value |
| Intention to treat | Aspirin vs AP | 0.63 (0.34–1.19) | 0.16 | 0.63 (0.34–1.16) | 0.14 |
| Per protocol analysis | $\geq$2 years AP[b] | 1.0 | | 1.0 | |
| | <2 years AP[b] | 0.96 (0.40–2.34) | 0.94 | 0.82 (0.35–1.96) | 0.66 |
| | <2 years aspirin[b] | 1.11 (0.46–2.68) | 0.82 | 0.90 (0.38–2.14) | 0.81 |
| | $\geq$2 years aspirin[b] | 0.47 (0.21–1.06) | 0.07 | 0.49 (0.23–1.05) | 0.07 |
| Cumulative aspirin dose | Units of 100 aspirin[d] | 0.96 (0.93–1.00) | 0.03 | 0.96 (0.93–1.00) | 0.03 |

[a] Cox proportional hazards analysis based on 40 case : HR = hazard ratio (95 % confidence interval)
[b] The threshold for 2 years intervention was consumption of more than 1,400 aspirin tablets; rounded down from a 2-year total of 1,461 tablets to allow for early scheduling of the exit colonoscopy and/or occasional missed dosage
[c] Incidence rate ratio (95 % Confidence Interval) from poisson regression
[d] Units of 100 aspirin = the total number of aspirin taken divided by 100

The planned secondary analysis with other LS cancers as the secondary outcome also showed a trend to protection with aspirin; 18 participants developed endometrial cancer of whom 5 were randomized to aspirin and 13 to AP. In total, 38 participants developed cancer at a site other than the colorectum (additionally 2 participants had CRC and another LS cancer) of whom 16 were randomized to aspirin and 22 to AP (Supplementary Table 5). The HR for those randomized to aspirin was 0.63 (CI 0.34–1.19 $p = 0.16$, Table 7) and IRR was 0.63 (CI 0.34–1.16 $p = 0.14$) compared with AP group. Per Protocol analysis showed that the HR for those who had taken aspirin for $\geq$2 years was 0.47 (CI 0.21–1.06 $p = 0.07$) with IRR = 0.49 (CI 0.23–1.05 $p = 0.07$) (Table 7).

Table 8 gives the combined analysis of all LS cancers including CRC. On intention to treat analysis, the HR was 0.65 (CI 0.42–1.00 $p = 0.05$ and IRR was 0.59 (CI 0.39–0.90 $p = 0.01$) while the Per Protocol analysis HR was 0.45 (CI 0.26–0.79 $p = 0.005$,) and IRR was 0.42 (CI 0.25–0.72, $p = 0.001$) supporting the protective effect of aspirin. Cox proportional hazards models analysis by cumulative aspirin consumption suggested a dose–response effect which was significant for non-CRC LS cancers ($p = 0.03$), LS cancers overall ($p = 0.007$) and a trend for CRC ($p = 0.06$, Tables 6, 7 and 8). Corresponding outcomes from the Poisson regression analysis were also significant ($p = 0.03$ for non-CRC LS cancers, $p = 0.002$ for LS cancers overall and $p = 0.03$ for CRC).

**Table 8** Cox proportional hazards analysis and poisson regression for all Lynch Syndrome (LS) cancers (adjusted for gender) based only on those randomized to aspirin or aspirin placebo (AP)

| | Estimate of effect of | All LS cancers | | All LS cancers | |
|---|---|---|---|---|---|
| | | HR (95 % CI)[a] | *p*-value | IRR[c] (95 % CI) | *p*-value |
| Intention to treat | Aspirin vs AP | 0.65 (0.42–1.00) | 0.05 | 0.59 (0.39–0.90) | 0.01 |
| Per protocol analysis | ≥2 years AP[b] | 1.0 | | 1.0 | |
| | <2 years AP[b] | 0.79 (0.42–1.49) | 0.47 | 0.76 (0.43–1.37) | 0.36 |
| | <2 years aspirin[b] | 1.13 (0.62–2.06) | 0.69 | 0.90 (0.51–1.59) | 0.71 |
| | ≥2 years aspirin[b] | 0.45 (0.26–0.79) | 0.005 | 0.42 (0.25–0.72) | 0.001 |
| Cumulative aspirin dose | Units of 100 aspirin[d] | 0.97 (0.95–0.99) | 0.007 | 0.96 (0.94–0.99) | 0.002 |

[a] Cox proportional Hazards analysis based on 86 participants with LS cancers involving a total of 93 cancer diagnoses: *HR* = hazard ratio (95 % confidence interval)
[b] The threshold for 2-years' intervention was consumption of more than 1,400 aspirin tablets; rounded down from a 2-year total of 1,461 tablets to allow for early scheduling of the exit colonoscopy and/or occasional missed dosage
[c] Incidence rate ratio (95 % Confidence Interval) from poisson regression
[d] Units of 100 aspirin = the total number of aspirin taken divided by 100

Where possible, details of adenoma development were collected in the post-intervention period. While incomplete, these data, gathered by blinded contributors' revealed no apparent effect of aspirin on numbers of participants who developed adenomas subsequent to the intervention phase i.e. 51 and 48 in the aspirin and AP groups respectively. The data were analysed according to the underlying MMR gene defect. Overall, there was no evidence of difference in CRC incidence by presence of proven germ-line mutation (Chi-squared (2) = 3.1, $p = 0.38$).

Eighteen (34 %) of 53 CRC diagnosed in aspirin or AP arms were Dukes stage A, 21 (39.6 %) Dukes B, 10 (18.9 %) had Dukes C and D, and 4 (7.5 %) were unknown. Twenty-seven (51 %) tumours were located in the ascending colon, transverse colon and splenic flexure, 6 (11.3 %) in the descending colon, 12 (22.6 %) in the sigmoid and rectum, and 8 (15.1 %) were unknown. There was no significant difference in staging (Chi-squared (3) = 2.92, $p = 0.40$) and tumour location (Chi-squared (3) = 0.08, $p = 0.99$) between aspirin and AP groups.

## 3.5 CAPP2 Toxicity

During the intervention phase adverse events in the aspirin and placebo groups were similar (Burn et al. 2008) with 11 significant gastrointestinal bleeds or ulcers in the aspirin group and 9 in the placebo group. No details of adverse events were available for the post-intervention phase. There was also no significant difference in compliance (i.e. proportion of scheduled tablets not taken during the intervention phase) between the aspirin and AP groups for those with complete intervention phase data (Chi-squared (1) = 1.27, $p = 0.20$).

## 3.6 CAPP2 Discussion

The CAPP2 Study is the first double blind RCT of aspirin chemoprevention with cancer as primary endpoint. The outcome is consistent with over two decades of observational data (Cuzick et al. 2009) and recent long-term follow-up of aspirin trials for cardiovascular disease (Rothwell et al. 2010, 2011). This concept of delayed cancer chemoprevention was apparent in observational studies (Chan et al. 2011), where protection against cancer among regular aspirin users took approximately 10 years to emerge. It was presumed that this effect was dependent on continued aspirin exposure but in the CVD trials trial medication ended at mean 6 years. Analysis of cancer-related death in eight trials revealed significant protection in those allocated aspirin for ≥4 years but only when followed for a further 5 years. Our observations support this hypothesis of a delayed effect of aspirin on CRC by showing that aspirin reduced CRC incidence with the effect becoming apparent after 3–4 years from beginning aspirin intervention, a difference consistent with faster cancer development in those with LS (Lynch et al. 1995; Vasen 2008).

In ITT analysis, Poisson regression analysis, which incorporates more of the follow-up information than the time-to-event analysis (i.e. total number of cancers in follow-up period *v.* time to first cancer), showed similar estimates of the protective effect but, as anticipated greater significance. The Per Protocol analysis showed a similar effect.

In keeping with our observed impact of aspirin on non-colonic LS cancers (endometrial cancer, ovarian cancer, pancreatic cancer, and cancer of the brain, small bowel, gall bladder, ureter, stomach and kidney) (Table 7), Rothwell et al. reported that aspirin treatment reduced risk of death from several non-colonic solid cancers including oesophageal, pancreatic, brain, lung, stomach and prostate. It is not clear whether LS cancers are more responsive to aspirin therapy. In CAPP2 "non-LS" extra-colonic cancers appeared unaffected by aspirin intervention (Table 5) but this group would be expected to show an effect later.

Our discovery of substantial protection by aspirin against CRC and other LS cancers is in striking contrast with our earlier report of no effect of aspirin on large bowel neoplasia. Taken together, these findings may help explain the marked disparity between the 50 % cancer reduction reported in observational studies and the outcomes of randomized adenoma prevention trials which have demonstrated, at best, a modest reduction effect; meta-analysis revealed a pooled risk ratio of any adenoma for any dose of aspirin versus placebo of 0.83 (95 % CI = 0.72–0.96) (Cole et al. 2009). Important questions include (1) does aspirin target the minority of adenomas with the greatest malignant potential, (2) do some LS CRCs arise from lesions other than adenomas (Jass et al. 2002) and (3) why are some tumours aspirin "resistant"?

The mechanism by which aspirin suppresses cancer development long after cessation of exposure to the drug remains unclear. The assumption that the primary action of anti-inflammatories is on COX2 in colonic tumours is unlikely to be the primary mechanism. The rapid progression from adenoma to carcinoma in LS makes it likely that many screen-detected cancers would have begun to develop after aspirin intervention ended. Aspirin may be pro-apoptotic at early stages of CRC development, perhaps preceding adenoma formation. Ruschoff et al. (1998). reported reduced microsatellite instability and enhanced apoptosis in MMR-deficient cells exposed to aspirin and argued that aspirin may induce genetic selection for microsatellite stability in a subset of MMR-deficient cells. Aspirin may delete those aberrant stem cells most likely to progress rapidly to cancer. Analysis of the conditional MSH2 knockout mouse, reported recently to survive significantly longer when exposed to aspirin (McIlhatton et al. 2011). might shed light on the mechanism.

Despite regular colonoscopy, 1 in 14 of those not taking aspirin in CAPP2 developed CRC in under 5 years, emphasising the need for additional prevention strategies. Our results, taken in conjunction with the recent literature, provide a basis for recommending aspirin chemoprevention in LS as the standard of care.

## 4 CAPP3

The evidence is now sufficient to recommend aspirin to all gene carriers with the clear statement that we still do not know what dose is ideal. It is hoped that all clinicians will encourage their patients who carry a mismatch repair gene defect to sign up to the CAPP3 dose inferiority study.

CAPP3 (www.capp3.org) will aim to provide a blinded daily aspirin dose over a 5-year period with regular surveillance continued as usual and collection of detailed information on adverse events and gastrointestinal tumours.

There is a need to recruit 3,000 gene carriers in total and follow the three dose groups for 5–10 years in order to test whether 100 mg is inferior to 300 or 600 mg doses. Individuals with microsatellite unstable CRCs develop antibodies to the neopeptides, which may contribute to the improved prognosis. Antibodies are also detectable in carriers of MMR gene defects who have not been known to have a previous cancer (Schwitalle 2008). In CAPP3, we will collect regular samples to monitor the development of these neopeptide antibodies as a biomarker of the benefits of aspirin intervention.

## 5 Conclusion

Chemoprevention for gastrointestinal cancer is desirable but the many logistical challenges associated with evaluation of prevention using randomised trial structures make it difficult to get effective agents into clinical practice. After 25 years we now have sufficient evidence to recommend aspirin in people at high risk of colorectal cancer, particularly those with Lynch syndrome. We must continue to explore the underlying mechanisms and combine this with efforts to refine the optimal dose.

## References


Bodmer WF, Bailey CJ et al (1987) Localization of the gene for familial adenomatous polyposis on chromosome 5. Nature 328: 614

Boland CR, Thibodeau SN et al (1998) The international workshop on microsatellite instability and rer phenotypes in cancer detection and familial predisposition. Cancer Research 58:5248–5257

Boland CR, Thibodeau SN et al (1997) The international workshop on microsatellite instability and rer phenotypes in cancer detection and familial predisposition: 1–35

Burn J, Bishop DT et al (2011a) A randomized placebo-controlled prevention trial of aspirin and/or resistant starch in young people with familial adenomatous polyposis. Cancer Prev Res (Phila) 4(5):655–665

Burn J, Gerdes AM et al (2011b) Long-term effect of aspirin on cancer risk in carriers of hereditary colorectal cancer: an analysis from the CAPP2 randomised controlled trial. Lancet 378:2081–2087

Burn J, Bishop DT et al (2008) Effect of aspirin or resistant starch on colorectal neoplasia in the lynch syndrome. N Engl J Med 359(24):2567–2578

Burn J, Chapman P et al (1991) The UK Northern Region genetic register for familial adenomatous polyposis coli: use of age of onset, congenital hypertrophy of the retinal pigment epithelium, and DNA markers in risk calculations. J Med Genet 28:289–296

Cassidy A, Bingham SA et al (1994) Starch intake and colorectal cancer risk: an international comparison. Br J Cancer (London) 69:937–942

Chan AT, Arber N et al (2011) Aspirin in the chemoprevention of colorectal neoplasia: an overview. Cancer Prev Res (Phila)

Clark S (ed) (2009) A guide to cancer genetics in clinical practice, tfm Publishing Ltd

Cole BF, Logan RF et al (2009) Aspirin for the chemoprevention of colorectal adenomas: meta-analysis of the randomized trials. J Natl Cancer Inst 101(4):256–266

Cruz-Correa M, Hylind LM et al (2002) Long-term treatment with sulindac in familial adenomatous polyposis: a prospective cohort study. Gastroenterology 122: 641–645

Cuzick J, Otto F et al (2009) Aspirin and non-steroidal anti-inflammatory drugs for cancer prevention: an international consensus statement. Lancet Oncol 10(5):501–507

de la Chapelle A (2004) Genetic predisposition to colorectal cancer. Nat Rev Cancer 4(10): 769–780

Dunstone GH, Knaggs TWL (1972) Familial cancer of the colon and rectum. J Med Genet 9:451–454

Fishel R, Lescoe MK et al (1993) The human mutator gene homolog MSH2 and its association with hereditary nonpolyposis colon cancer. Cell 75(Dec 3): 1027–1038

Giardiello FM, Hamilton SR et al (1993) Treatment of colonic and rectal adenomas with sulindac in familial adenomatous polyposis. N Engl J Med 328:1313–1316

Giardiello FM, Yang VW et al (2002) Primary chemoprevention of familial adenomatous polyposis with sulindac. New England J Med 346(14):1054–1059

Giovannucci E, Egan KM et al (1995) Aspirin and the risk of colorectal cancer in women. N Engl J Med 333(10):609–614

Grubben M, Braak CVD et al (2001) Effect of resistant starch on potential biomarkers for colonic cancer risk in patients with colonic adenomas: a controlled trial. Dig Dis Sci 46(4):750–756

Hampel H, Frankel WL et al (2008) Feasibility of screening for Lynch syndrome among patients with colorectal cancer. J Clin Oncol 26(35):5783–5788

Herrera L, Kakati S et al (1986) Gardner syndrome in a man with an interstitial deletion of 5q. Am J Med Genet 25:473–476
Huang K, Gutierrez LP et al (2011) Clinical characteristics and outcomes in familial adenomatous polyposis patients with a long-term treatment of celecoxib: a matched cohort study. Fam Cancer 10(2):303–308
Hylla S, Gostner A et al (1998) Effects of resistant starch on the colon in healthy volunteers: possible implications for cancer prevention. Am J Clin Nutr 67:136–142
Jaeger E, Leedham S, Lewis A et al (2012) Hereditary mixed polyposis syndrome is caused by a 40kb upstream duplication that leads to increased and ectopic expression of the BMPantagonist GREM1 Nature Genetics Epub 6 May doi:10.1038/ng2263
Jass JR, Walsh MD et al (2002) Distinction between familial and sporadic forms of colorectal cancer showing DNA microsatellite instability. Eur J Cancer 38(7):858–866
Kune GA, Kune S et al (1988) Colorectal cancer risk, chronic illness, operations, medications: case control results from the Melbourne colorectal cancer study. Cancer Res 48:4399–4404
Labayle D, Fischer D et al (1991) Sulindac causes regression of rectal polyps in familial adenomatous polyposis. Gastroenterology 101: 635–639
Lichtenstein DR, Wolfe MM (2000) COX-2-Selective NSAIDs. J Am Med Assoc 284(10): 1297–1299
Lynch HT, Krush AJ (1971) Cancer family "G" revisited: 1895–1970. ) Cancer 27: 1505–1511
Lynch HT, Smyrk T et al (1995) Hereditary nonpolyposis colorectal cancer and colonic adenomas: aggressive adenomas? Semin Surg Oncol 11(6):406–410
Lynch HT, Thorson AG et al (1995) Rectal cancer after prolonged sulindac chemoprevention. Cancer 75(4): 936–938
McIlhatton MA, Tyler J et al (2011) Aspirin and low dose nitric oxide-donating aspirin increase life span in a lynch syndrome mouse model. Cancer Prev Res 4(5):684–693
Mills SJ, Mathers JC et al (2001) Colonic crypt cell proliferation state assessed by whole crypt microdissection in sporadic neoplasia and familial adenomatous polyposis. GUT 48:41–46
Nugent KP, Farmer KC et al (1993) Randomized controlled trial of the effect of sulindac on duodenal and rectal polyposis and cell proliferation in patients with familial adenomatous polyposis. Br J Surg 80(12):1618–1619
Rothwell PM, Fowkes FG et al (2011) Effect of daily aspirin on long-term risk of death due to cancer: analysis of individual patient data from randomised trials. Lancet 377(9759):31–41
Rothwell PM, Wilson M et al (2010) Long-term effect of aspirin on colorectal cancer incidence and mortality: 20-year follow-up of five randomised trials. Lancet 376(9754):1741–1750
Ruschoff J, Wallinger S et al (1998) Aspirin suppresses the mutator phenotype associated with hereditary nonpolyposis colorectal cancer by genetic selection. Proc Natl Acad Sci U S A 95(19):11301–11306
Steinbach G, Lynch PM et al (2000) The effect of celecoxib, a cyclooxygenase-2 inhibitor, in familial adenomatous polyposis. New England J Med 342(26):1946–1952
Schwitalle Y, Kloor M (2008) Immune response against frameshift-induced neopeptides in HNPCC patients and healthy HNPCC mutation carriers. Gastroenterology 134:988-997
Thun MJ, Namboodiri MM et al (1991) Aspirin use and reduced risk of fatal colon cancer. N Engl J Med 325:1593–1596
Tomlinson IP, Carvajal-Carmona LG et al (2011) Multiple common susceptibility variants near BMP pathway loci GREM1, BMP4, and BMP2 explain part of the missing heritability of colorectal cancer. PLoS Genet 7(6):e1002105
van Munster IP, Tangerman A et al (1994) Effect of resistant starch on colonic fermentation, bile acid metabolism, and mucosal proliferation. Dig Dis Sci 39(4):834–842
Vasen HF (2008) Can the identification of high risk groups increase the effectiveness of colon cancer screening programmes? Z Gastroenterol 46(Suppl 1):S41–S42
Vasen HF, Moslein G et al (2007) Guidelines for the clinical management of Lynch syndrome (hereditary non-polyposis cancer). J Med Genet 44(6):353–362

Williams EA, Coxhead JM et al (2003) Anti-cancer effects of butyrate: use of micro-array technology to investigate mechanisms. Proc Nutr Soc 62(1):107–115

Young G, Leu RL (2004) Resistant starch and colorectal neoplasia. J AOAC Int 87(3):775–786

Lynch HT, Thorson AG et al (1995) Rectal cancer after prolonged sulindac chemoprevention. Cancer 75(4): 936–938